# ATLAS OF DIAGNOSTIC CYTOLOGY

in Small Animals

Plaza Antonio Beltrán Martínez nº 1, planta 8 - letra I
(Centro empresarial El Trovador)
50002 Zaragoza - Spain

First printing: July 2019

This book was originally published in Spanish under the title:
*Atlas de diagnóstico citológico en animales de compañía*
© 2018 Grupo Asís Biomedia, SL
ISBN Spanish edition: 978-84-17225-51-3

Translation:
Owen Howard

ISBN: 978-84-17640-61-3
DL: Z 1257-2019

Design, layout and printing:
Servet editorial - Grupo Asís Biomedia, SL
www.grupoasis.com
info@grupoasis.com

GRUPO asis

Servet is the publishing house of Grupo Asís



Warning:

Veterinary science is constantly evolving, as are pharmacology and the other sciences. Inevitably, it is therefore the responsibility of the veterinary surgeon to determine and verify the dosage, the method of administration, the duration of treatment and any possible contraindications to the treatments given to each individual patient, based on his or her professional experience. Neither the publisher nor the author can be held liable for any damage or harm caused to people, animals or properties resulting from the correct or incorrect application of the information contained in this book.

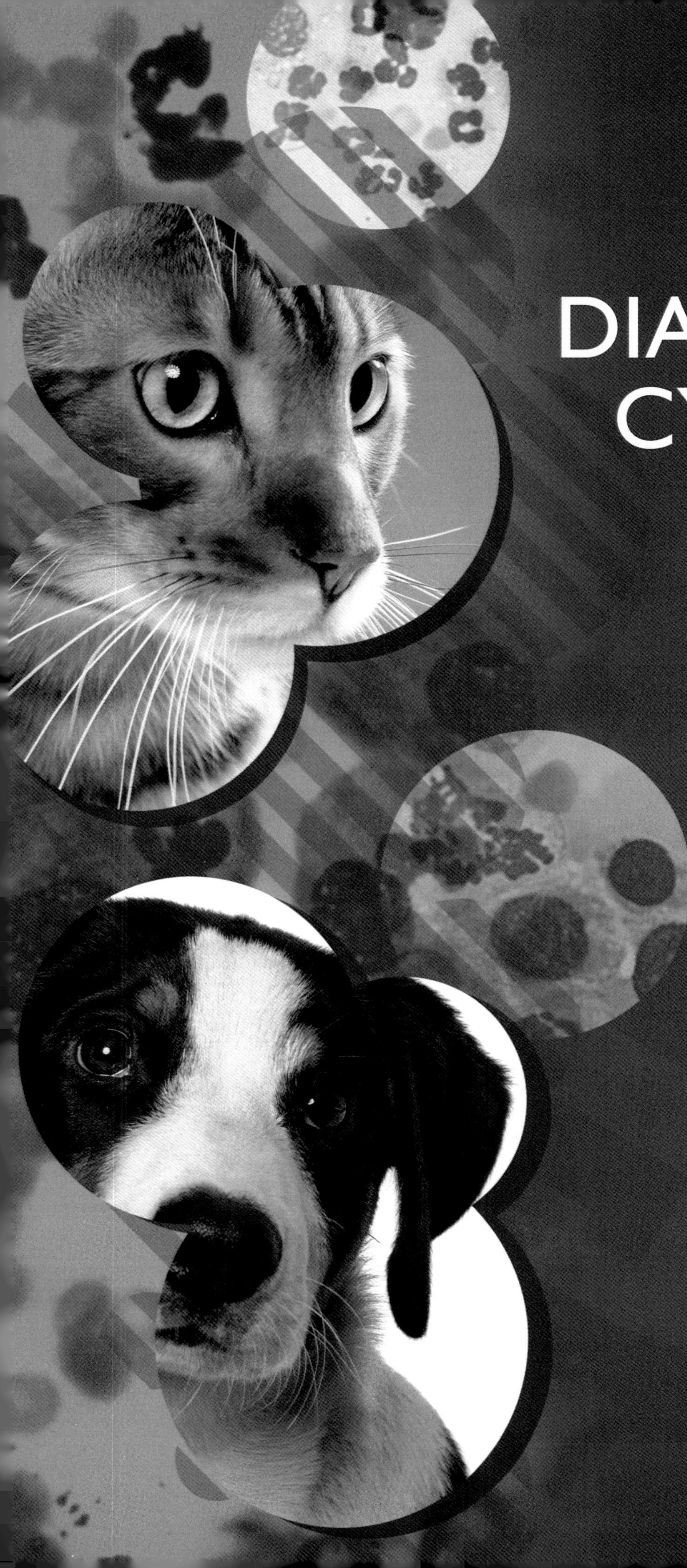

# ATLAS OF DIAGNOSTIC CYTOLOGY

## in Small Animals

Elena Martínez de Merlo

SERVET

# The author

## ELENA MARTÍNEZ DE MERLO

Elena Martínez de Merlo graduated in veterinary medicine from the Complutense University of Madrid (UCM) in 1987, and earned her PhD in veterinary medicine from the same university in 1993. Since 1998 she has worked as a professor at the UCM's Department of Medicine and Animal Surgery. Elena is a veterinary surgeon at the UCM's Veterinary Teaching Hospital, where she heads the Oncology and Cytological Diagnosis units of the Clinical Biopathology Service. She is the author of two books: *Atlas de citología clínica del perro y del gato* (Atlas of Clinical Cytology in Dogs and Cats), published by Editorial Servet in 2008, and *Manual Práctico de Oncología en Pequeños Animales* (Manual of Practical Small Animal Oncology) (2011 and 2014). Elena directs the UCM's Continuous Education Diploma in cytological interpretation in small animals (60 teaching hours), a course now in its 11th edition. She is certified in oncology by the Spanish Small Animal Veterinary Association (AVEPA) and served as the president of GEVONC, AVEPA's specialist veterinary oncology group, from its establishment in 2011 until April 2014. She has presented at numerous national and international congresses, and has given courses, lectures, and practical workshops in oncology and cytological diagnosis. She has authored and coauthored many articles on oncology and clinical applications of cytological diagnostic techniques in both Spanish and international journals.

# Preface and acknowledgments

It has been 10 years since the publication of the *Atlas de citología clínica del perro y del gato* (Atlas of Clinical Cytology in Dogs and Cats, Servet, 2008), in which myself and my coauthors sought to promote the use of cytology as a general diagnostic technique and provide a general overview of cytological interpretation, and ultimately to encourage veterinary surgeons working with small animals to establish their own diagnoses.

A few months ago, Servet once again contacted me to ask me to write a second edition of the atlas. While basic cytological interpretation has not changed over the last decade, concepts have been updated and new criteria established to improve the performance of cytological techniques. After giving it some thought, we agreed that it would be better to begin a new project than simply extending the content of the previous atlas.

Cytology can only be explained with images, and therefore we agreed that the atlas format was essential. However, the most notable feature of this book is that, unlike the previous atlas (and most published cytology atlases), it focuses on diseases rather than organs or tissues. Thus, in each chapter readers will find multiple images reflecting different aspects of the most frequently encountered conditions, regardless of lesion location.

Without doubt, the two atlases complement one another. The first atlas covers the fundamentals of cytological interpretation required to establish a diagnosis of specific conditions, while this book provides more in-depth information on each condition and explains how to obtain maximum information from each cytological preparation. When the reader suspects a specific condition they can directly consult the corresponding chapter, where they will find multiple images reflecting all relevant cytological pictures, allowing them to confirm or rule out diagnostic suspicions and ensure greater diagnostic accuracy. Because cytological diagnosis often hinges on small details, we have specifically focused on differential diagnoses, providing images of other diseases with similar cytological pictures in order to highlight distinguishing features. Owing to the limitations of cytology, diagnosis is not always possible. Nonetheless, our objective as authors is to provide readers with the necessary tools (in this case, images) in order to limit, to the extent possible, diagnostic errors.

This atlas was put together after consulting numerous published texts (including the atlases that we all keep next to our microscopes), as well as information published on websites devoted to cytological diagnosis. However, the bibliography only lists specific publications focused on the description of specific cytological concepts, which must be understood to ensure that the cytological diagnosis is as detailed and precise as possible.

This atlas is also the product of many years of first-hand experience: 30 years working in the field of cytology provides many learning opportunities. We have attempted to provide readers with the tools necessary to answer the many questions that they will face when sitting alone at the microscope examining a cytological preparation from a specific patient. Cytology can only be understood by devoting considerable time to its study. However, if the information provided in this atlas can help to reduce the time required to establish a diagnosis, in addition to improving performance and ultimately benefitting the patient, we will have fulfilled our objective.

From the outset, our intention was that the "atlas" component would outweigh the text; no matter how many times a cell is described, you will not recognise it until you actually see it, and the more times you see it, the better. Virtually all the cytological preparations shown in this atlas are stained with the May–Grünwald–Giemsa stain. Most have been photographed at intermediate magnification (40×), but in some cases microscopic fields are presented at lower (20×) or higher (60×) magnification in order to provide more general or more detailed information.

Although I am the sole author, this atlas could not have been completed without the help of others. Most of the images contained within were obtained from the slide library of the Clinical Biopathology Laboratory of the UCM's Veterinary Teaching Hospital. I would like to thank all my colleagues at the hospital, who continuously send me samples from their patients (I must have taught them well!), forcing me to face new cytological challenges every day. Sincere thanks also to everyone at the Biopathology Laboratory and, above all, to the staff who work so hard to ensure that samples are well prepared, stained, and preserved, even if this interrupts their other laboratory activities. I want to express my gratitude to technicians Ana Angulo, Eva Manceras, and Pilar Torrecilla for their fine work.

I am also grateful to my veterinary colleagues who requested my help with cytological diagnoses and provided me with challenging preparations, allowing me to expand my library. Thanks also to the entire "cytologist by day, gamer by night" team (Víctor, Eva, Mamen, Ricardo, and Noemí); our daily WhatsApp exchanges of experiences, images, and cytological knowledge has proved enormously helpful.

This atlas could not have been completed without the assistance of my colleagues who allowed me to use and abuse their microscope cameras and spend many hours photographing the images included in this book. While they always insisted that I never bothered them, I know this was not always true. Thanks, Eduardo, Nines, and Rosa.

And, of course, thanks to Editorial Servet for putting their trust in me, and for inviting me to once again collaborate with them.

Finally, thanks to all my colleagues who have made sure that the *Atlas de citología clínica del perro y del gato* was so well received; that was the greatest motivation when devoting myself to this new project. I hope you can now enjoy this atlas as much as I enjoyed compiling it.

**Elena M. Martínez de Merlo**

February 2018

# Table of contents

# 01

# Cytology of inflammation

# Cytology of inflammation

The cytological diagnosis of inflammation, regardless of location, is based on the detection of a predominant population of inflammatory cells.

Inflammatory cytology should always be interpreted with caution and no diagnosis established based on this methodology should be considered definitive. Many neoplastic processes are accompanied by the presence of an inflammatory cell population (e.g. reactive cells or cells generated in response to necrosis or ulceration) that can mask tissue cells and appear to predominate (Figs. 1 and 2). Even the presence of microorganisms does not rule out the possibility that the primary process may be neoplastic and that the infection is a secondary or opportunistic process (Figs. 3 and 4). If the predominant population is inflammatory, the cytological diagnosis should be "inflammation", although other clinical data should be taken into account when making this interpretation.

Evaluation of a cytological preparation in which an inflammatory cell population predominates involves the following steps:

1. Identification of the inflammatory cells present.
2. Definition of the inflammatory pattern.
3. Search for and identification of microorganisms, if applicable.
4. Assessment of the relevance of tissue cells, if present.

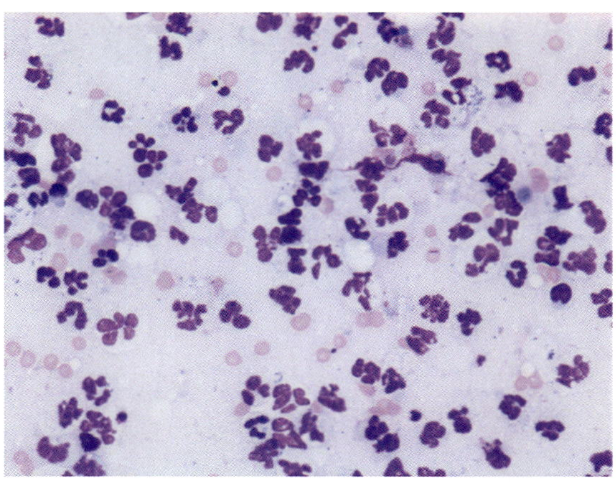
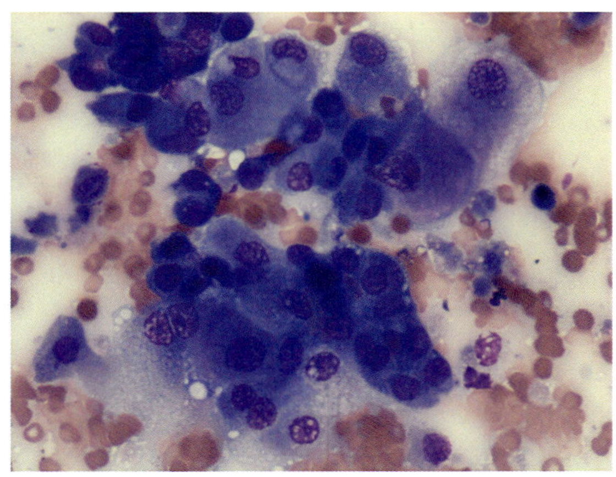

Figures 1 and 2. Prostate cytology. After treatment of inflammation (1), neoplastic cells are observed (2).

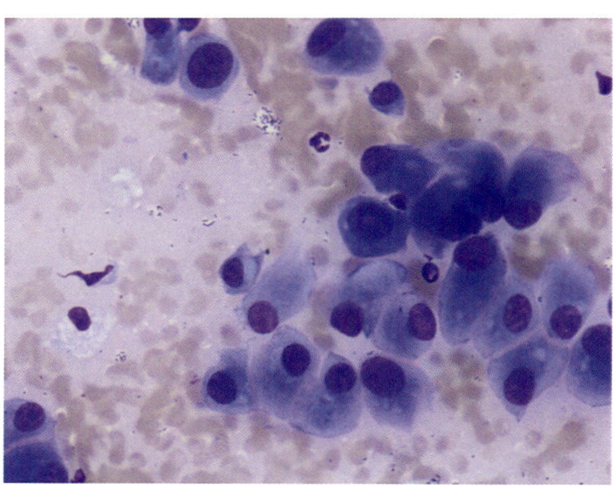
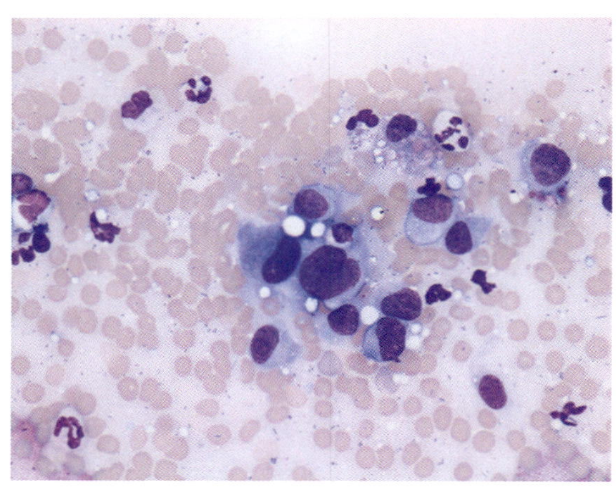

Figures 3 and 4. Neoplastic cytology. The tissue cell population is accompanied by contaminating bacteria (3) and bacteria associated with an inflammatory reaction (4).

# IDENTIFICATION OF INFLAMMATORY CELLS

## NEUTROPHILS

Neutrophils are the predominant nucleated blood cells. It is therefore necessary to assess the relevance of their presence in highly haemodiluted samples; if their number exceeds that expected based on the degree of blood contamination, an inflammatory origin be considered (Fig. 5).

In aseptic inflammation, neutrophil levels are similar to those seen in circulating blood, although age-associated changes (Figs. 6 and 7), such as hypersegmentation (lobes are joined by a very thin nuclear band), pyknosis (retraction of the nucleus, which has a rounded shape due to chromatin condensation), and karyorrhexis (the condensed chromatin is fragmented into small, intensely stained round structures) may be observed. By contrast, in septic conditions neutrophils undergo toxic or degenerative changes due to karyolysis, and contain swollen and pale nuclei with poorly defined lobes. In cases involving very marked toxic changes it can be very difficult to recognise the cells as neutrophils (Figs. 8–10).

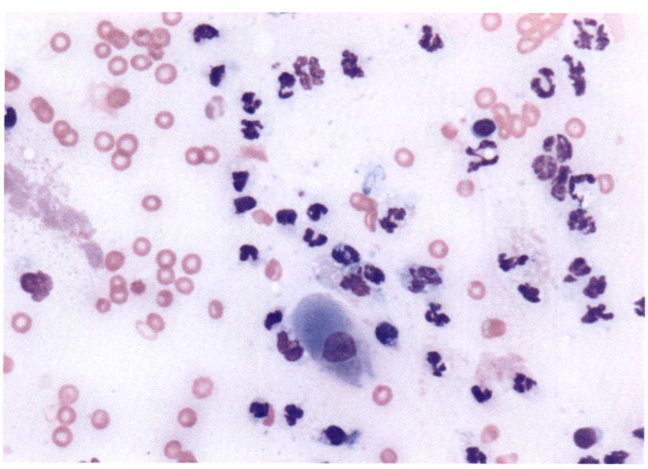

Figure 5. Very haemodiluted renal cytology preparation. It is necessary to determine whether the neutrophil presence is relevant. Their number and morphology (degenerate) point to an inflammatory origin.

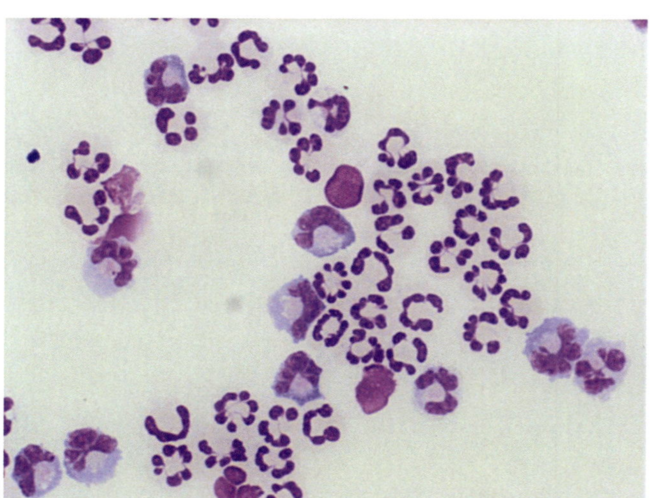

Figure 6. Cerebrospinal fluid sample containing hypersegmented neutrophils (steroid responsive meningitis).

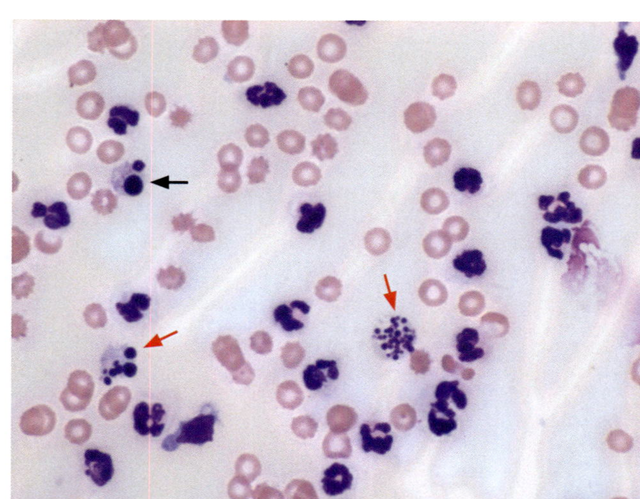

Figure 7. Neutrophils exhibiting pyknosis (black arrow) and karyorrhexis (red arrows).

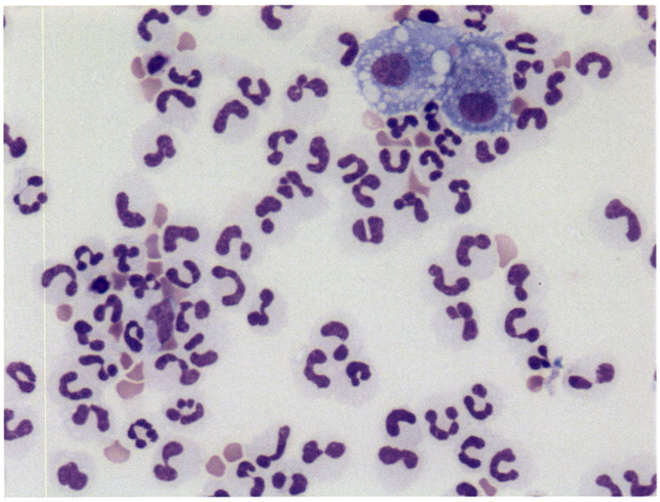

Figure 8.

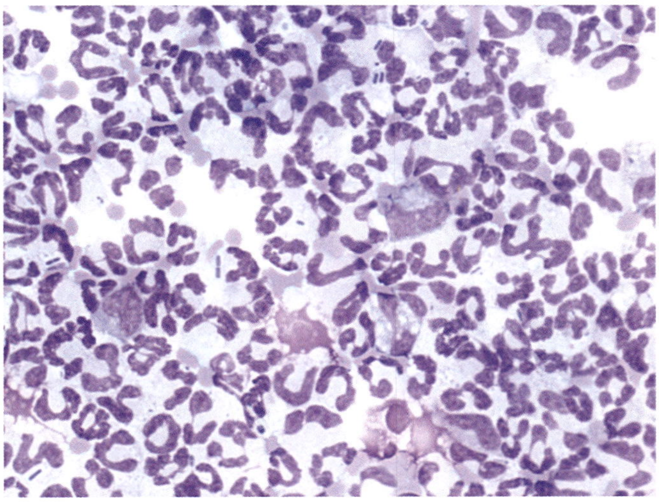

Figure 9.

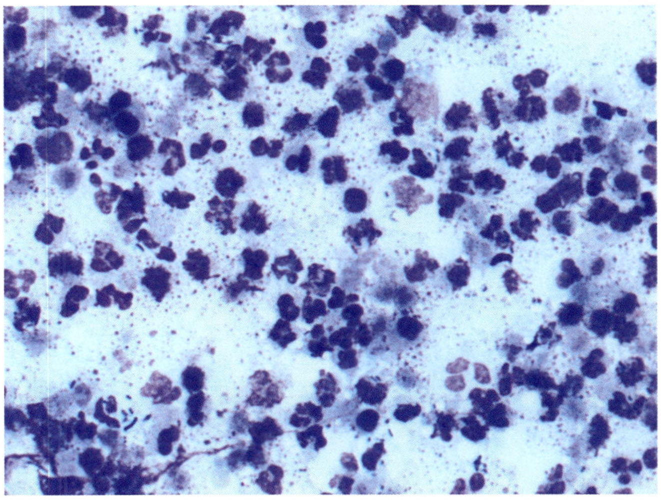

◀ Figure 10.

Figures 8–10. Neutrophils exhibiting karyolysis and other nuclear degenerative changes in pleural fluid (8), abdominal fluid (9), and an intestinal abscess (10).

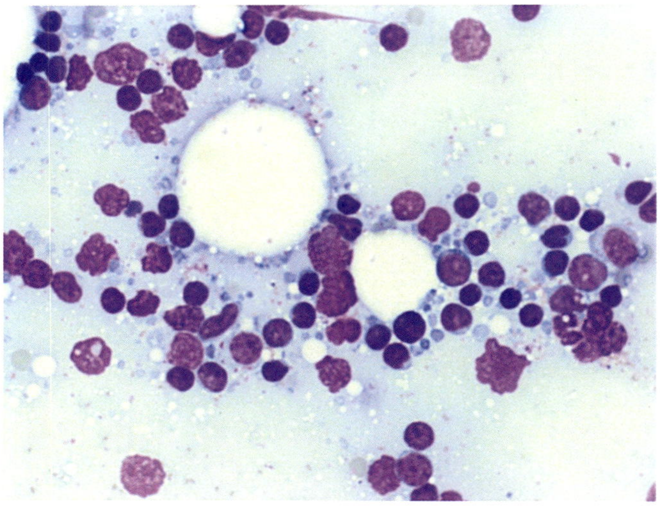

Figure 11. Lymphocytic panniculitis (cat).

## LYMPHOCYTES

Heterogeneous populations of lymphocytes are commonly observed in inflammatory reactions. Although mature lymphocytes predominate, reactive lymphocytes or even lymphoblasts can be observed (Fig. 11).

Although uncommon, if lymphocytes are the sole or predominant inflammatory population then differential diagnosis from lymphoma is necessary, especially in samples containing monomorphic cell populations.

## EOSINOPHILS

Eosinophils are considered relevant in inflammatory cytology when they account for more than 10–15 % of the cell population, although in some feline conditions (e.g. asthma) they must account for over 25 % of the cell population to be considered diagnostically relevant (Fig. 12). In these cases, inflammation should be considered eosinophilic in nature even if these cells do not constitute the predominant population. In some samples, including cerebrospinal fluid (CSF) and conjunctival/corneal samples, the presence of a single eosinophil is considered pathological (assuming the samples are not contaminated with blood) (Fig. 13).

In general, eosinophil morphology is similar to that observed in blood, although cells with pyknotic nuclei may be observed (Fig. 14).

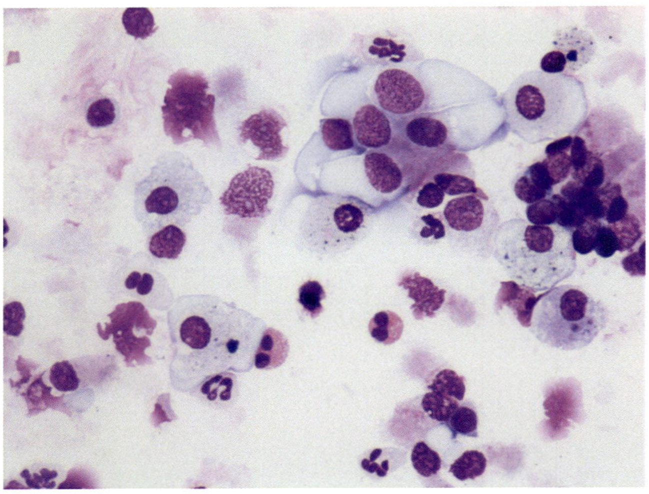

Figure 12. Tracheal wash (cat). Isolated eosinophils are not indicative of eosinophilic inflammation.

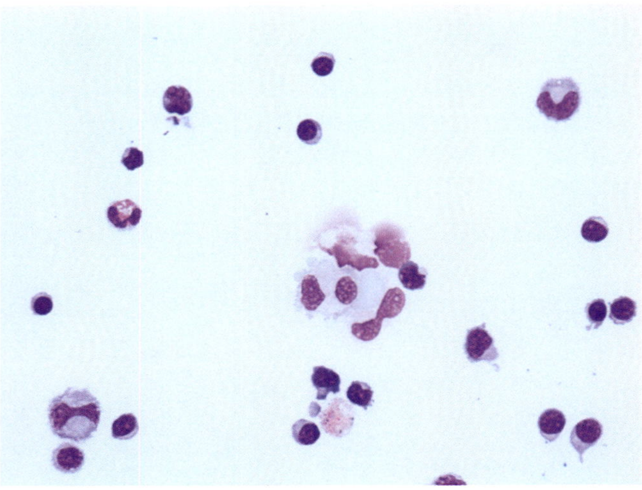

Figure 13. Cerebrospinal fluid sample. The presence of a single eosinophil is considered pathological (lymphocytic pleocytosis).

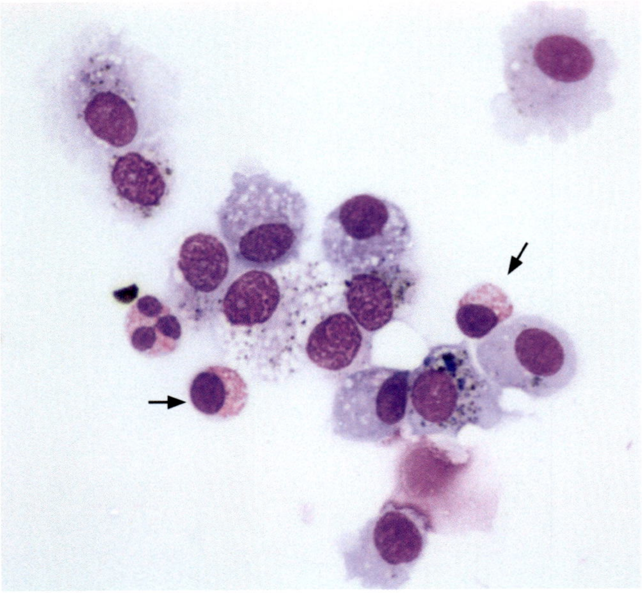

Figure 14. Tracheal wash sample containing pyknotic eosinophils (arrows).

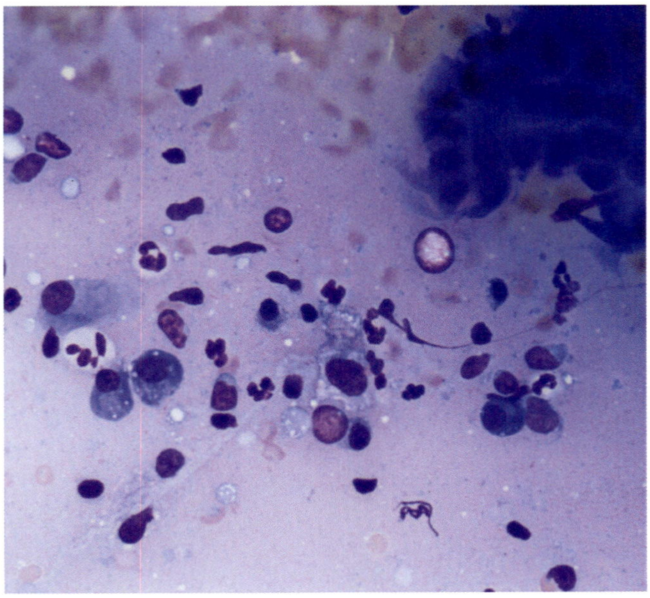

Figure 15. Nasal wash sample (lymphoplasmacytic rhinitis).

## MAST CELLS

These cells may be observed in cases of allergic inflammation, albeit infrequently. High numbers of mast cells are suggestive of a diagnosis of mast cell tumour, as opposed to inflammation.

## PLASMA CELLS

The presence of plasma cells during an inflammatory process indicates chronicity and, above all, a strongly allergenic cause (Fig. 15). Although potentially abundant, plasma cells rarely constitute the predominant population, in which case plasmacytoma should be suspected.

## MACROPHAGES

Macrophages lack a characteristic morphology, since these cells undergo marked changes that are dependent on their activation. Macrophages are derived from monocytic or histiocytic cells that evolve and undergo morphological changes: their cytoplasm becomes vacuolated and increases in size and quantity, and the nucleus becomes rounded and eccentric. The most active forms (Figs. 16–18) include foamy macrophages, in which the entire cytoplasm is occupied by small vacuoles; signet-ring macrophages, which contain a single large vacuole that occupies the entire cytoplasm and displaces the nucleus to the periphery; and multinucleated giant cells. Typically, the same cytological sample contains macrophages in different phases of activation, and therefore of different shapes and sizes and with varying numbers of vacuoles (Fig. 19). Macrophages are predominantly defined by their phagocytic activity (Fig. 20).

In granulomas, they may acquire an epithelioid morphology (Fig. 21), i.e. large cells with a round or oval nucleus and abundant cytoplasm, in some cases lacking vacuoles. Unlike epithelial cells, these cells tend not to form clusters.

Macrophages form part of the normal population of numerous structures, particularly those covered by mesothelial cells (Figs. 22–24). Therefore, they are the predominant population in synovial fluid, CSF, and the pulmonary alveoli. In these locations, increases in their number and/or activity, as opposed to their mere presence, are indicative of inflammation.

In cystic glandular structures (e.g. salivary, mammary, or apocrine glands), foamy macrophages predominate, but are not indicative of inflammation (Fig. 25).

Mesothelial cells are observed in cytological preparations of pleural, peritoneal, or pericardial effusion fluid. These cells are initially at rest, and can be activated even in the absence of inflammatory stimuli (Fig. 26). In these cases, the presence of neutrophils is indicative of inflammation and potentiates the activation of mesothelial cells until they acquire phagocytic capacity.

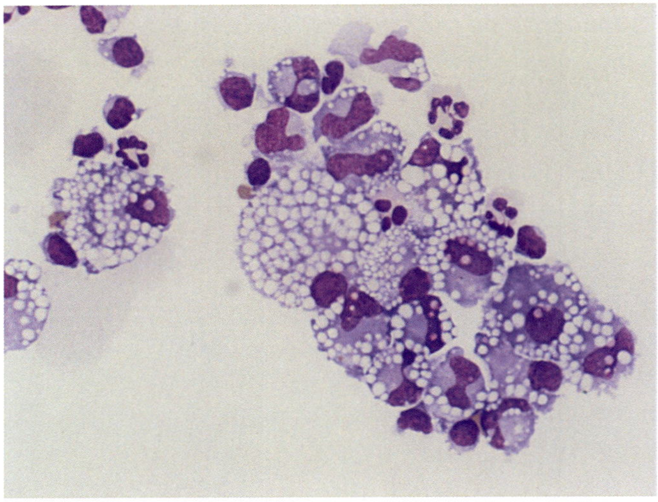

Figure 16.

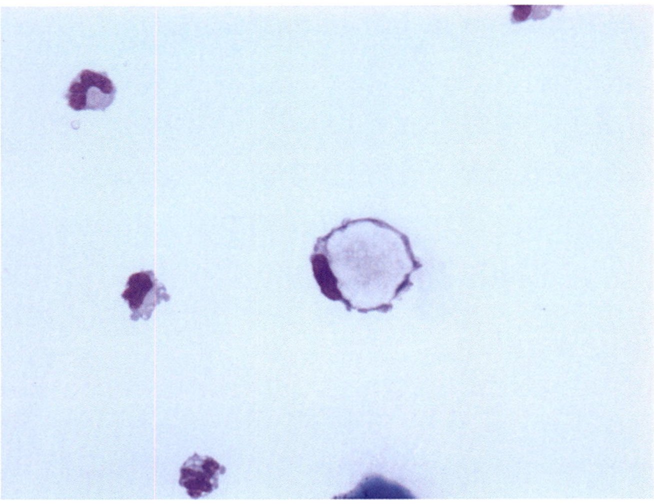

Figure 17.

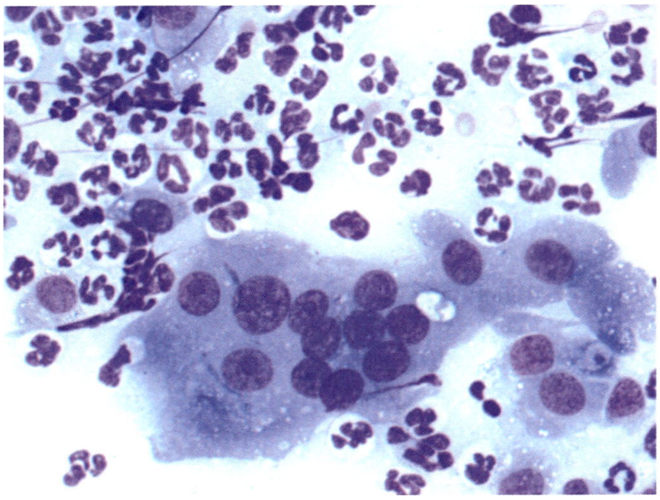

Figure 18.

Figures 16–18. Foamy macrophages (abdominal fluid, 16); signet-ring macrophages (cerebrospinal fluid, 17); and giant multinucleated cells (pyogranuloma, 18).

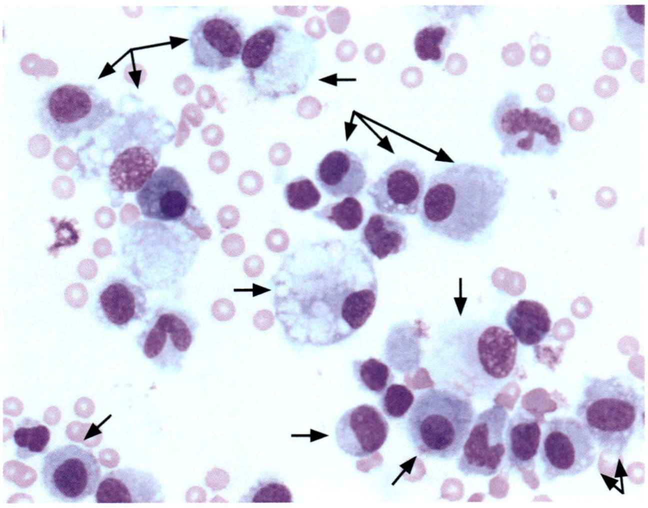

Figure 19. Synovial fluid. The macrophages (arrows) exhibit varying morphologies depending on their degree of activation.

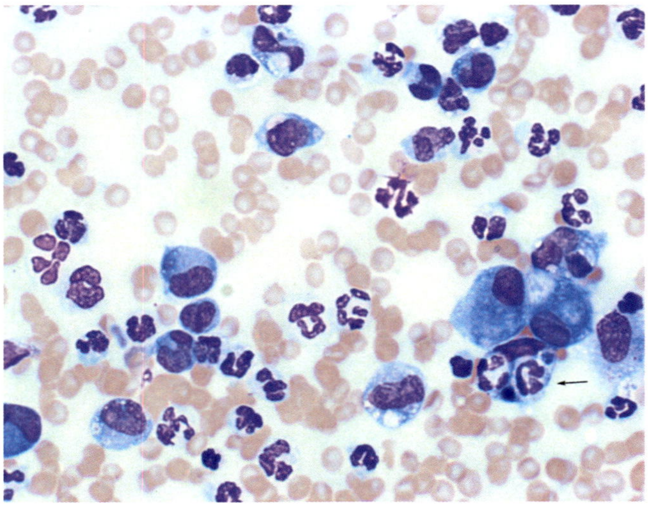

Figure 20. Pyogranuloma. Macrophage displaying leukophagocytosis (arrow).

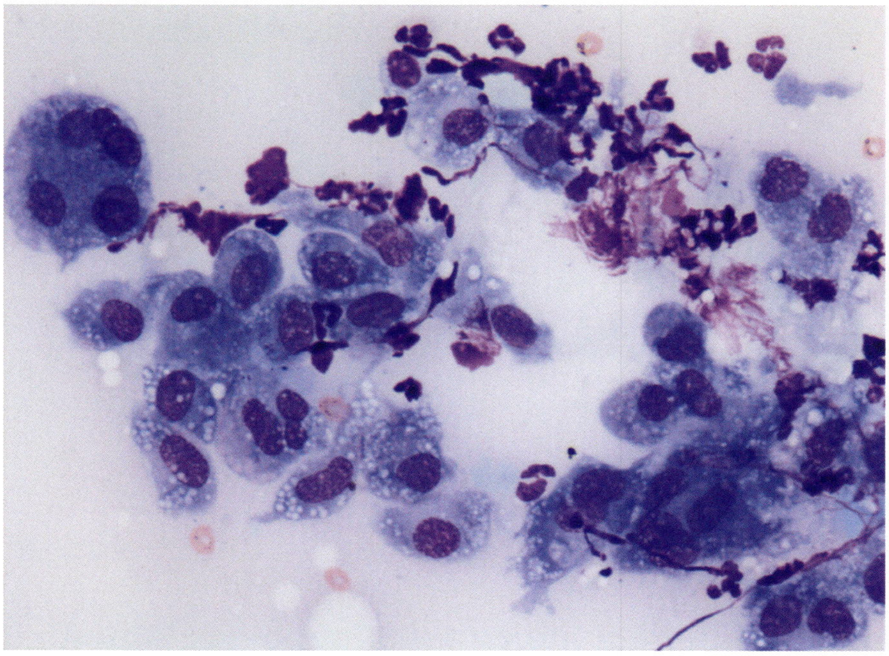

Figure 21. Granuloma. Epithelioid macrophages.

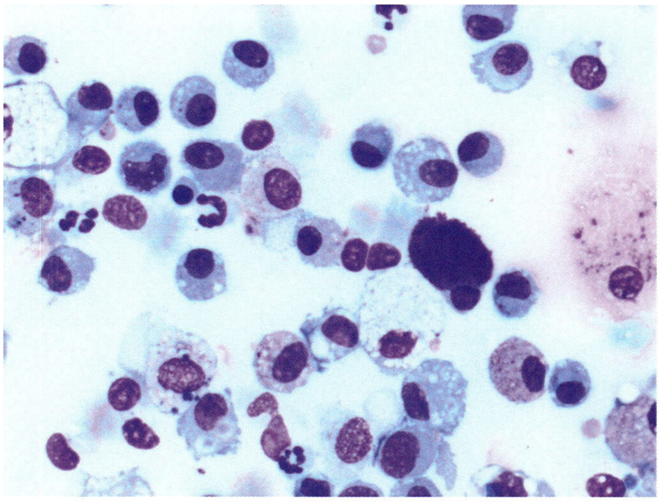

Figure 22.

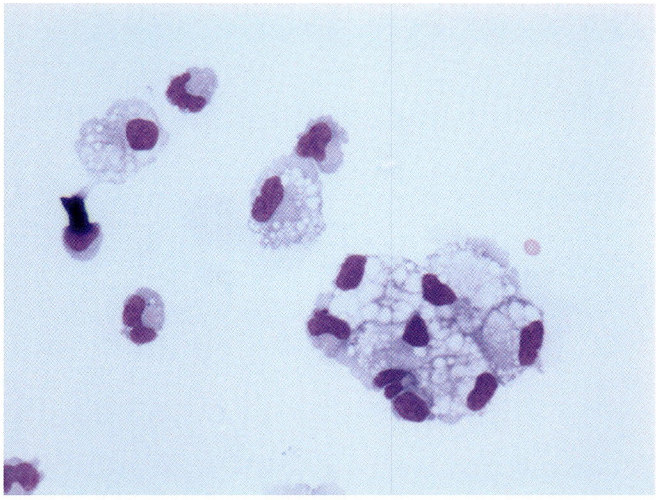

Figure 23.

Figure 24. ▶

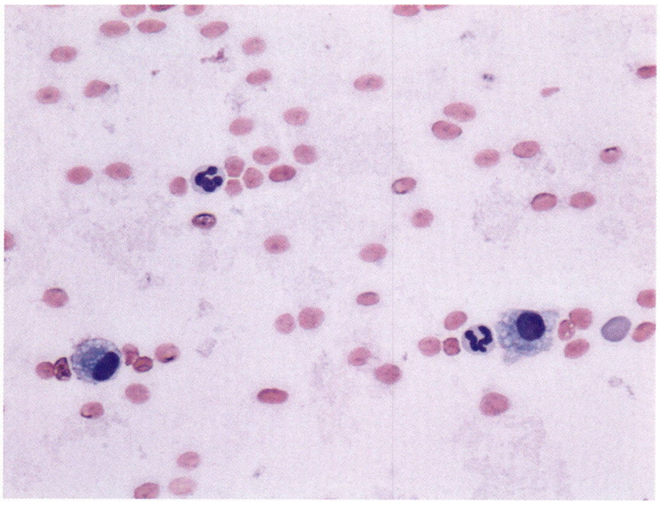

Figures 22–24. Macrophage cells are found in the normal cellular population of the pulmonary alveolus (tracheal wash, 22), cerebrospinal fluid (23), and synovial fluid (24). Increases in their degree of activation are indicative of inflammation.

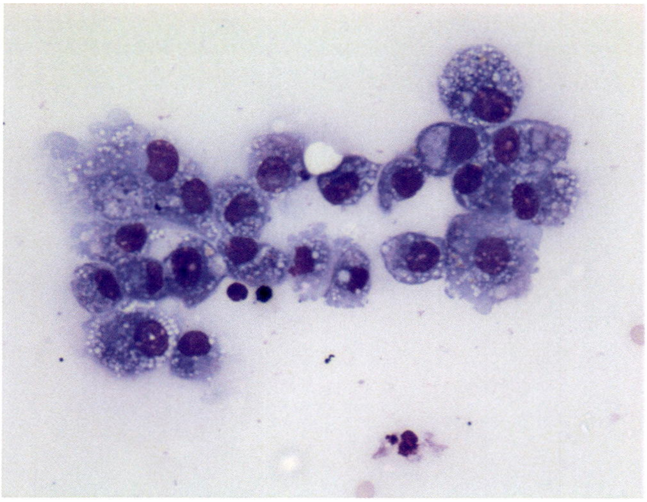

Figure 25. Foamy macrophages in mammary cytology.

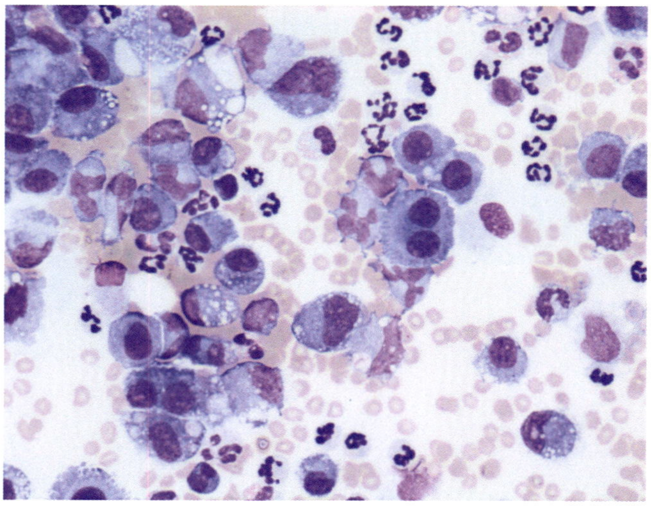

Figure 26. Abdominal fluid sample containing numerous mesothelial/macrophage cells in different stages of activation.

## DEFINING INFLAMMATORY PATTERNS

In most cases, inflammatory processes are characterised by a mixture of several cell types, with the predominant cell population varying depending on the origin and chronicity of the lesion (Figs. 27–33).

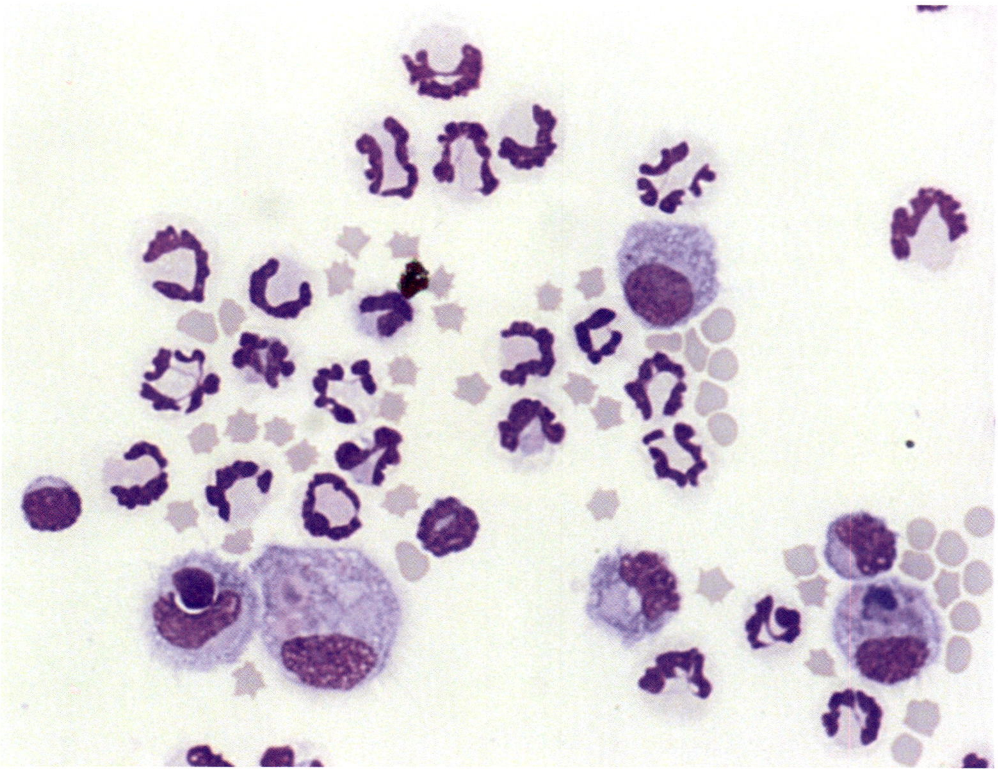

◀ Figure 27.

Figures 27–33. Aseptic pleuritis due to feline infectious peritonitis (27); immune-mediated lymphadenitis (28); foreign body-associated pyogranuloma (29); panniculitis (30); hepatic lymphocytic inflammation (31); mixed pleocytosis (32) and allergic bronchitis (33) in cerebrospinal fluid samples.

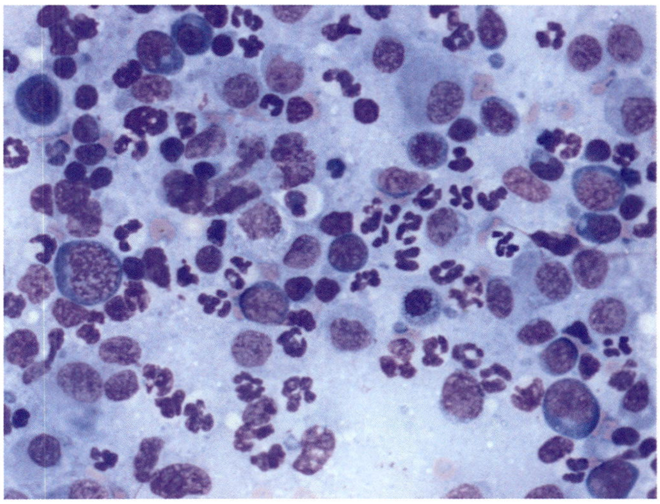
Figure 28.

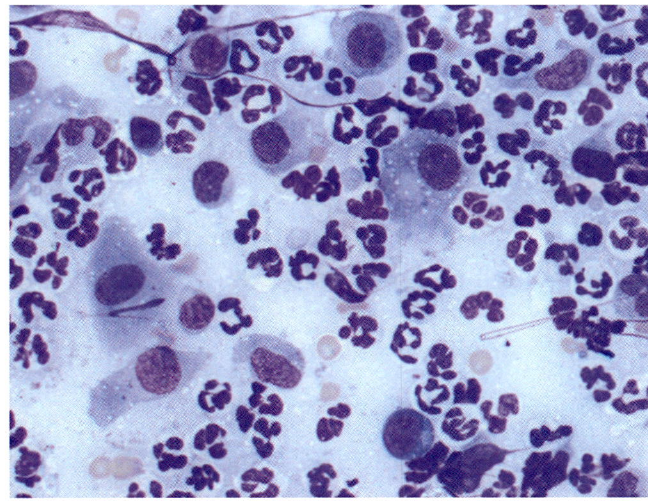
Figure 29.

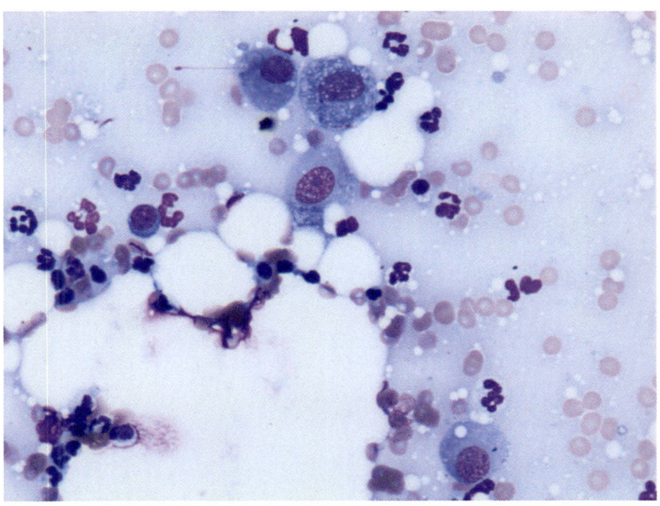
Figure 30.

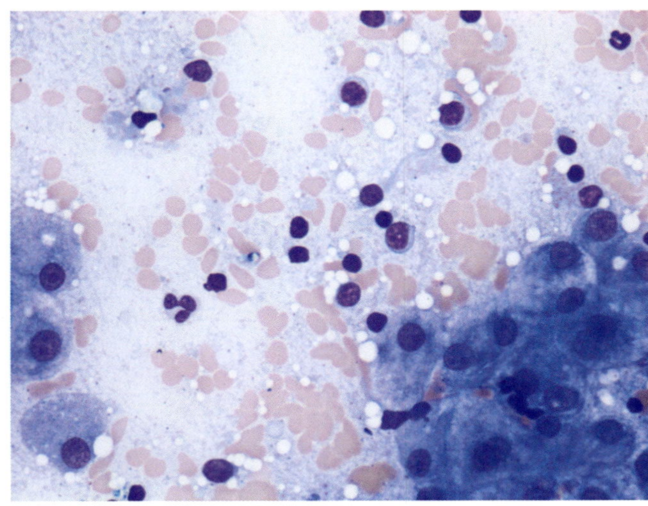
Figure 31.

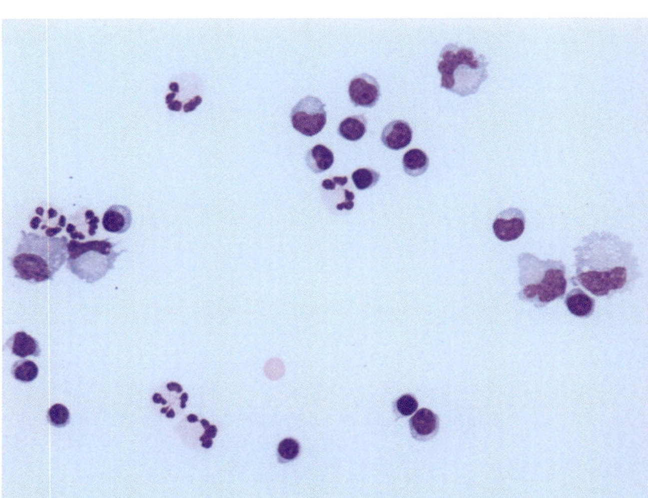
Figure 32.

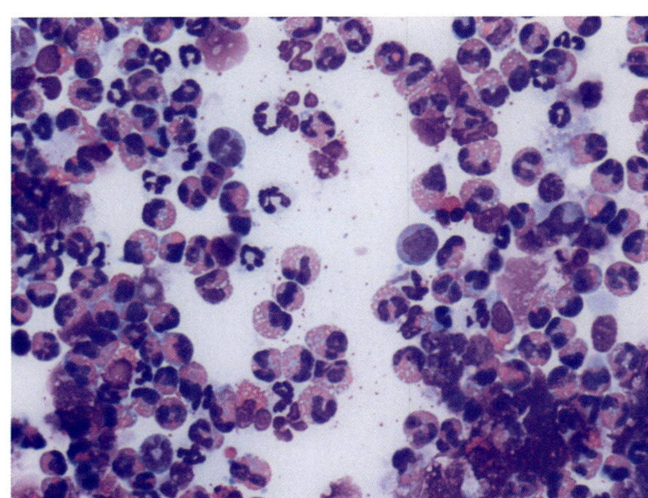
Figure 33.

The following table shows the most common inflammatory patterns (Table 1):

**TABLE 1. Classification of the most common inflammatory patterns.**

| Predominant population | Morphology | Possible origin |
|---|---|---|
| Neutrophils (<70 %): acute inflammation | May display age-associated alterations | ■ Immune-mediated processes<br>■ FIP<br>■ Sterile lesions<br>■ Cancer-associated |
| | With degenerative changes | ■ Septic bacterial processes |
| Neutrophils (50–70 %) + mononuclear cells (30–50 %): pyogranulomas | | ■ Chronicity<br>■ Foreign bodies<br>■ Fungal processes<br>■ Panniculitis |
| Mononuclear cells (>50 %): chronic inflammation | Lymphocytes* | ■ Lymphocytic inflammation (liver)<br>■ Early-stage viral processes (except FIP)<br>■ Feline panniculitis (postvaccination reaction) |
| | Plasma cells | ■ Allergenic component (leishmaniasis) |
| | Macrophages* | ■ Granuloma due to mycobacteria<br>■ Foreign bodies<br>■ Fungal processes<br>■ Panniculitis |
| >10–15 % eosinophils | | ■ Allergic processes<br>■ Parasitic processes<br>■ Fungal processes<br>■ Eosinophilic granuloma**<br>■ Cancer-associated |

FIP, feline infectious peritonitis; * an increase in lymphocytes and monocytes/macrophages in cerebrospinal fluid indicates meningoencephalitis of unknown origin; ** predominant population.

## IDENTIFICATION OF MICROORGANISMS

In inflammatory cytology, the possibility of an infectious origin should be evaluated. In some cases microorganisms are observed, but in others their presence can be deduced based on the cytological pattern or the changes that the inflammatory population undergoes.

Infectious inflammation is most often bacterial in origin. It is important to keep in mind that the presence of bacteria is not synonymous with infection. To demonstrate a potentially septic origin, a reaction to the microorganisms must be observed (e.g. an increase in the number of neutrophils, the presence of phagocytised intracellular bacteria, and/or degenerative changes in neutrophils) (Fig. 34). In the absence of these alterations, the bacterial population should be considered contaminant (Figs. 35–37).

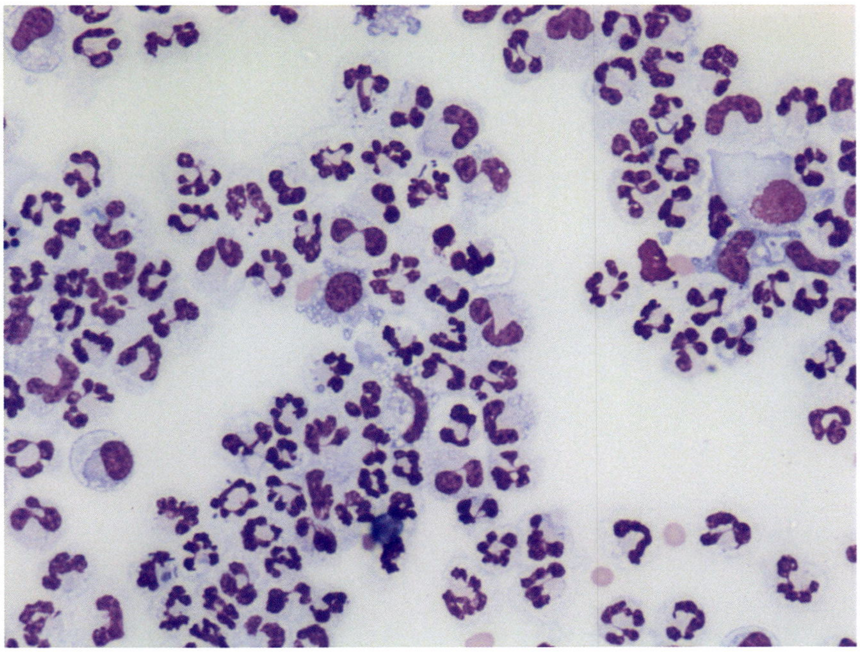

Figure 34. Septic peritonitis. The increase in the number of neutrophils, their degenerative characteristics, and the presence of intracellular bacteria are indicative of infection.

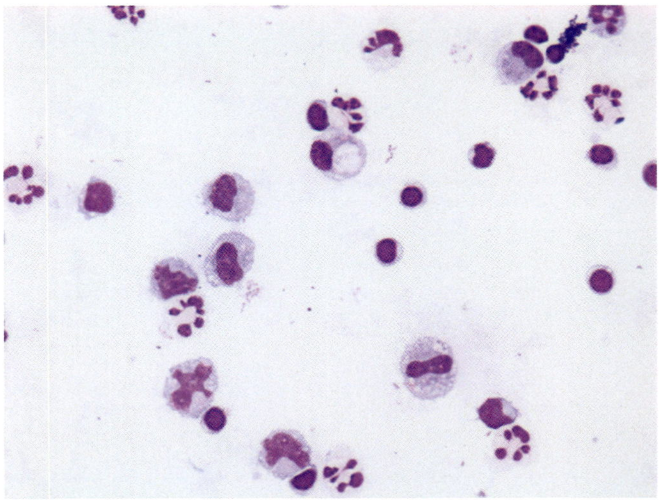

Figure 35.

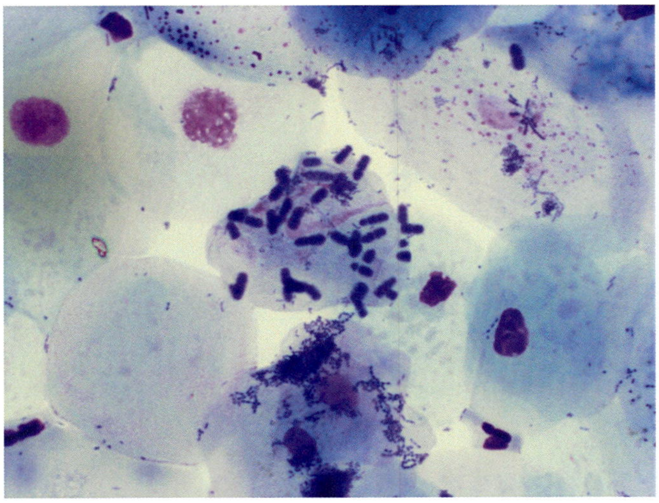

Figure 36.

Figure 37. ▶

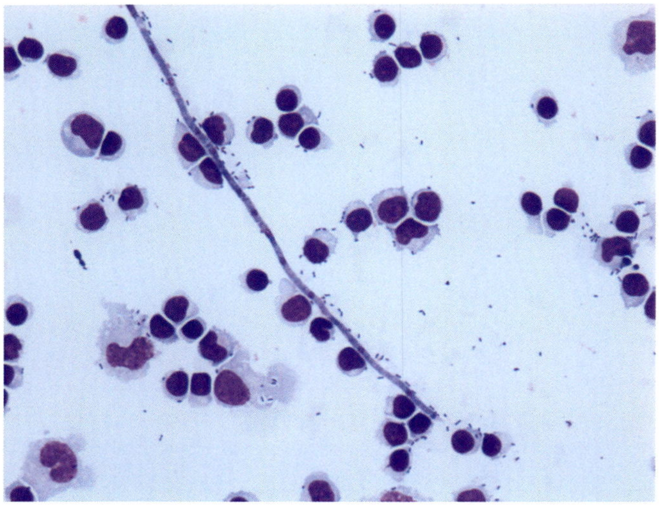

Figures 35–37. Bacterial contamination in abdominal fluid (35), and tracheal wash (38) samples, and bacterial/fungal contamination in a cerebrospinal fluid sample (37). Despite the abundant bacteria, there is no increase in the number of neutrophils and no evidence of phagocytosed microorganisms.

Filamentous bacteria (*Actinomyces, Nocardia*) can be mistaken for cell debris (Fig. 38).

Mycobacteria can be observed inside the macrophages that phagocytose them in the form of a negative image, since they are not stained by routine haematological techniques (Fig. 39).

The majority of cytological reactions to viral diseases are lymphocytic; inclusion bodies are only occasionally observed (Fig. 40).

The presence of parasitic forms (Fig. 41) is usually associated with an increase in the number of eosinophils, although it may be accompanied by a nonspecific increase in neutrophils. In CSF cytology, the presence of eosinophils indicates the need to rule out toxoplasmosis/neosporosis. Filarias are commonly found in cytological analyses of different organs (Fig. 42), but usually as circulating parasitic forms introduced as a result of blood contamination, and not associated with an inflammatory tissue reaction.

Among other vector-borne diseases, only leishmaniasis induces a significant inflammatory tissue response, characterised by an increase in the number of mononuclear cells, especially lymphocytes and plasma cells, and an increased presence of macrophages that phagocytose amastigotes (Figs. 43 and 44). Very occasionally, *Ehrlichia* morulae may be observed in mononuclear cells (Fig. 45).

The incidence of fungal infections varies greatly according to geographical area (Figs. 46–48). Fungal structures, usually phagocytosed, are often observed in samples obtained from the respiratory tract, and are accompanied by a pyogranulomatous/granulomatous inflammatory reaction, which may include eosinophils.

Owing to their size, the granules of large granular lymphocytes can be mistaken for fungal structures. Their location inside lymphoid cells (not macrophages) is the main distinguishing criterion (Fig. 49).

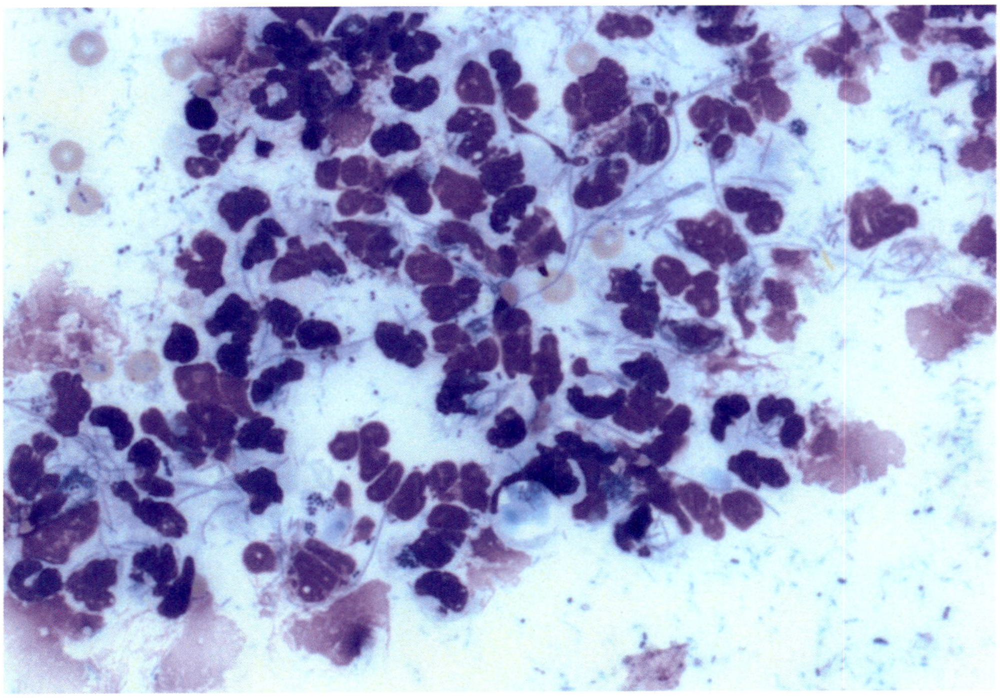

Figure 38. Urethral inflammation with the presence of filamentous bacteria.

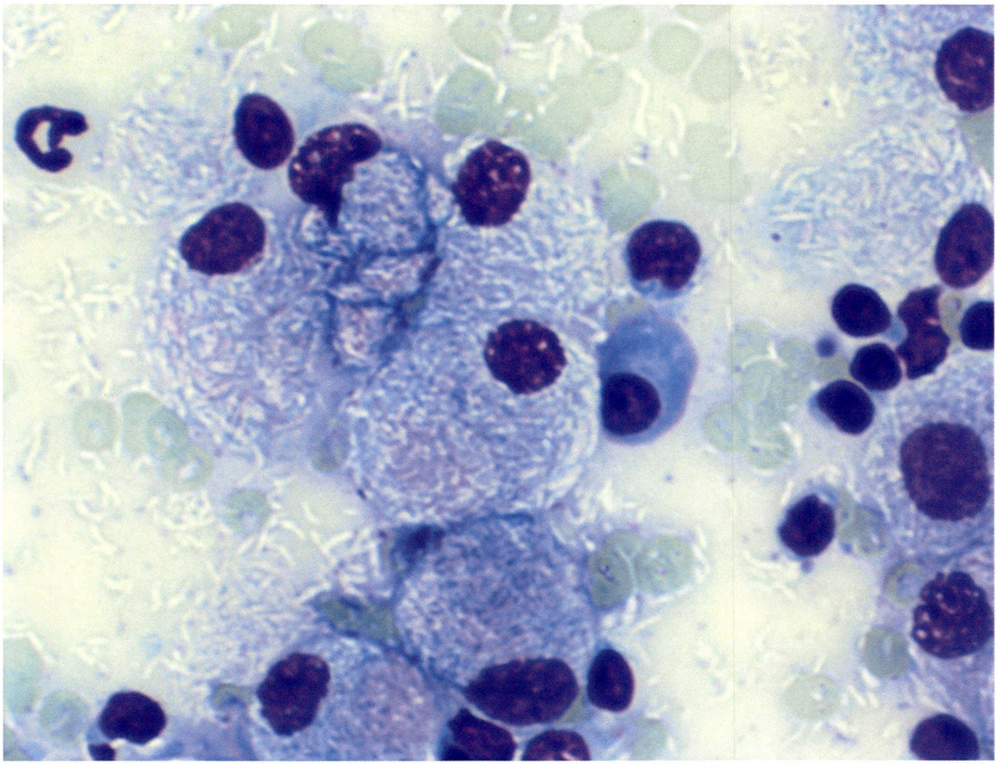

Figure 39. Granulomatous lymphadenitis due to mycobacteria.

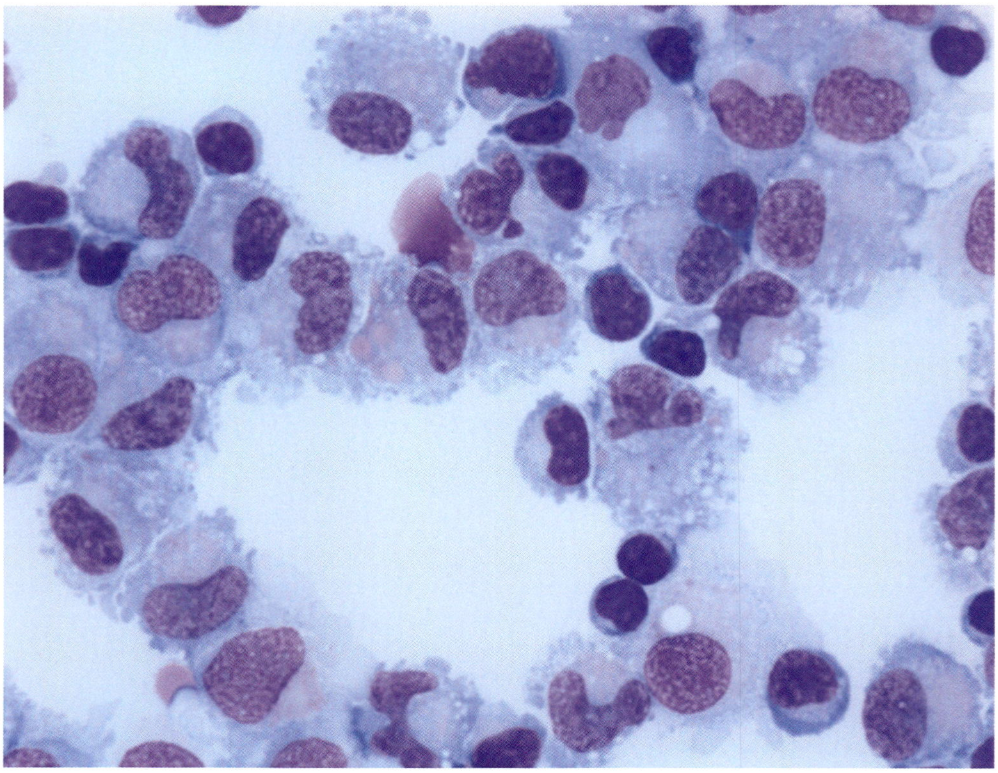

Figure 40. Cerebrospinal fluid sample. Inclusion bodies in a case of distemper.

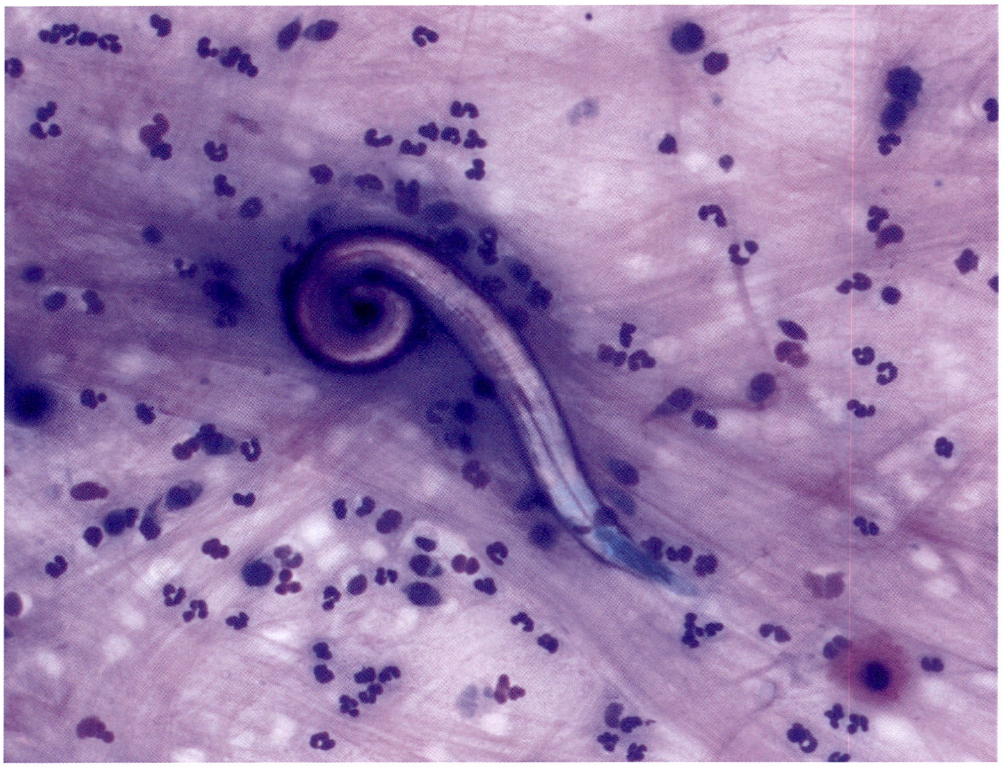

Figure 41. Tracheal wash sample containing a parasitic form.

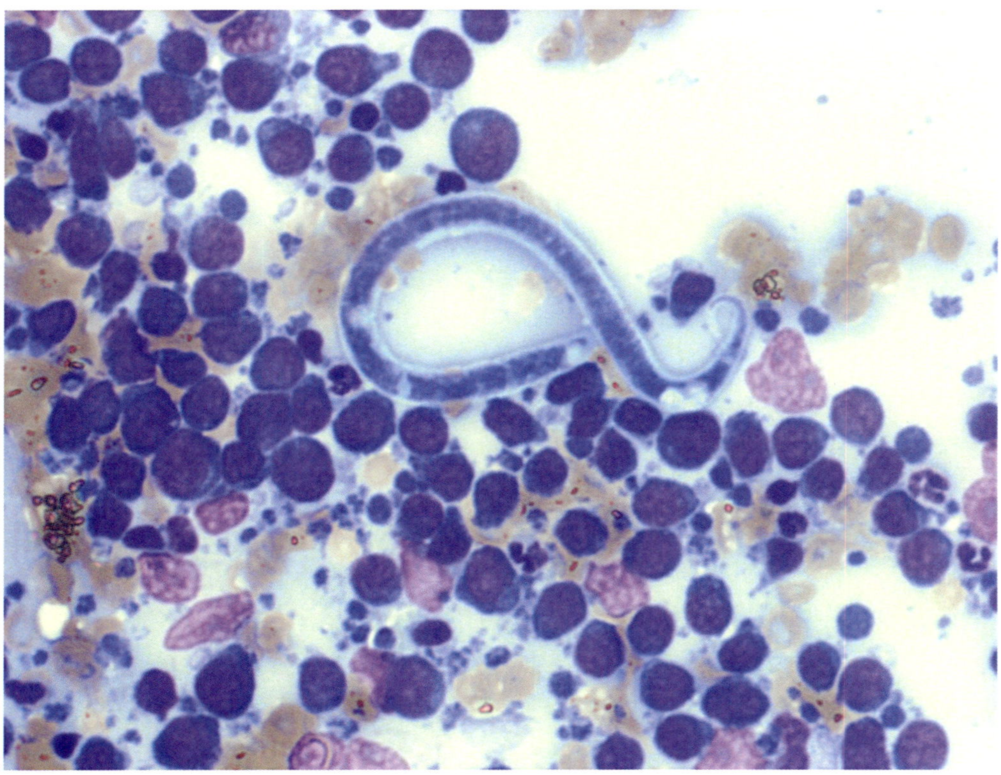

Figure 42. Filaria in lymph node cytology in a case of lymphoma.

Figures 43 and 44. Leishmaniasis. Amastigotes in lymph node (43) and cutaneous granuloma (44) samples.

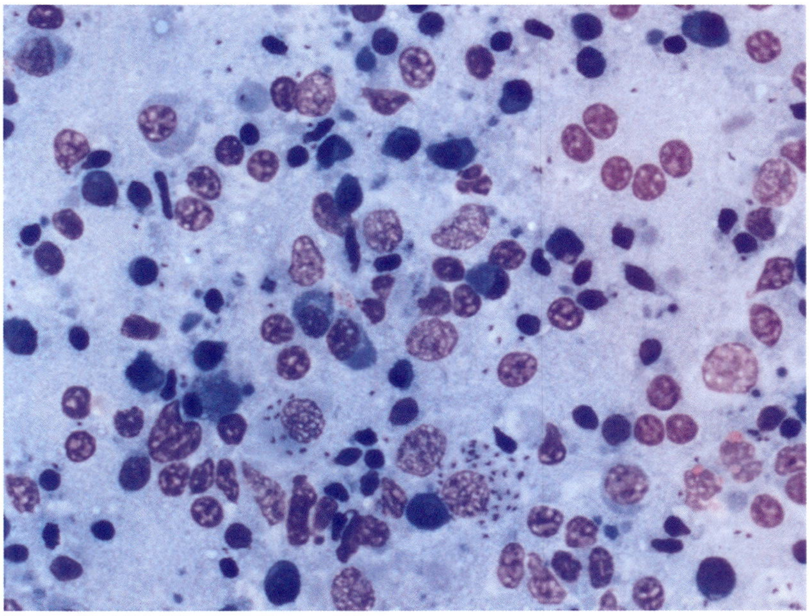

Figure 43.

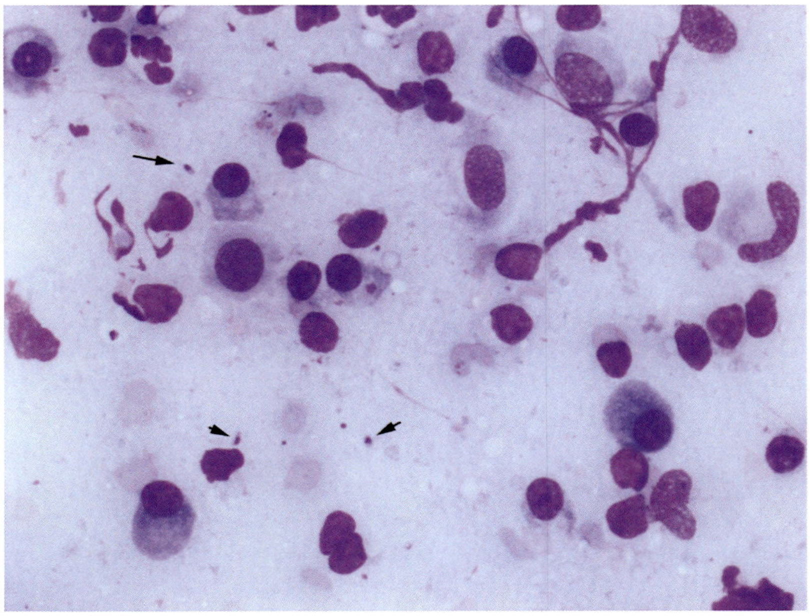

Figure 44.

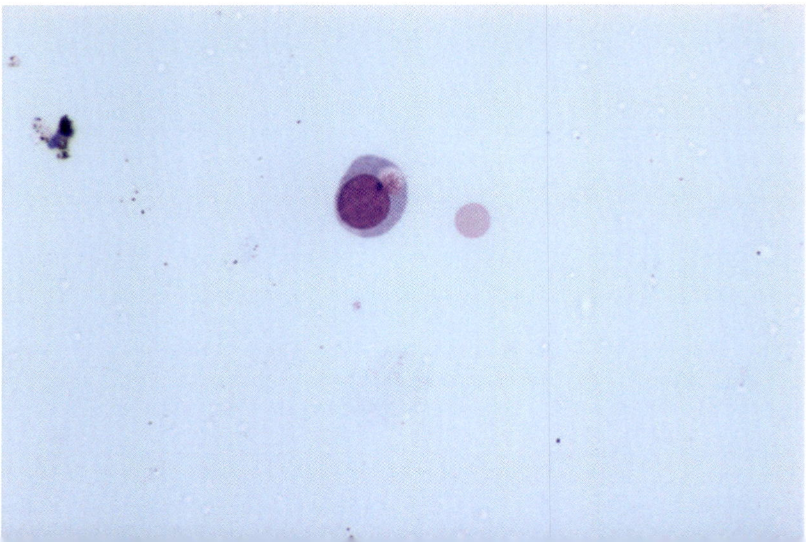

Figure 45. Cerebrospinal fluid sample containing *Ehrlichia* morula.

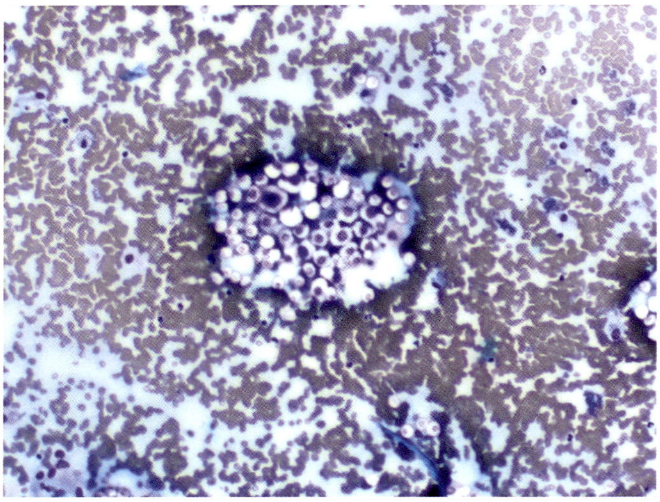

Figure 46.

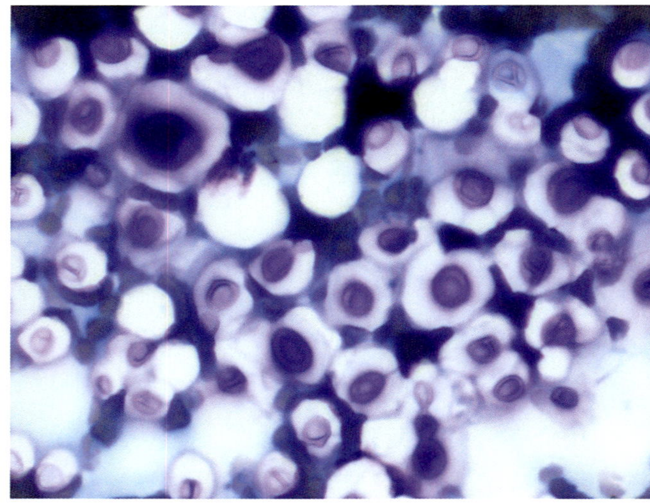

Figure 47.

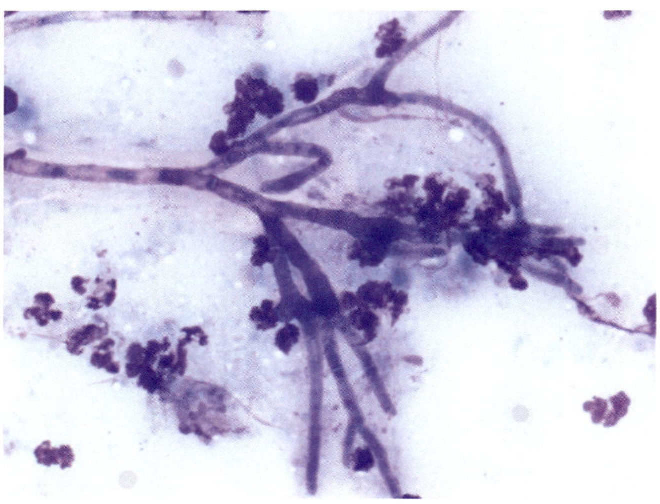

Figure 48.

Figures 46–48. Nasal wash samples: cryptococcosis (46, 47) and aspergillosis (48).

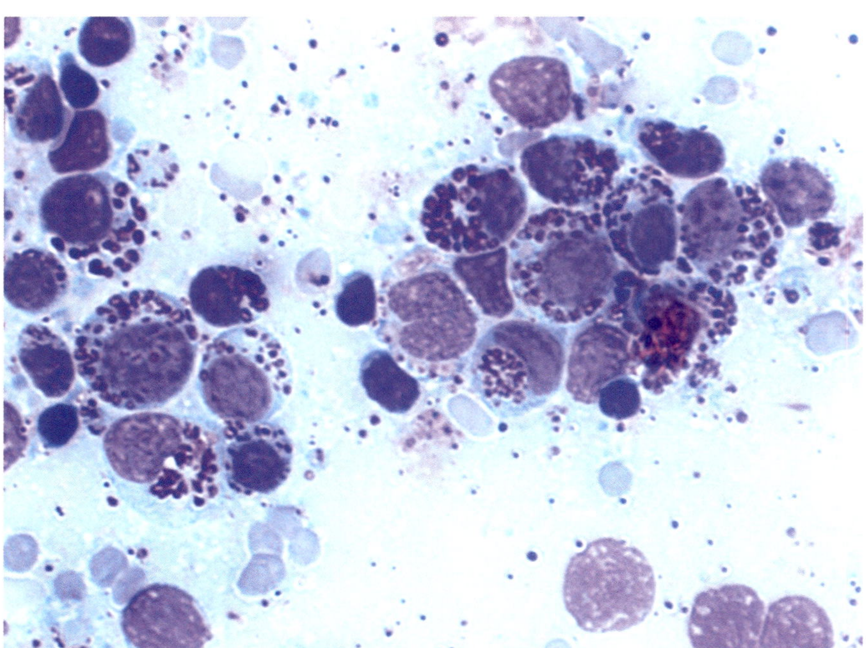

Figure 49. Large granule cell lymphoma (cat). The granules resemble fungal structures.

## PRESENCE OF TISSUE CELLS IN INFLAMMATORY CYTOLOGY

In cases in which a predominantly inflammatory cytological specimen contains tissue cells (usually derived from the inflamed organ), it can be difficult to determine whether the inflammatory process is primary or is secondary to another (generally neoplastic) process (Figs. 50 and 51). It is important to keep in mind that in response to inflammation tissue cells can undergo dysplastic changes that resemble malignant changes. In these cases, establishing diagnosis is more challenging. It is difficult to determine whether the primary process is the inflammation or the tissue activation (neoplasia). Neoplasia can only be confirmed if these changes are maintained once the inflammatory reaction ceases.

Figures 50 and 51. Tissue cells associated with an inflammatory process (nasal and bladder samples). It is difficult to determine whether the cells are dysplastic or neoplastic.

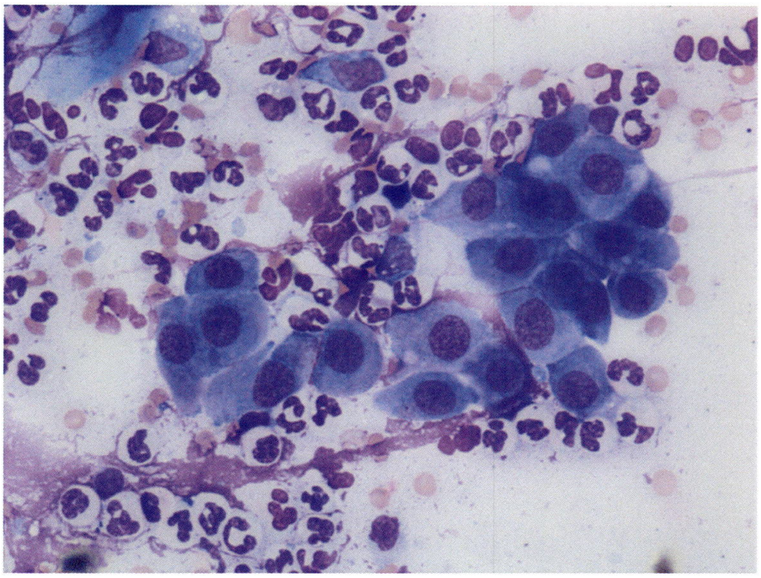

Figure 50.

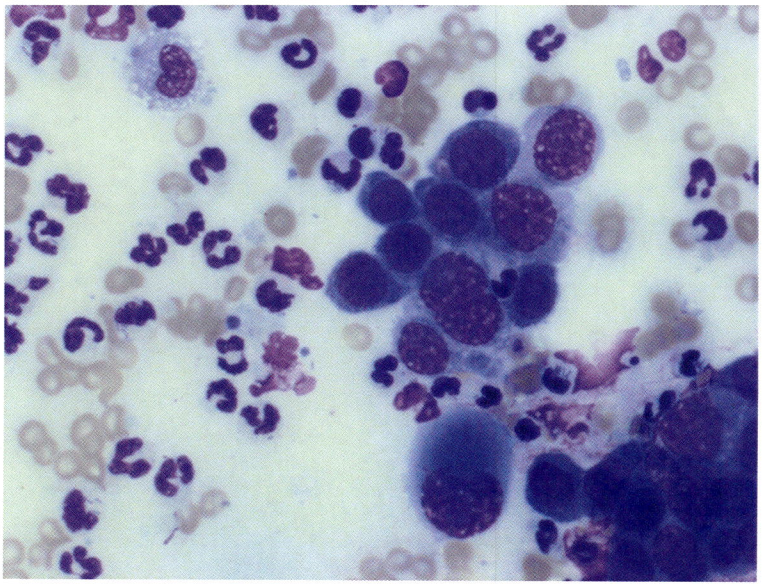

Figure 51.

# 02

# Cytology of noninflammatory/ nonneoplastic lesions

# Cytology of noninflammatory/ nonneoplastic lesions

There are numerous noninflammatory/nonneoplastic lesions that can affect a variety of structures. In this chapter, we will discuss three different types, owing to their clinical importance and diagnostic ambiguity: hyperplastic processes, degenerative processes, and extramedullary haematopoiesis (EH).

## HYPERPLASTIC CHANGES

Hyperplasia involves an increase in the number of cells in nonneoplastic tissue (Fig. 1). Common characteristics of all hyperplastic changes include increased cell volume and mild signs of nuclear activation, such as an increase in the nucleus:cytoplasm ratio and anisokaryosis.

Although cytology is commonly used to initiate the diagnostic process, in this particular context it offers less than reliable results. In most cases, the cytological picture cannot be distinguished from that of normal tissue or of a well-differentiated benign/malignant neoplasm. Therefore, the results should always be interpreted with caution and only considered suggestive of a diagnosis.

The most clinically important forms of hyperplasia are hyperplasia of the sebaceous glands, squamous cells, prostate, liver, and lymphoid tissue.

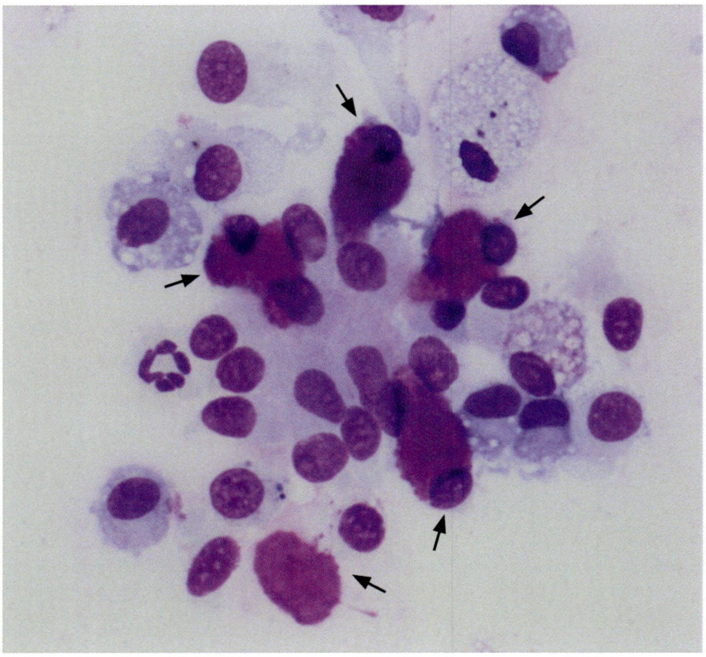

Figure 1. Tracheal wash sample. Goblet cell hyperplasia (arrows) in a case of chronic bronchitis. In normal conditions, numbers of these cells are very low.

Sebaceous hyperplasia is cytologically indistinguishable from adenoma. Consequently, it is common to reach a diagnosis of hyperplasia/sebaceous adenoma (Fig. 2).

Squamous cell hyperplasia can be confused with benign papillomatous lesions, metaplasia, and well-differentiated carcinoma (Figs. 3 and 4). In general, the cells do not exhibit marked atypia, and therefore aggressive carcinoma can be ruled out in most cases. Metaplasia is uncommon and usually restricted to prostatic tissue (Fig. 5) that has been exposed to high concentrations of oestrogen.

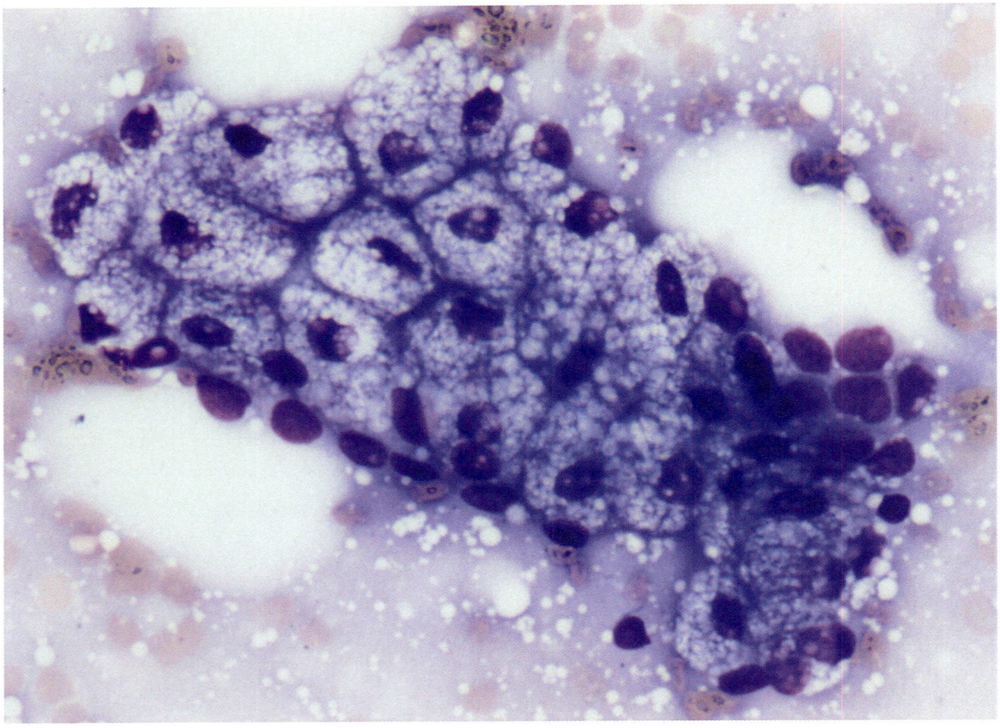

Figure 2. Group of sebaceous cells. It is impossible to determine whether this is indicative of hyperplasia or adenoma.

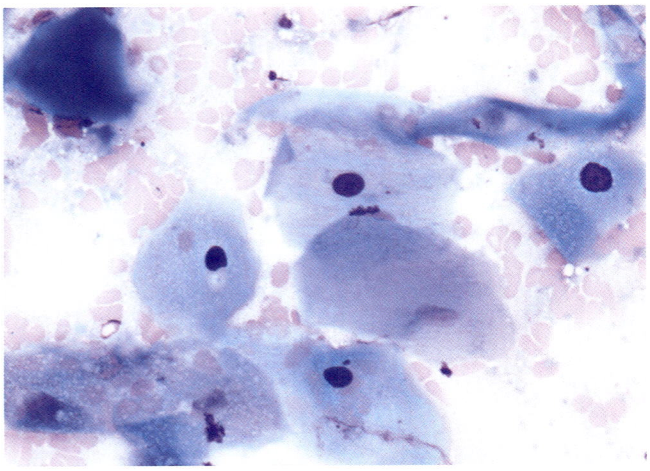

Figure 3. Squamous cell hyperplasia associated with a follicular cyst.

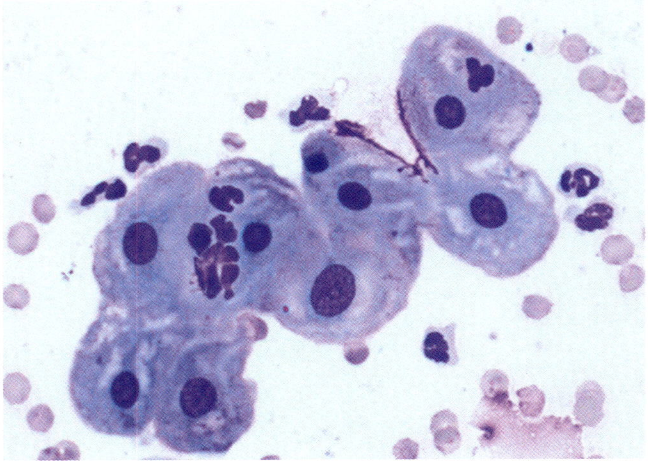

Figure 4. Papillomatous lesion on the foreskin. Squamous cell hyperplasia (histopathological diagnosis). Cytologically, this should be differentiated from well-differentiated squamous cell carcinoma.

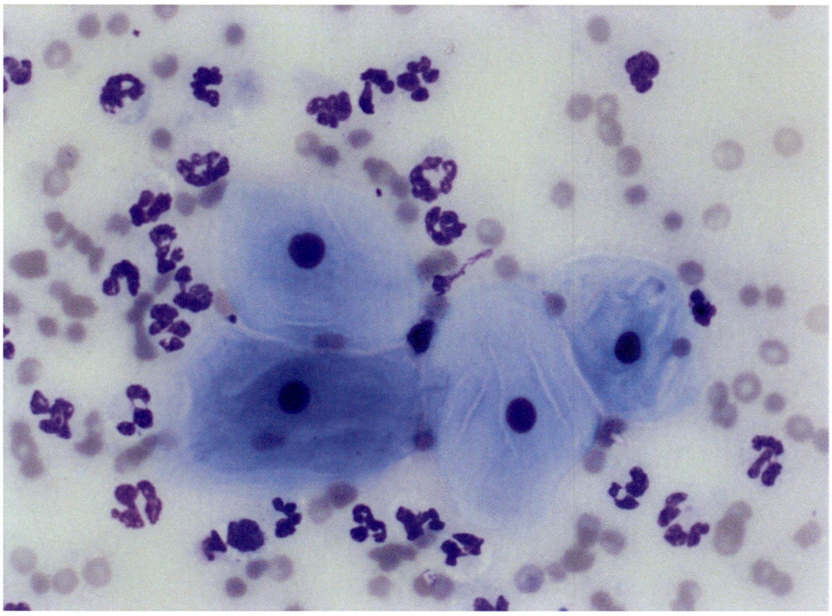

Figure 5. Prostate cytology. Squamous metaplasia associated with inflammation in a patient with a Sertoli cell tumour.

Benign prostatic hyperplasia is one of the most common diseases in dogs. The cytological picture is similar to that of normal prostatic tissue (Fig. 6). Prostate tumours usually display marked cellular and nuclear atypia (Fig. 7), facilitating differentiation of these two processes.

Hyperplasia phenomena are common in the liver (benign nodular hyperplasia). In addition to the generic features described above, these processes are characterised by an increase in the number of binucleated hepatocytes. In most cases, there are insufficient differential features to distinguish hyperplasia from a well-differentiated benign or malignant hepatocellular tumour (Figs. 8–11).

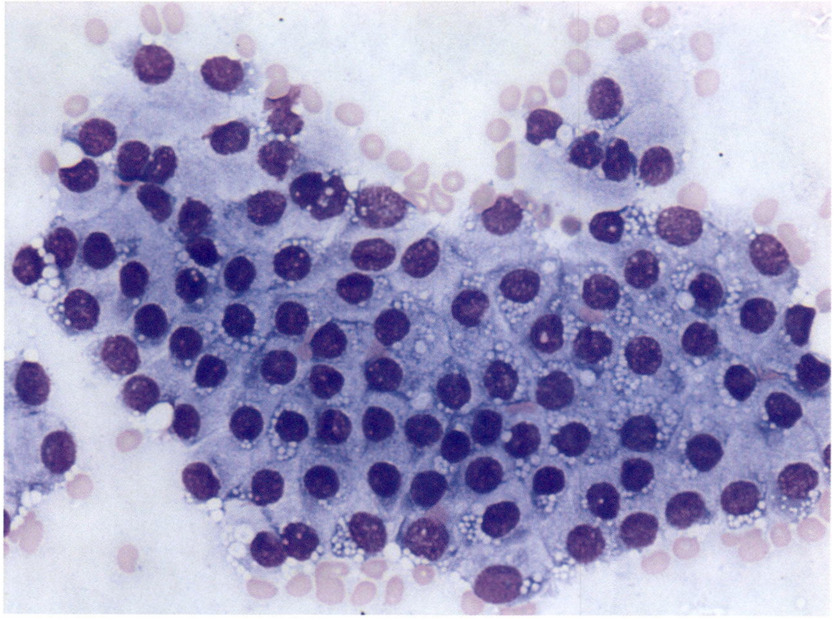

Figure 6. Benign prostatic hyperplasia. The cells exhibit increased vacuolisation and mild signs of nuclear activation.

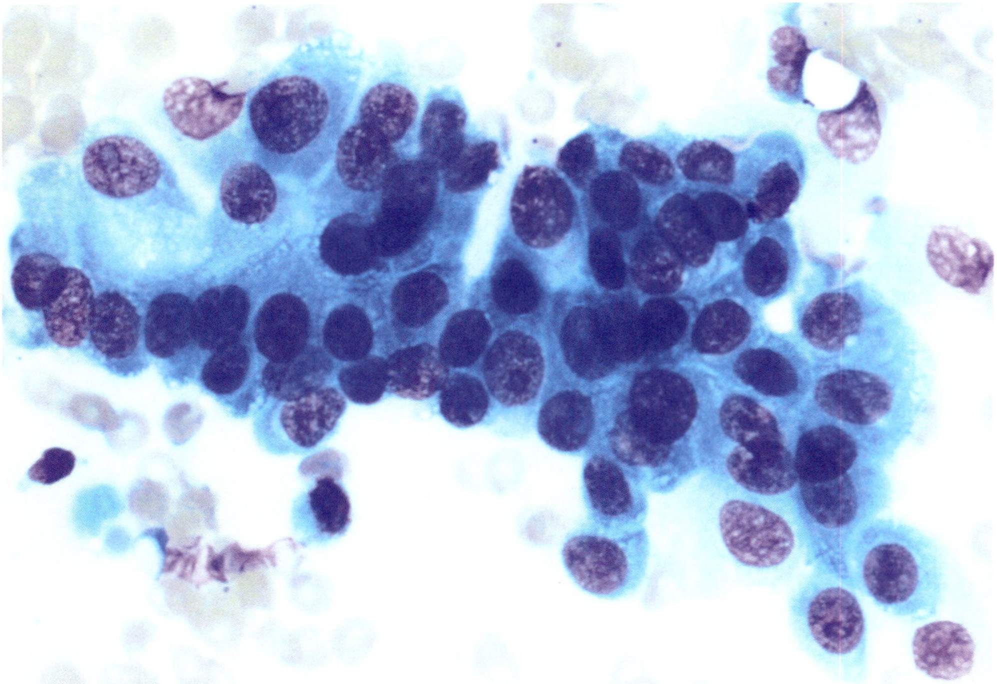

Figure 7. Prostate carcinoma. This cytological picture cannot be confused with that of hyperplasia.

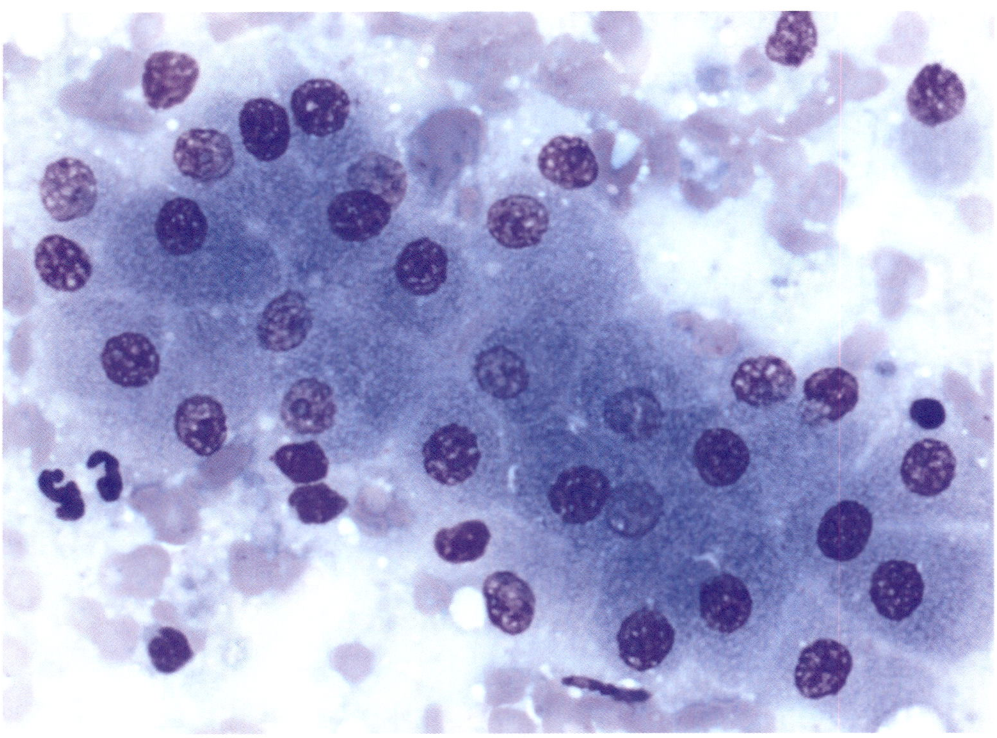

Figure 8. Hepatic cytology. Group of hepatocytes showing very mild signs of hyperplasia. This cytological picture cannot be distinguished from that of normal tissue.

Figures 9–11. Hepatic cytology in which the hepatocytes show the following signs of hyperplasia: increased cellular volume, increased nucleus:cytoplasm ratio, mild anisokaryosis, binucleated cells. The images could correspond to well-differentiated benign or malignant tumours.

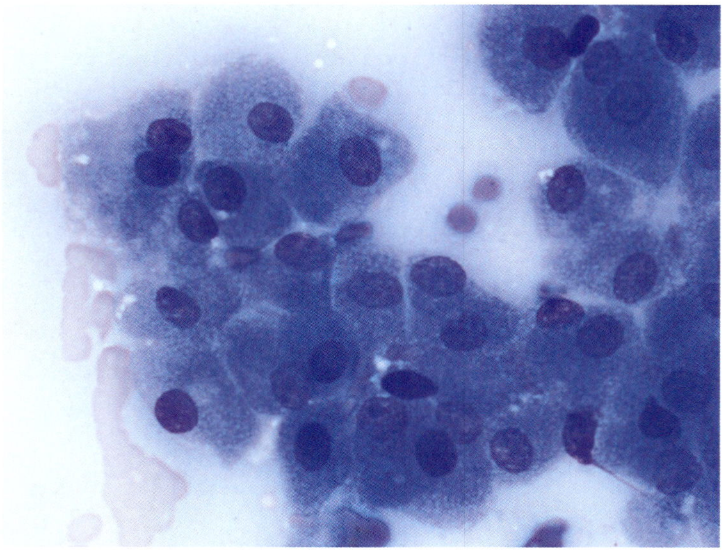

Figure 9.

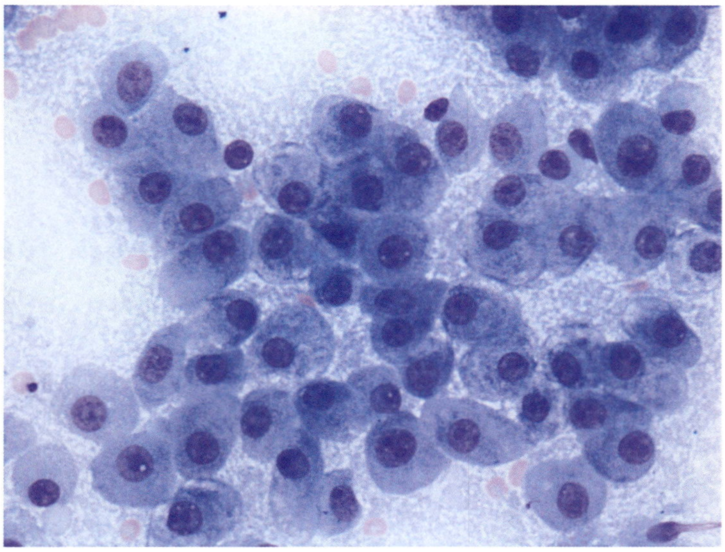

Figure 10.

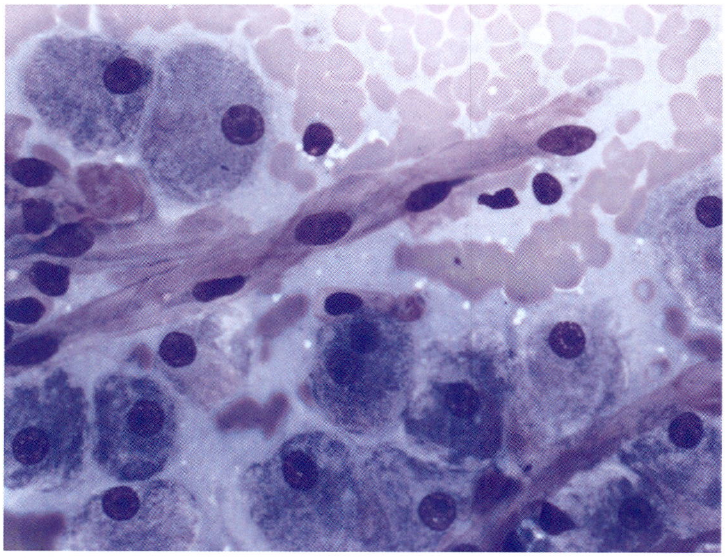

Figure 11.

Cytological diagnosis of lymphoid hyperplasia in the lymph nodes and spleen in response to different antigenic stimuli is very common. Characteristics of hyperplasia and reactive tissue tend to coexist, resulting in increases in the numbers of prolymphocytes and lymphoblasts (usually in different stages), as well as plasma cells. Increases in the proportions of macrophages and mast cells are also common. Together, these alterations give rise to a heterogeneous cytological picture, which allows easy differentiation of reactive/hyperplastic tissue from lymphoma (Figs. 12–14). Plasma cells are activated, as evidenced by the presence of Russell bodies (plasma cells with vacuoles or Mott cells), flame cells, and binucleated cells. In addition, there is an increase in the number of immature plasma cells, which are larger than mature cells and contain greyish cytoplasm (Figs. 15–20). The increase in the number of plasma cells can be very marked, requiring differentiation from plasma cell neoplasm. However, in the case of reactive tissue, the observed cellular changes do not include marked nuclear atypia (Figs. 21 and 22).

Intense lymphoid hyperplasia without an increase in the number of plasma cells can be confused with lymphoma. It is therefore necessary to differentiate between these two processes using histology, immunohistochemistry, cytometry, or clonality tests. This situation is more common in cats, especially young cats (idiopathic benign hyperplasia) or those with viral infections, although in dogs it can also occur in cases of ehrlichiosis or in response to other antigenic stimuli (Figs. 23–26).

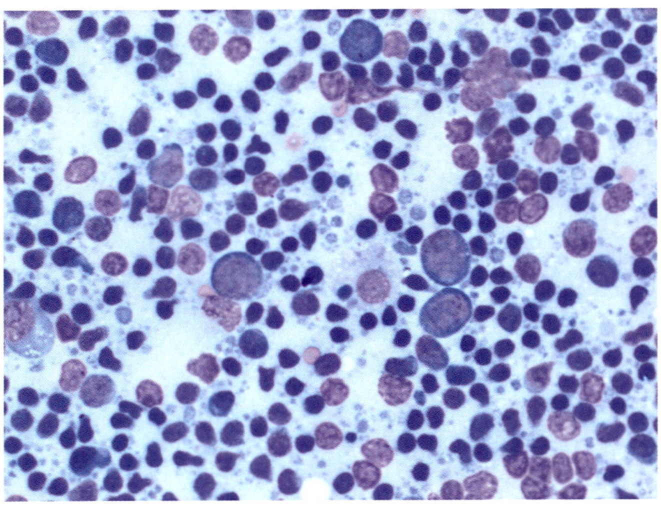

Figure 12.

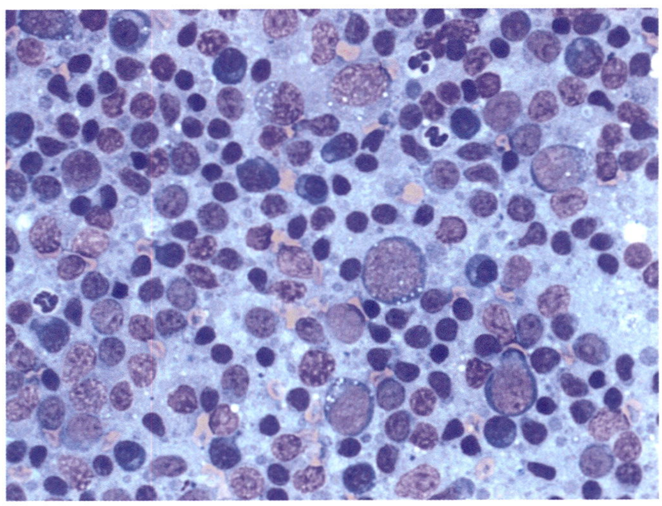

Figure 13.

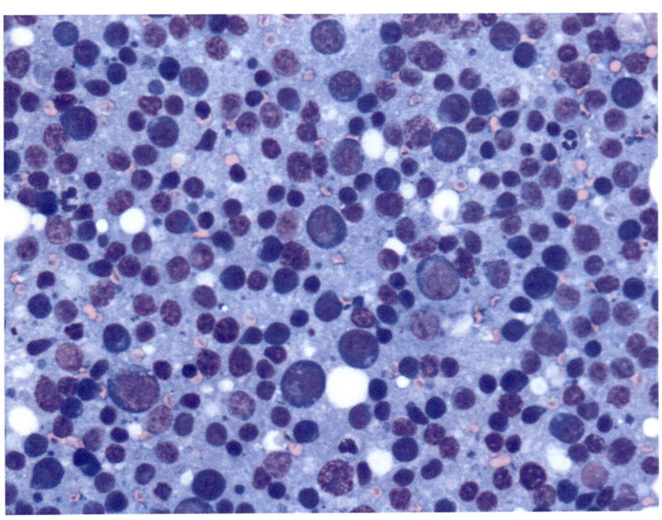

◂ Figure 14.

Figures 12–14. Hyperplastic/reactive lymph node and spleen lymphoid tissue showing a heterogeneous picture, with an increase in the number of blasts and plasma cells.

Figures 15–20. Hyperplastic/reactive lymph node and spleen lymphoid tissue with activated plasma cells. Russell bodies (15, 16), flame cells (17, 18), immature cells (19, 20, black arrows), and binucleated cells (20). Red arrows in image 19 indicate erythroid precursors.

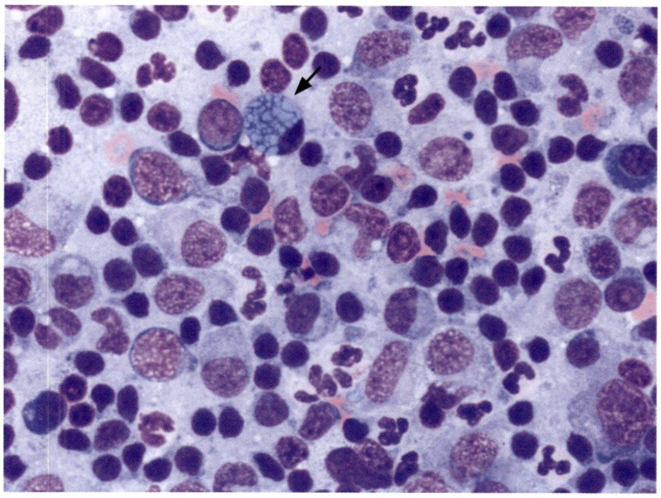

Figure 15.

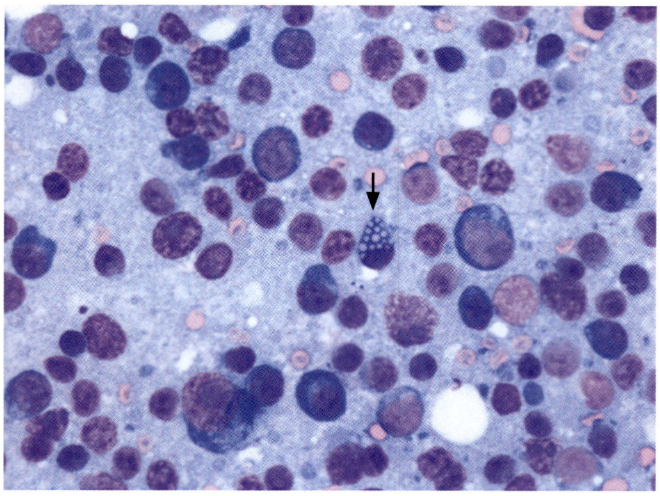

Figure 16.

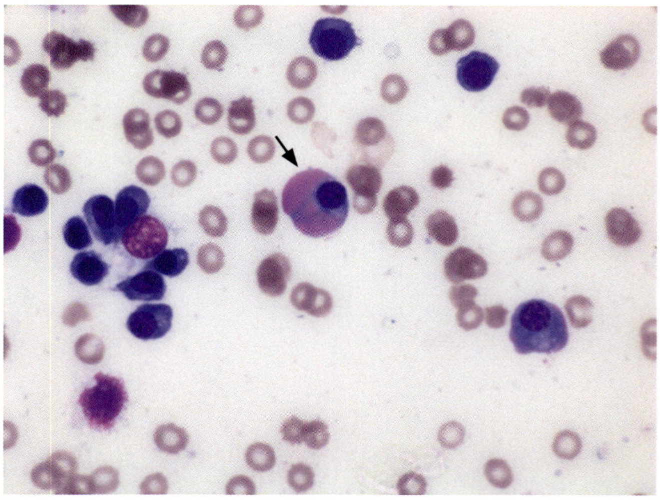

Figure 17.

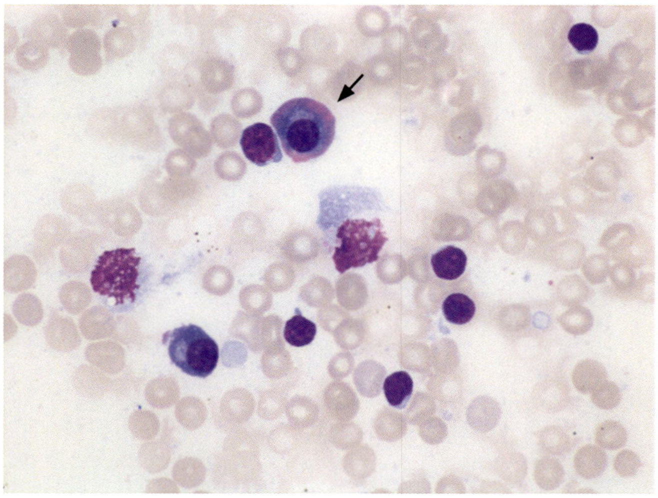

Figure 18.

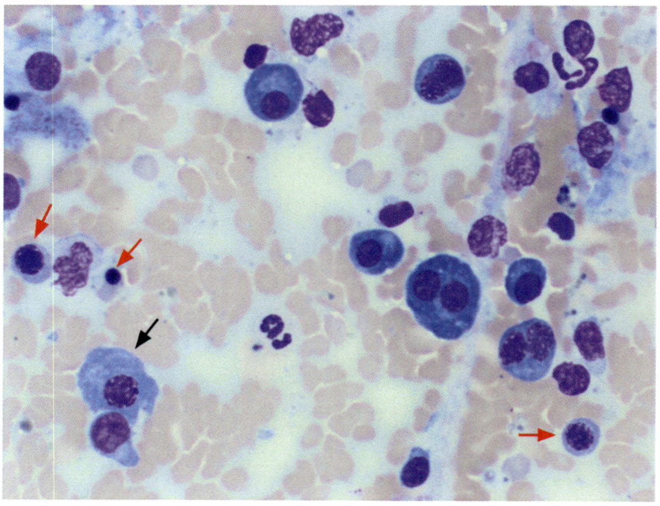

Figure 19.

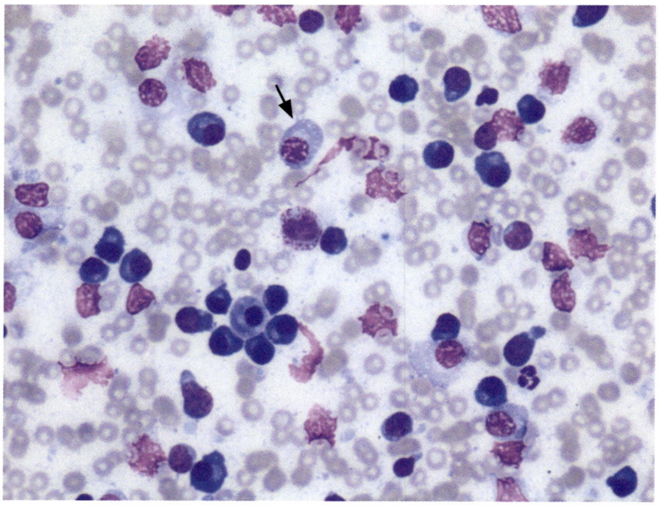

Figure 20.

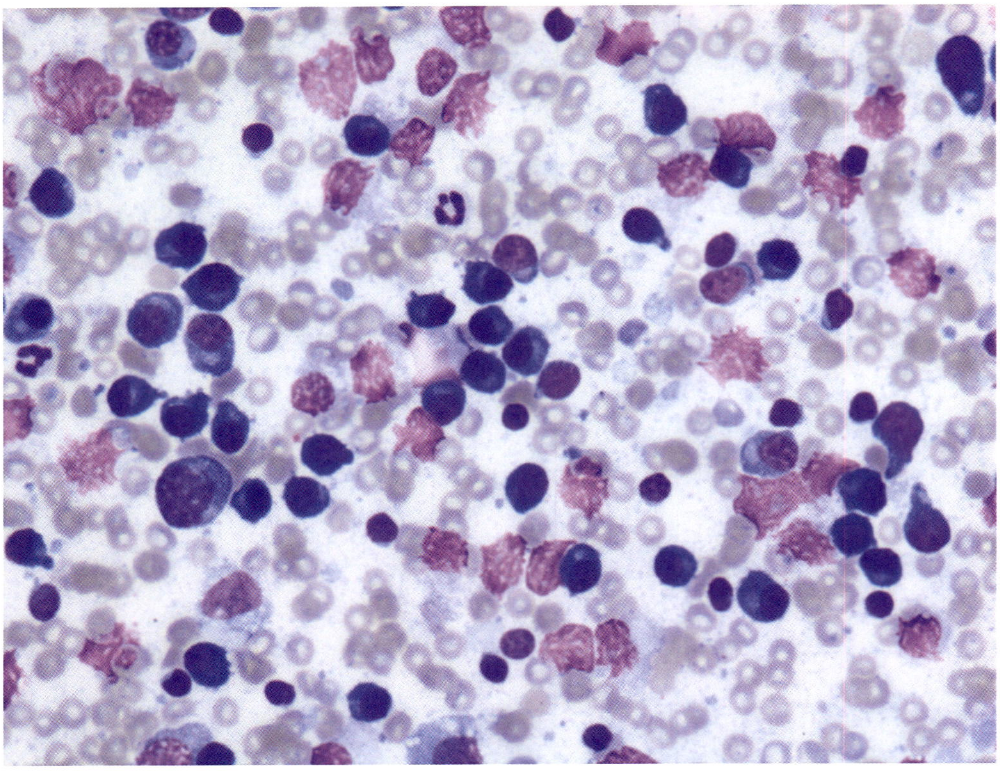

Figures 21. Lymph node exhibiting intense plasma cell hyperplasia. Despite the abundant plasma cells, the cytological picture cannot be confused with that of a neoplasm.

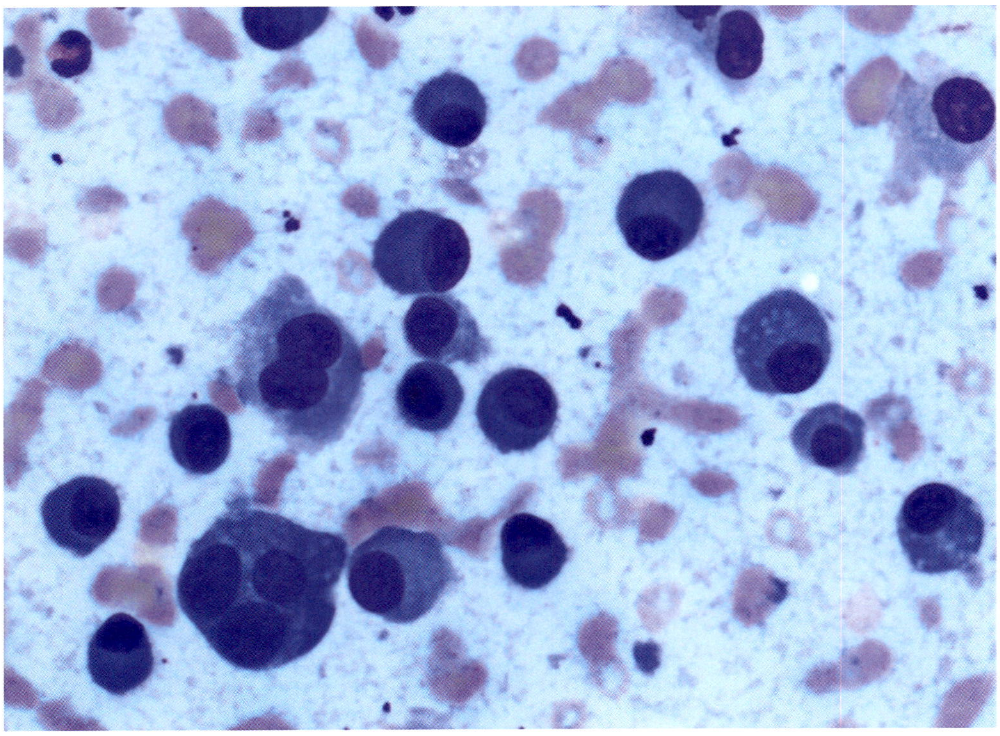

Figure 22. Lymph node in which atypical plasma cells are evident (plasmacytoma metastasis).

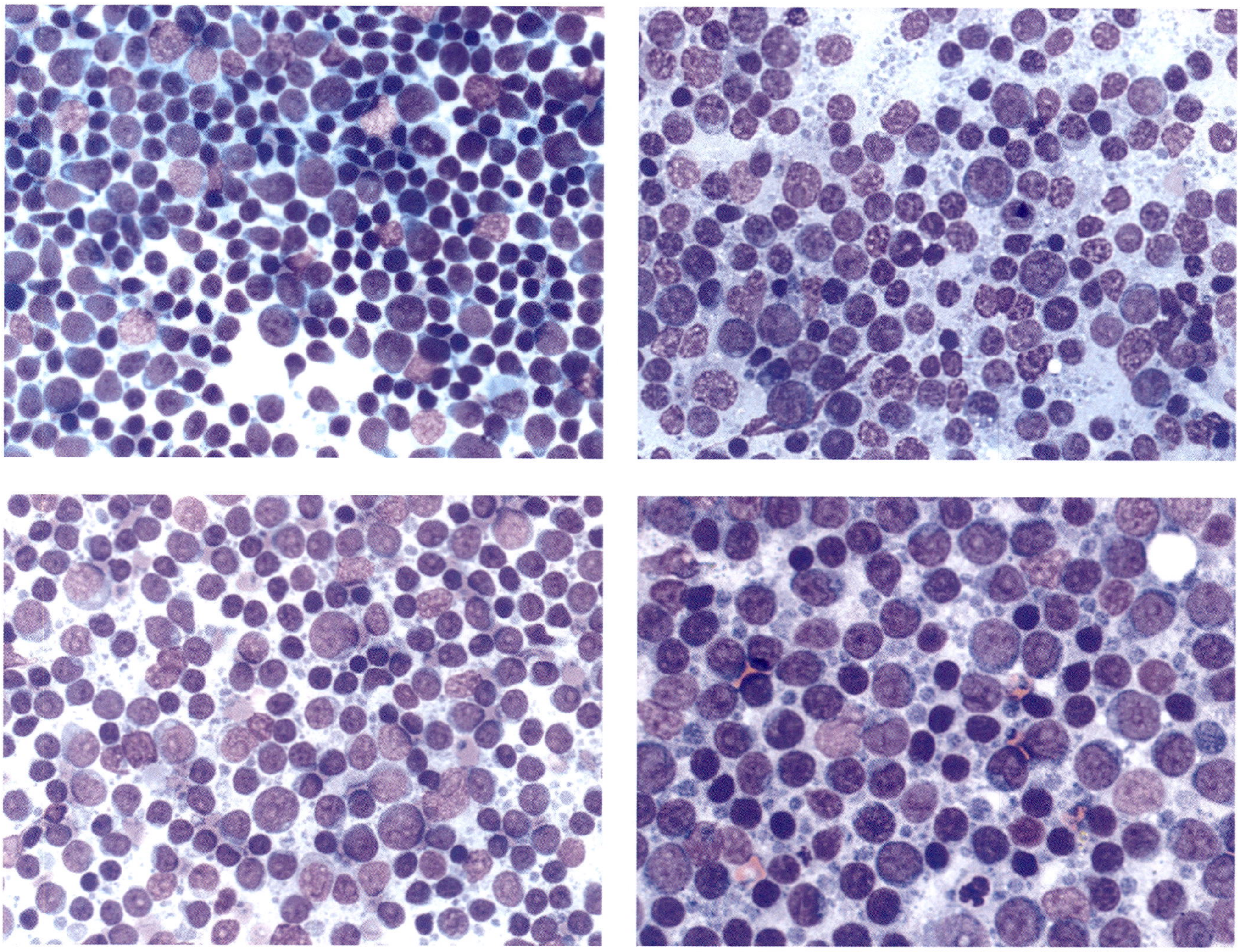

Figures 23–26. Lymphoid hyperplasia with no increase in plasma cell number. Although the cytological picture is heterogeneous, it may ultimately resemble a lymphoma.

# DEGENERATIVE CHANGES

In this section we will focus on the two types of degenerative changes that are most commonly diagnosed cytologically: degenerative hepatic and articular changes. We will not discuss the degenerative changes that cells may undergo in a sample (e.g. CSF or other body fluids) or in response to infection (e.g. neutrophil degeneration, tissue necrosis).

## DEGENERATIVE HEPATIC CHANGES

These changes are very common and characterised by the formation of macrovacuoles in the microvacuolated cytoplasm of hepatocytes. Of all pathological changes in the liver, the greatest concordance between the cytological and histopathological diagnosis is observed for vacuolar degeneration, although it can be difficult to determine the primary cause.

The degree of degeneration is established based on the number of affected hepatocytes and the intensity of the changes in each cell. Associated hyperplastic alterations are common.

The cytological picture of vacuolar changes allows easy differentiation between lipid and non-lipid degeneration.

The former (which is most common in cats) manifests with the presence of clear, round, well-defined vacuoles of varying sizes. In some cases the cytoplasm becomes completely filled with vacuoles (or with a single vacuole), making it difficult to recognise the cells as liver cells (they more closely resemble adipocytes) (Figs. 27–29). Cytology is a very reliable means of diagnosing lipidosis, and is considered the diagnostic tool of choice in cases in which lipidosis is suspected based on clinical signs or ultrasound findings.

Figures 27–29. Mild, moderate, and intense hepatic lipid degeneration.

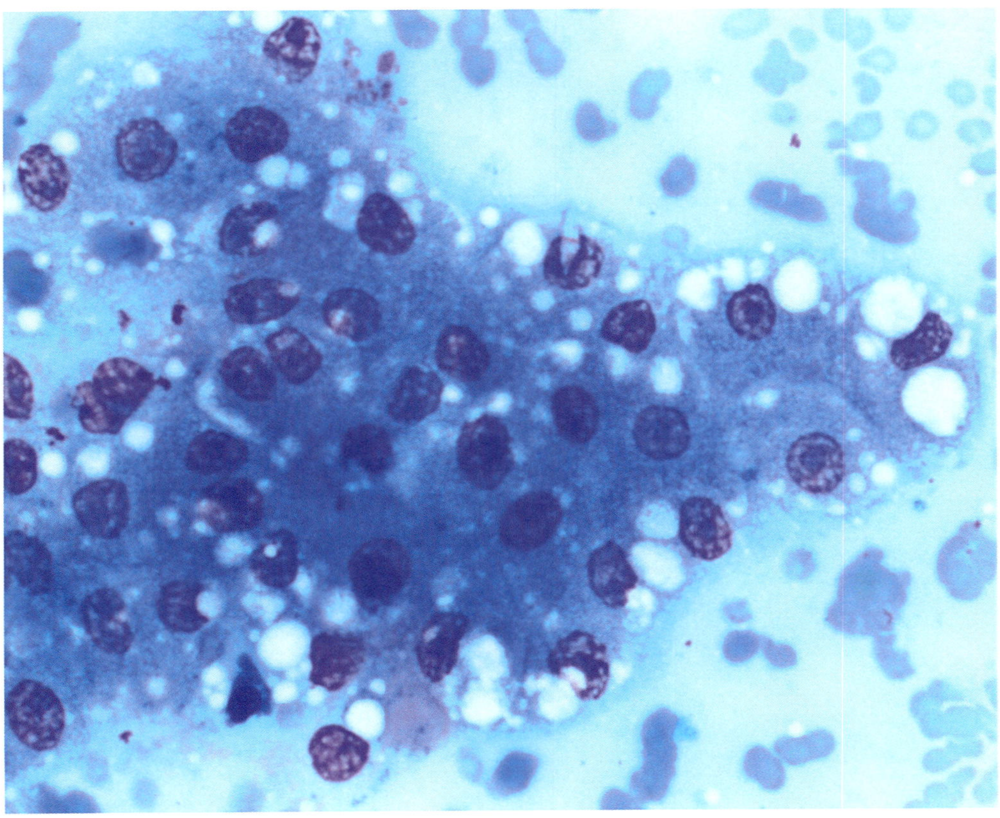

Figure 27.

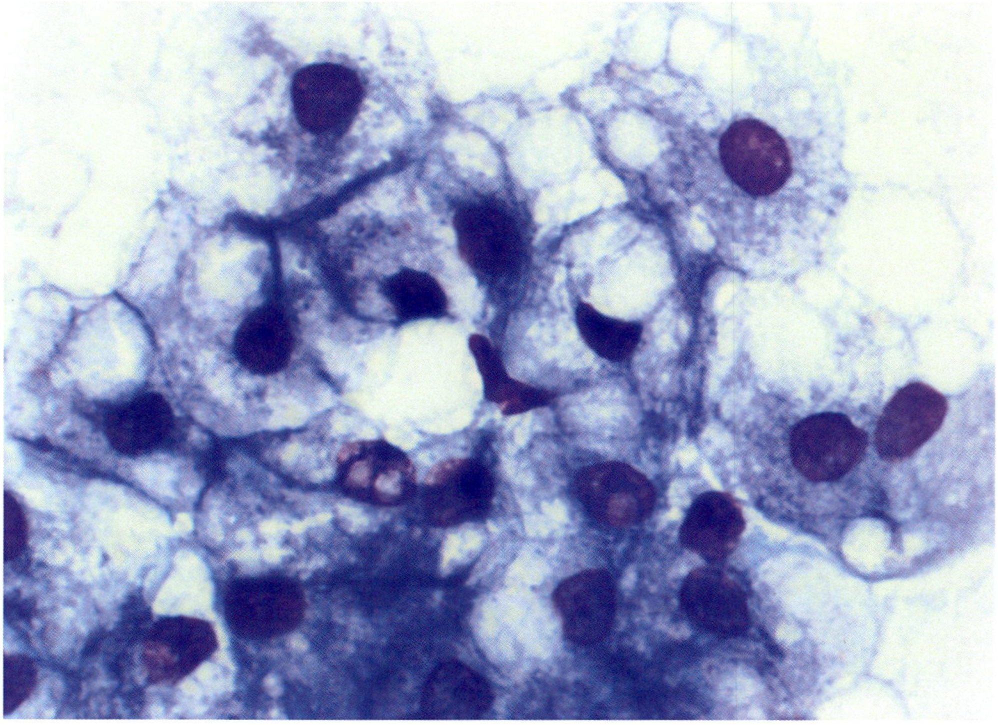

Figure 28.

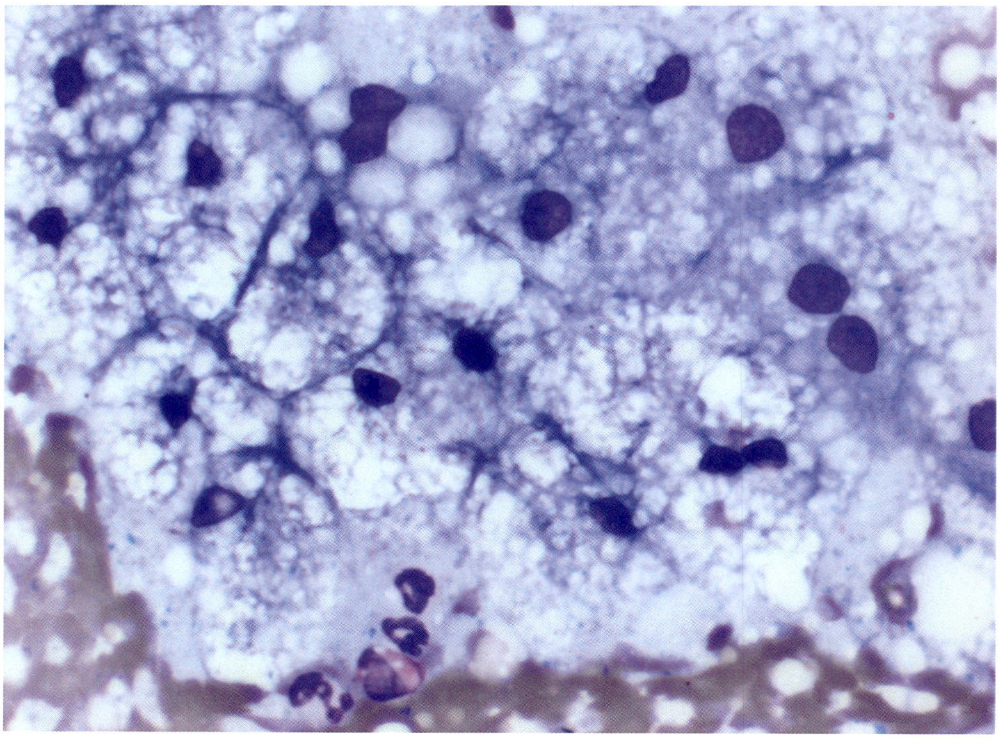

Figure 29.

Nonlipid degeneration is more common in dogs, and can be associated with hydropic changes or the accumulation of glycogen. Although the structures observed are considered vacuoles, they actually form as a result of cytoplasmic rarefaction (a decrease in the density of the cytoplasm), which gives rise to areas of cytoplasmic clearing with poorly defined borders that extend from the periphery to the nucleus (Figs. 30–32).

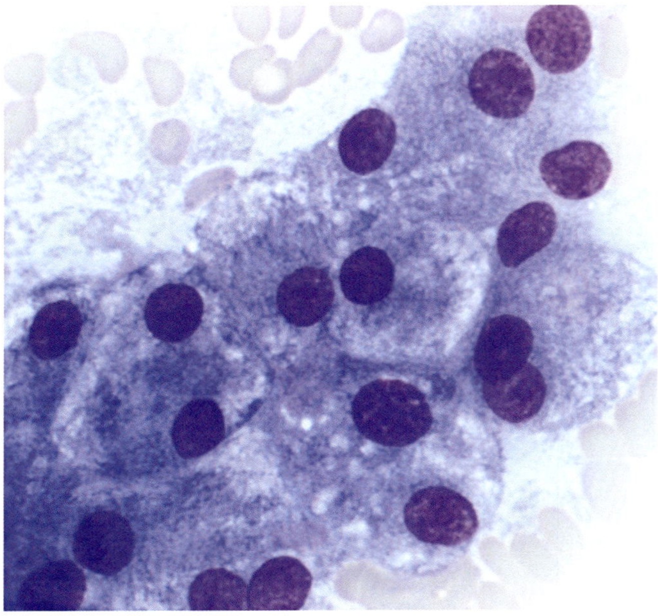

Figure 30.

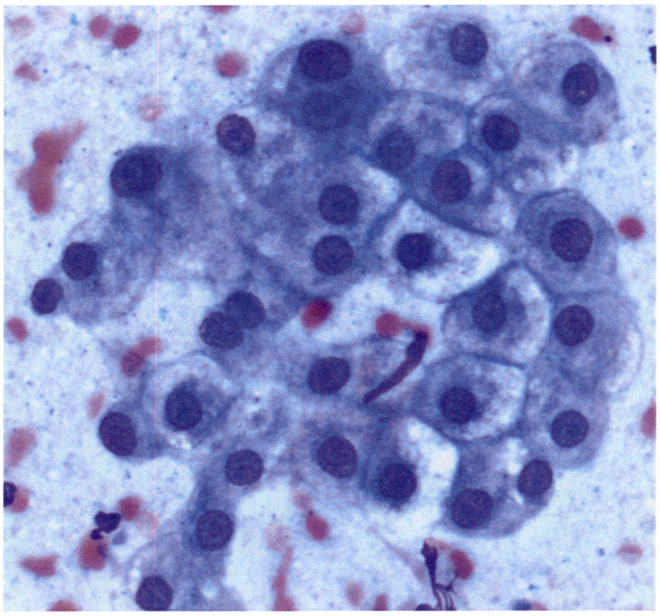

Figure 31.

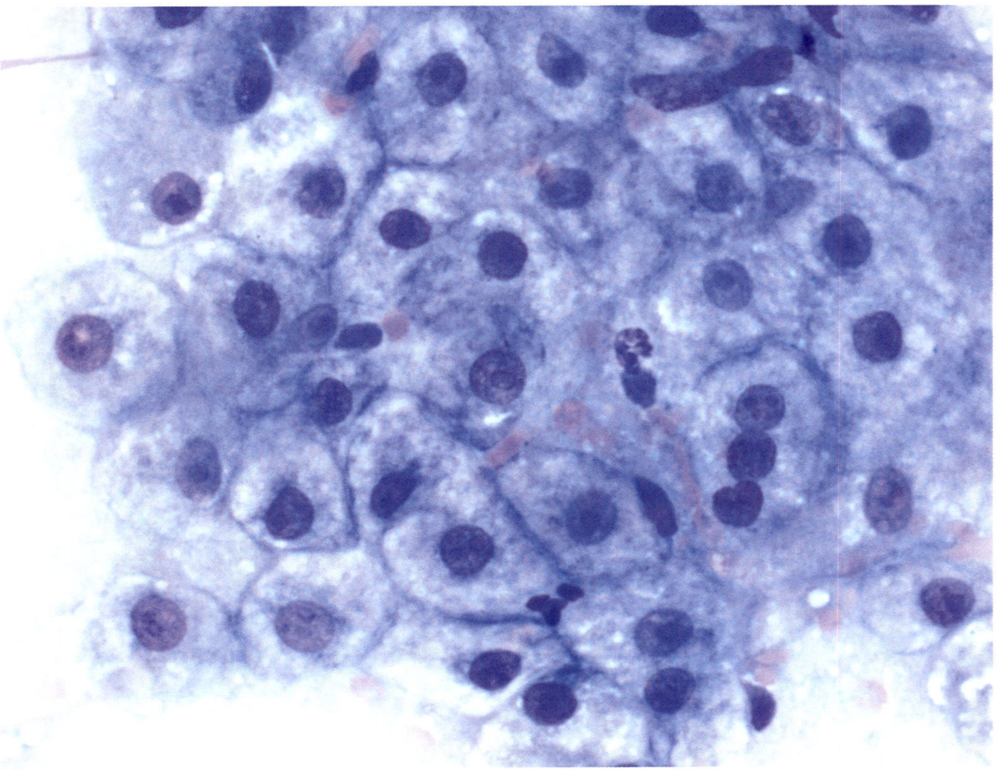

Figure 32.

Figures 30–32. Mild, moderate, and intense hepatic nonlipid degeneration.

## DEGENERATIVE ARTICULAR CHANGES

Synovial fluid cytology in degenerative diseases allows easy differentiation from inflammatory processes. The cytological picture is characterised by an increase in the activation of large mononuclear cells, which, under resting conditions, constitute the predominant population in normal synovial fluid. The diagnosis of degeneration is based not only on the increase in cellularity (although increases may be observed), but also on the presence of macrophagic cells identifiable by their abundant vacuolated cytoplasm (Fig. 33).

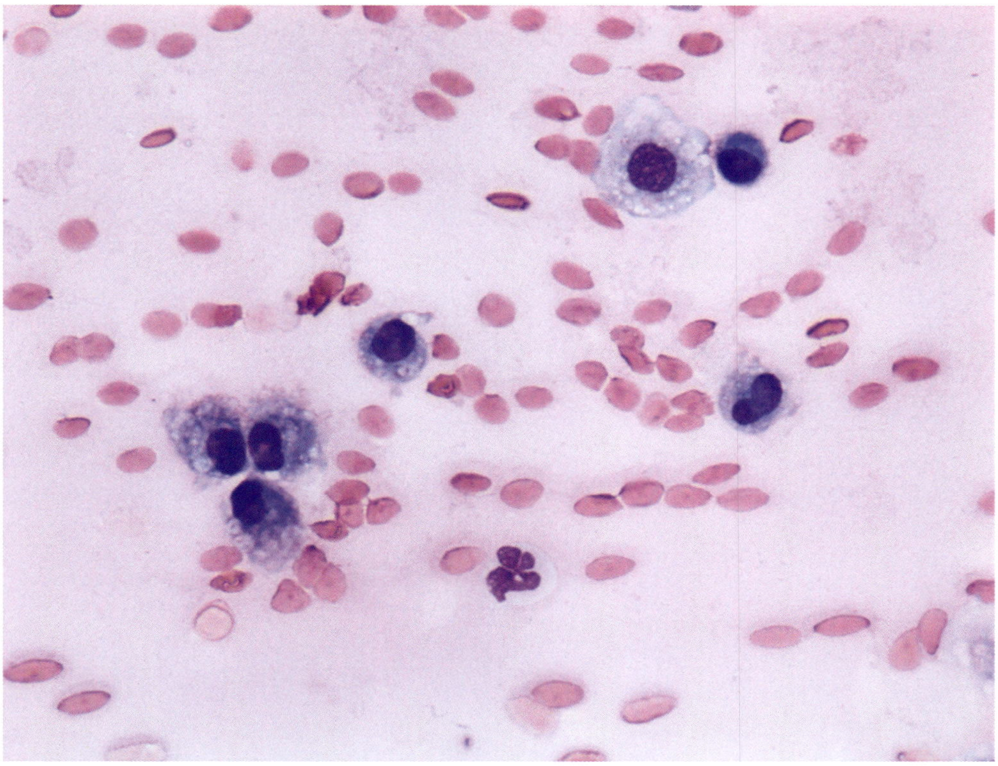

Figure 33. Synovial fluid cytology (very haemodiluted sample) in a case of degenerative arthropathy, with activation of mononuclear cells.

## EXTRAMEDULLARY HAEMATOPOIESIS

Extramedullary haematopoiesis (EH) is the result of the formation and development of hematopoietic cells outside the bone marrow. It is a common finding in splenic and hepatic cytological preparations, although it can occur in any organ (Fig. 34). It most often occurs in response to an intense cellular demand (which may or may not be associated with a failure in marrow production).

In EH, precursors of the three cell lineages are typically observed (Fig. 35), although one may predominate depending on the primary pathology. One characteristic feature is an ordered sequence of cell maturation, whereby the most mature cells are the most abundant (Fig. 36).

Increases in the number of megakaryocytes are easily visible owing to their large size (Fig. 37). The presence of these cells enables orientation of the cytological diagnosis towards EH.

Signs of mild EH can be observed in any splenic (or hepatic) cytological sample, but do not necessarily indicate that EH is the primary pathological process (Fig. 38). However, when very intense, haematopoietic precursors may constitute the predominant population. This situation can lead to confusion.

- Immature erythroid precursors are morphologically very similar to lymphoblasts. Therefore, if this cell population predominates a diagnosis of lymphoma may be established erroneously (Fig. 39).
- In myeloproliferative processes, solid organs can be infiltrated, and therefore cytology may reveal a predominance of leukaemic cells. In these cases, only the neoplastic precursor is observed (there are no signs of ordered cell maturation), allowing distinction from EH (Fig. 40).

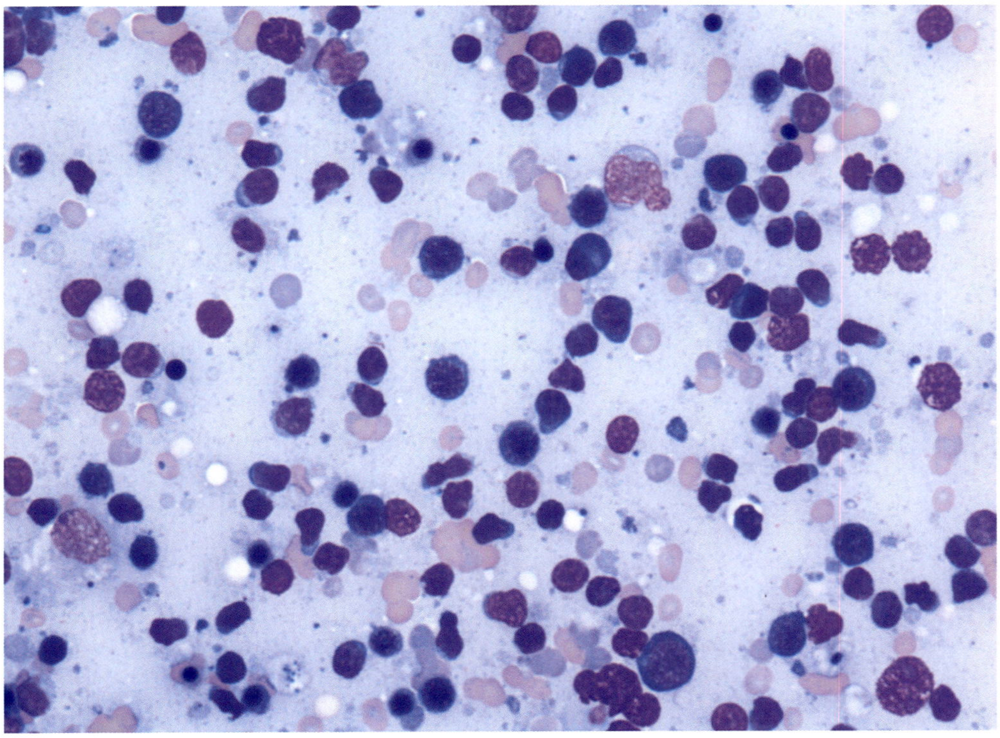

Figure 34. Extramedullary haematopoiesis of the lymph node in a cat with anaemia. Note the presence of numerous erythroid precursors.

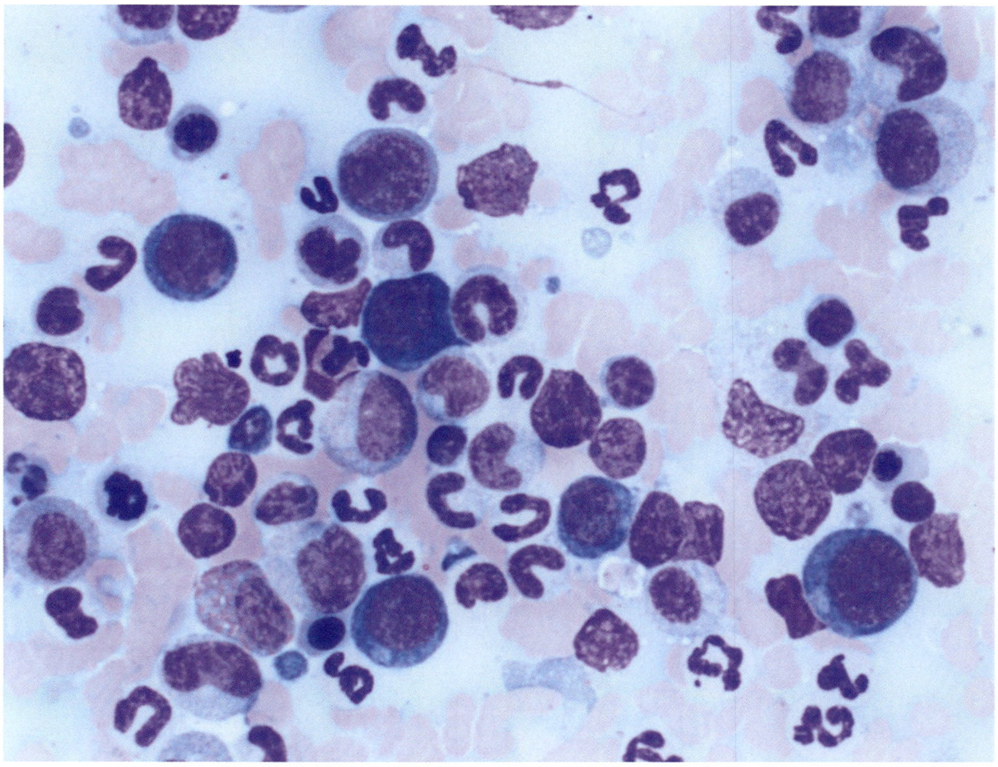

Figure 35. Extramedullary haematopoiesis of the spleen. Note the presence of erythroid and myeloid precursors.

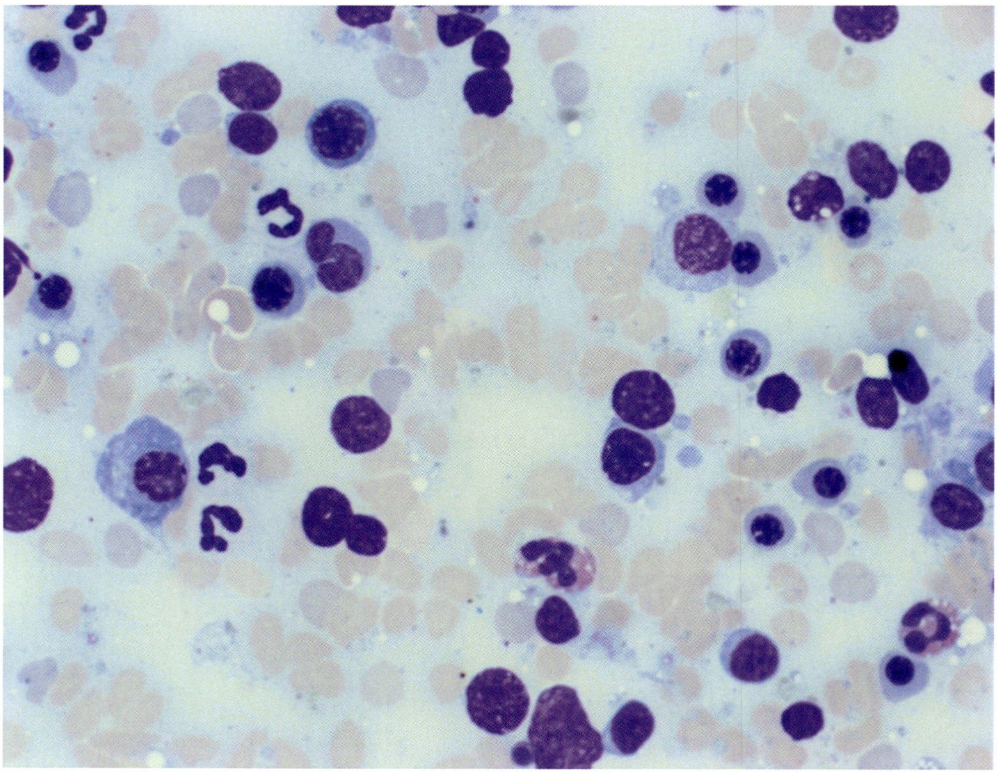

Figure 36. Extramedullary haematopoiesis of the spleen. Note the predominance of erythroid precursors in advanced stages of maturation.

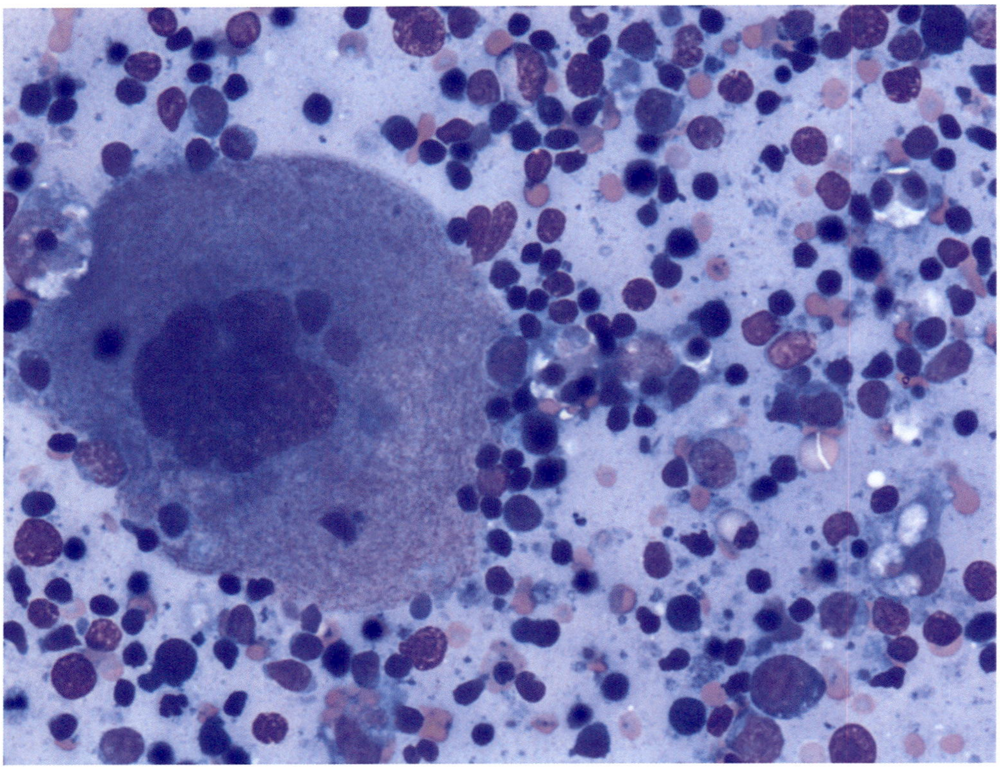

Figure 37. Extramedullary haematopoiesis of a lymph node. A megakaryocyte is easily visible owing to its large size.

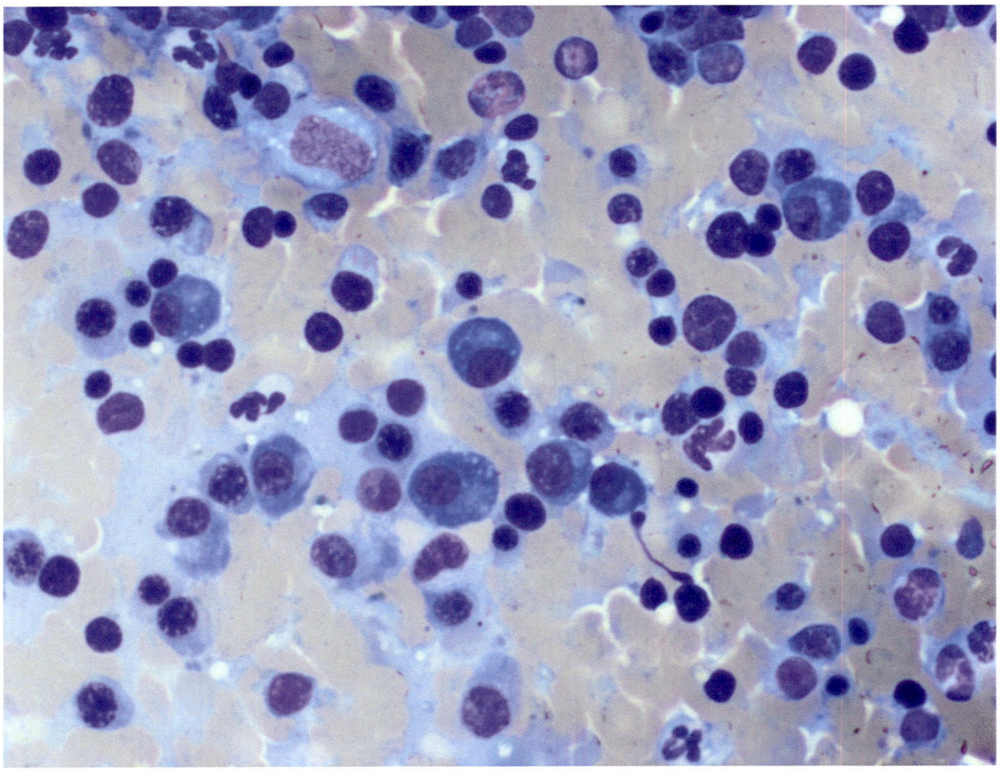

Figure 38. Spleen. Reactive changes and extramedullary haematopoiesis are simultaneously observed.

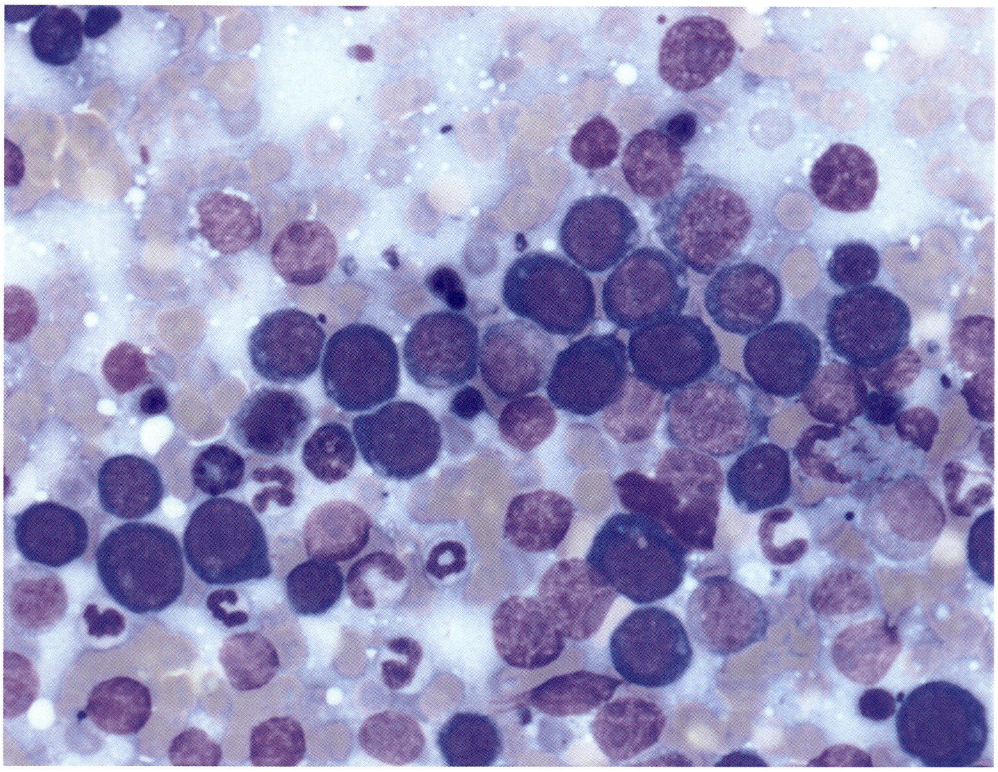

Figure 39. Extramedullary haematopoiesis of the spleen. The erythroid precursors resemble lymphoblasts, but can be identified by their more intense cytoplasmic basophilia and the presence of cytoplasm around the entire nucleus.

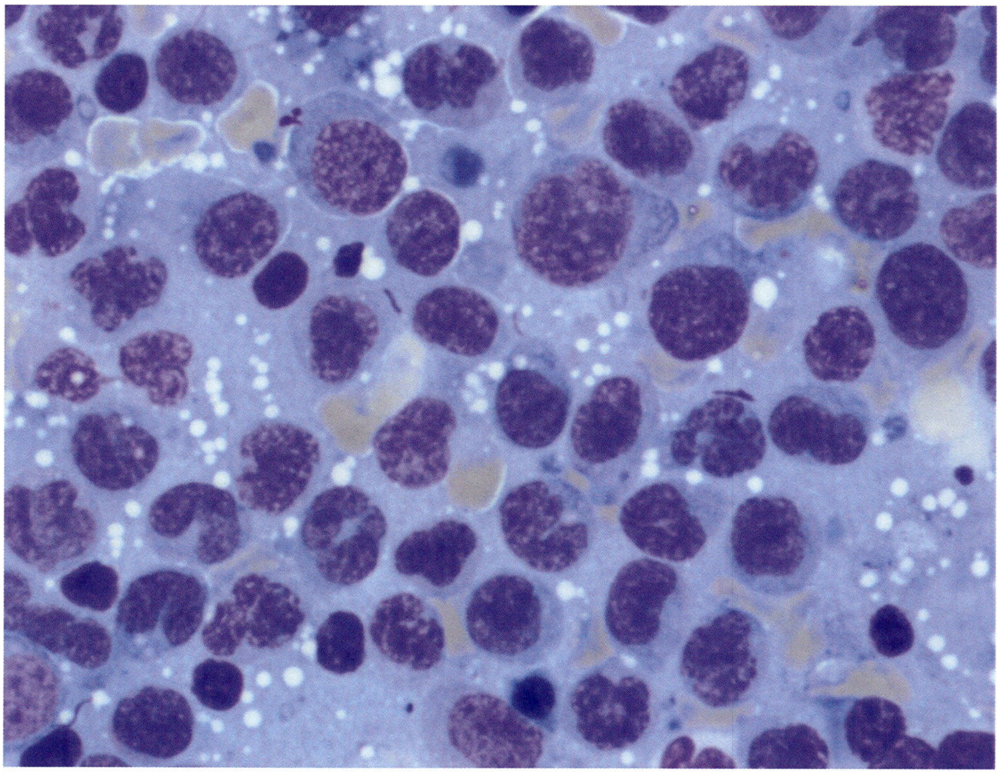

Figure 40. Spleen infiltrated by myeloblastic leukaemia cells. The absence of ordered maturation and of other precursors allows differentiation from extramedullary haematopoiesis.

# 03

# Cytology of mast cell tumours

# Cytology of mast cell tumours

Cutaneous mast cell tumours are very common in dogs. In cats, mast cell tumours affect the spleen and gastrointestinal tract in 50 % of cases. With this tumour type, cytology is sufficient to establish a definitive diagnosis (in 92–96 % of cases), since the characteristics of mast cells are easily identifiable.

The objectives of cytology in the diagnosis of these tumours are as follows:
1. Verify that the tumour is indeed a mast cell tumour.
2. Estimate the degree of differentiation.
3. Identify possible regional or distant metastases.

## DIAGNOSTIC CRITERIA FOR MAST CELL TUMOURS

Mast cells are small- to medium-sized round cells, with a round nucleus and abundant cytoplasm containing reddish-purple metachromatic granules. Degranulation phenomena occur in response to different stimuli, resulting in the release of vasoactive substances contained within the granules (Fig. 1).

The presence of cytoplasmic granules is the main criterion for identification of a mast cell. These cells should be distinguished from other cells that contain granules or pigment, particularly goblet cells (in tracheal washes) and large granular lymphocytes, both of which contain granules that are more pinkish-red than purple. While most goblet cells are elongated, they can occasionally be rounded, therefore generating confusion (Fig. 2). Granular lymphocytes can be distinguished by their greater nucleus:cytoplasm ratio and the morphology of the granules (Fig. 3).

Mast cells are widely distributed, and increase in number in numerous inflammatory and reactive processes. For a diagnosis of cutaneous mast cell tumour, the mast cell population should exceed 50 % of the total cell population.

In addition to mast cells, mast cell tumours contain other cell types, sometimes in large numbers:

- The second most commonly encountered cell type is the eosinophil. For this reason, it is necessary to determine which is the predominant cell type (eosinophilic lesion versus mast cell tumour) and which is secondary (Fig. 4). Although the percentage of eosinophils can be very high in mast cell tumours, mast cells must predominate. The percentage of eosinophils is not indicative of the degree of differentiation of a mast cell tumour. Their presence is very useful to orient the diagnosis when they accompany an undifferentiated population of round cells.
- Conjunctive cells are commonly observed in mast cell tumours. These are fibroblastic cells that are activated by mast cell mediators, and exhibit obvious dysplastic signs that should not be attributed to neoplastic changes. Although their number cannot be used as an indicator of tumour grade, they are more abundant in well-differentiated mast cell tumours (Figs. 5 and 6).

Degranulation can be very marked. Cytology of most well-differentiated mast cell tumours typically reveals numerous extracellular granules, which should not be confused with bacteria or other microorganisms (Figs. 7 and 8).

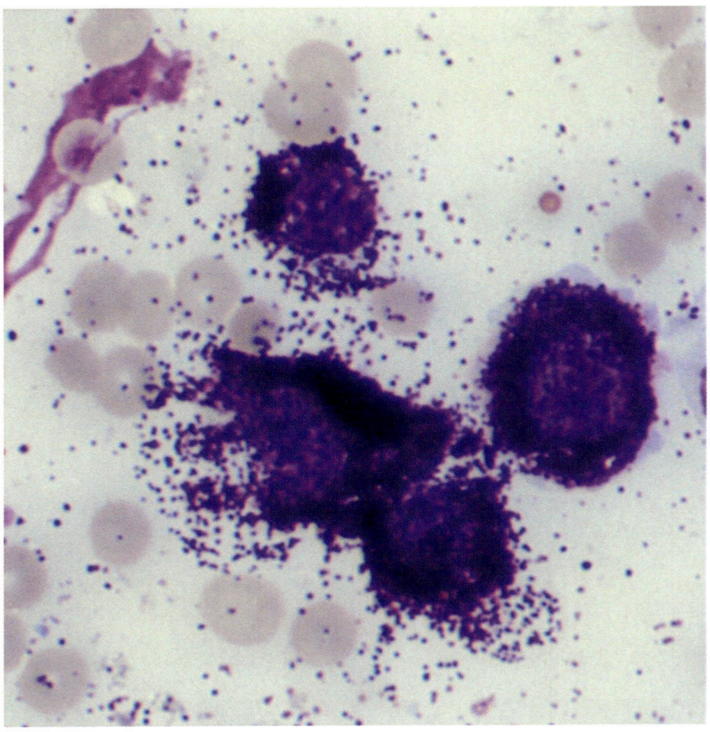

Figure 1. Mast cells. One is intact and three are degranulating.

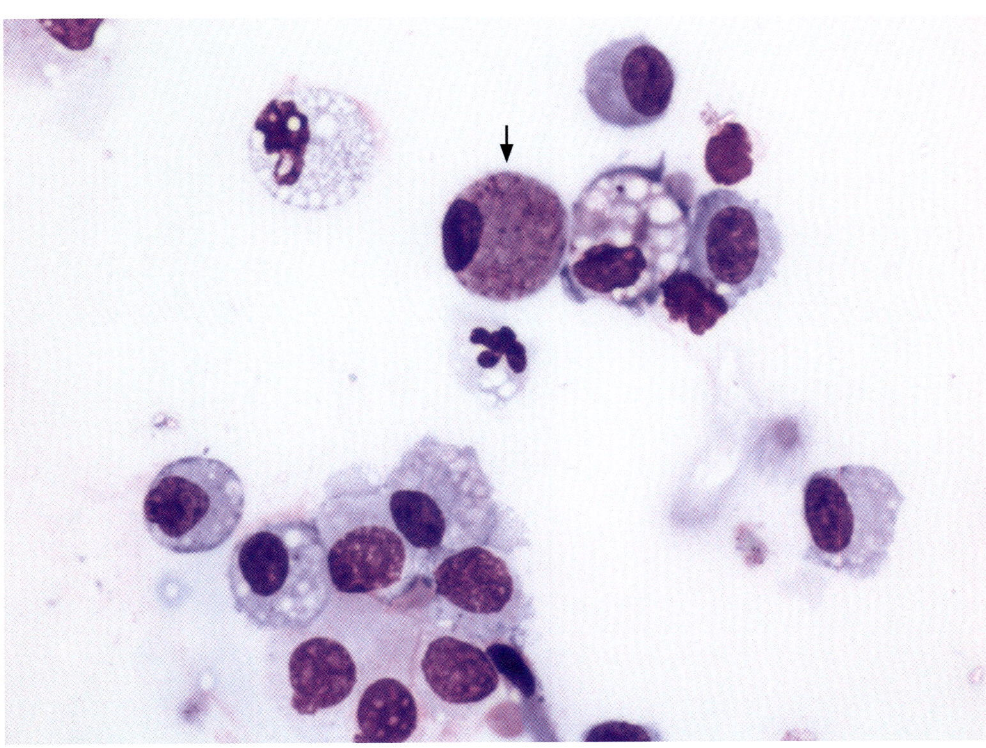

Figure 2. Goblet cell (arrow) in a tracheal wash sample (not to be confused with a mast cell).

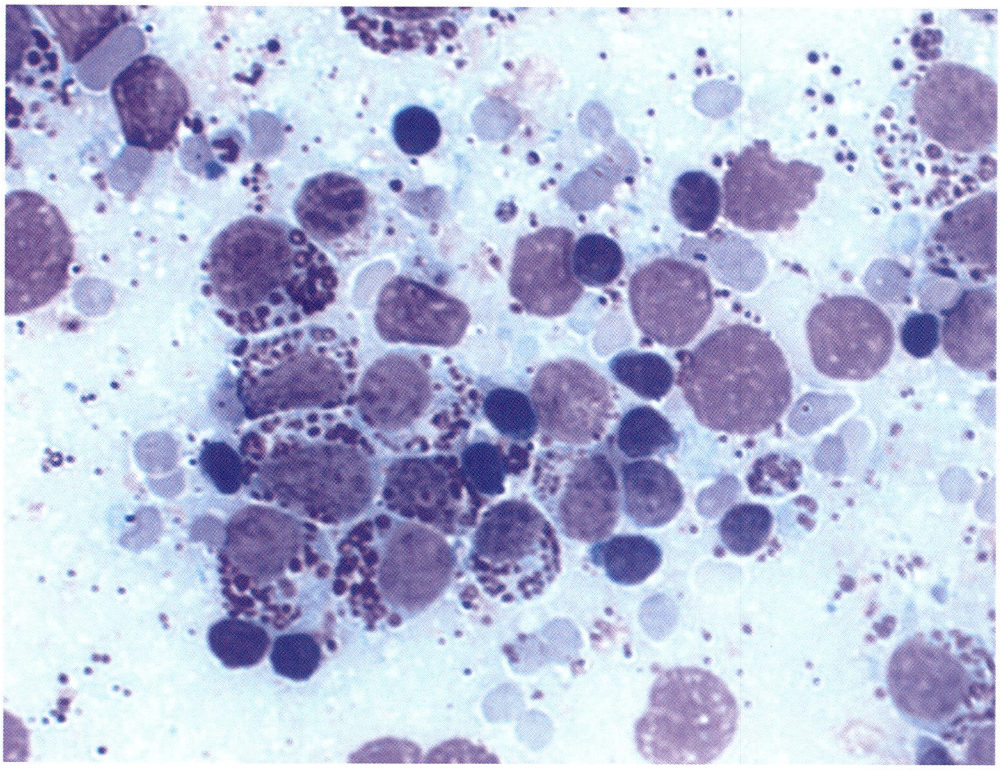

Figure 3. Large granular lymphocyte lymphoma (cat). The cell and granule type differ to those of mast cells.

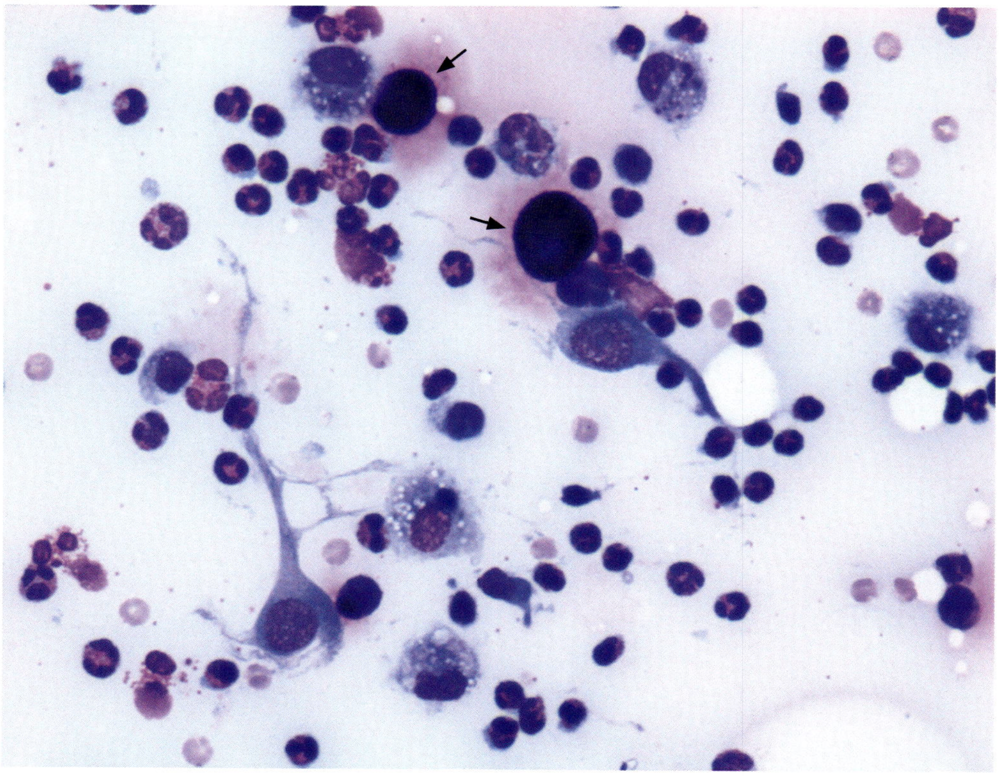

Figure 4. Eosinophilic inflammation. Although two very granulated mast cells are observed (arrows), the predominant cell population is eosinophilic (with macrophages and activated conjunctive cells).

Figures 5 and 6. Well-differentiated mast cells accompanied by eosinophils and conjunctive cells with dysplastic changes (which should not be attributed to malignancy).

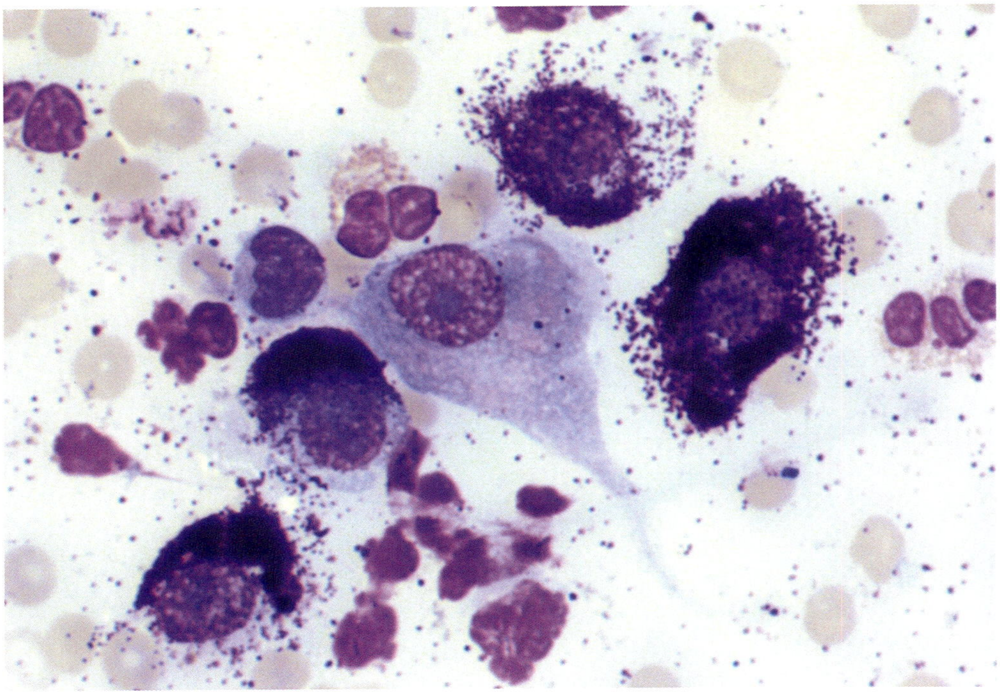

Figure 5.

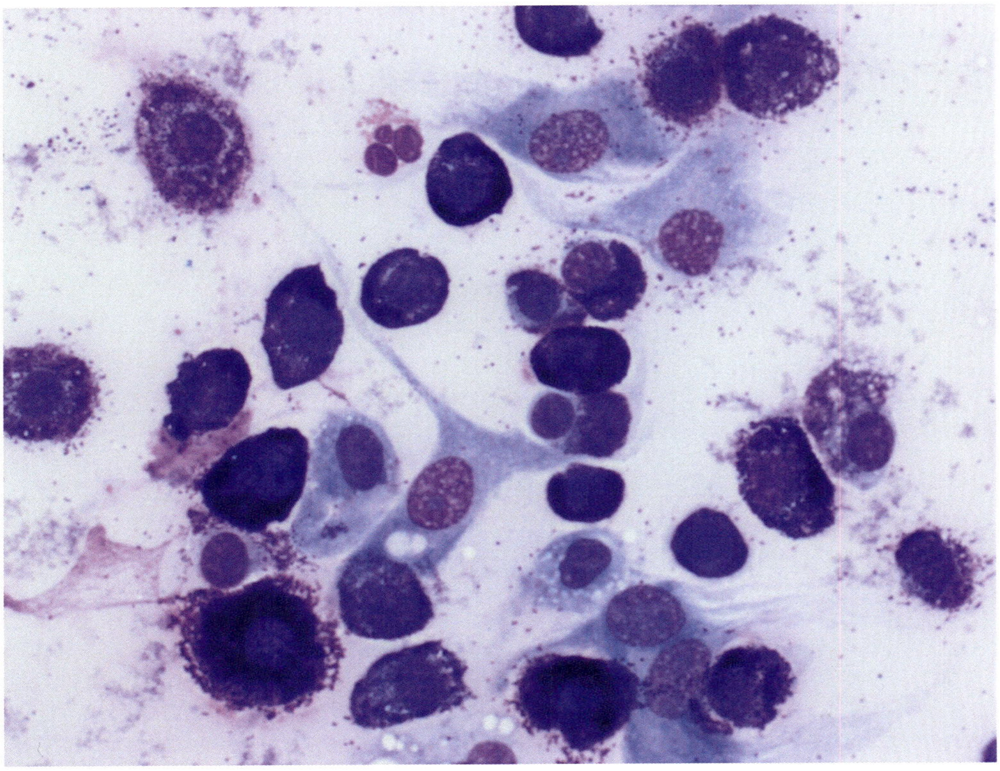

Figure 6.

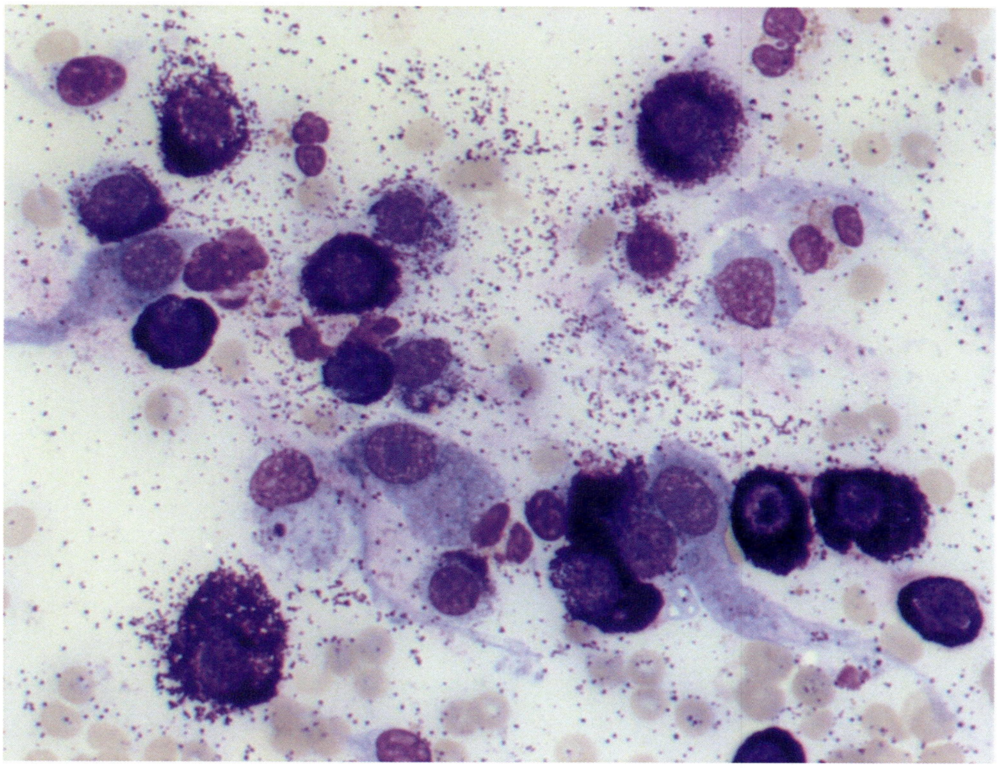

Figure 7. Well-differentiated mast cell tumour. Note the many extracellular granules resulting from cell degranulation.

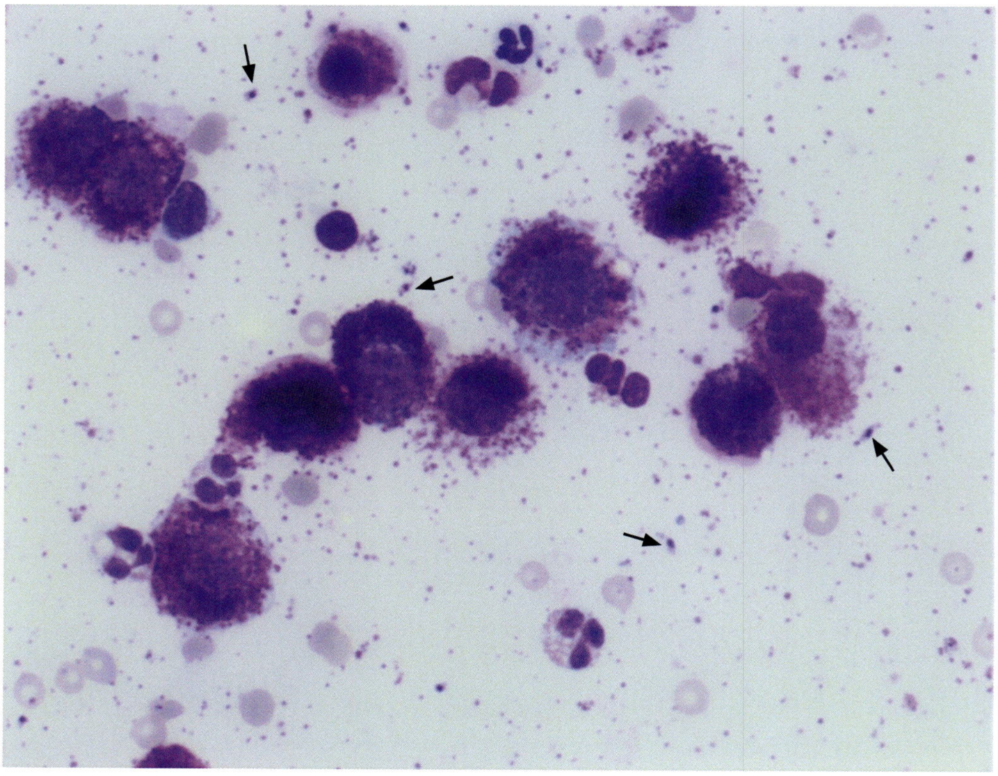

Figure 8. Well-differentiated mast cell tumour. Note the presence of *Leishmania* amastigotes (arrows), which can be confused with granules.

## ESTIMATION OF THE DEGREE OF DIFFERENTIATION

Although there is consensus on the role of cytology as a fundamental tool for the diagnosis of mast cell tumour, its use as a means of estimating the degree of differentiation is controversial. Histology is the only technique that can be used to grade mast cell tumours (Patnaik or Kiupel criteria), although cytology can be used to estimate the grade as a first step in the diagnostic protocol.

Estimation of the degree of differentiation can be based on the following criteria:[1]

- Number of granules (many, few, mixed).
- Absence or presence of nuclear pleomorphism (nonround nuclei).
- Absence or presence of mitotic figures.
- Absence or presence of binucleated or multinucleated cells.
- Absence or presence of karyomegaly (>50 % variation in nuclear size).

Based on the evaluation of these parameters a diagnostic algorithm can be established.

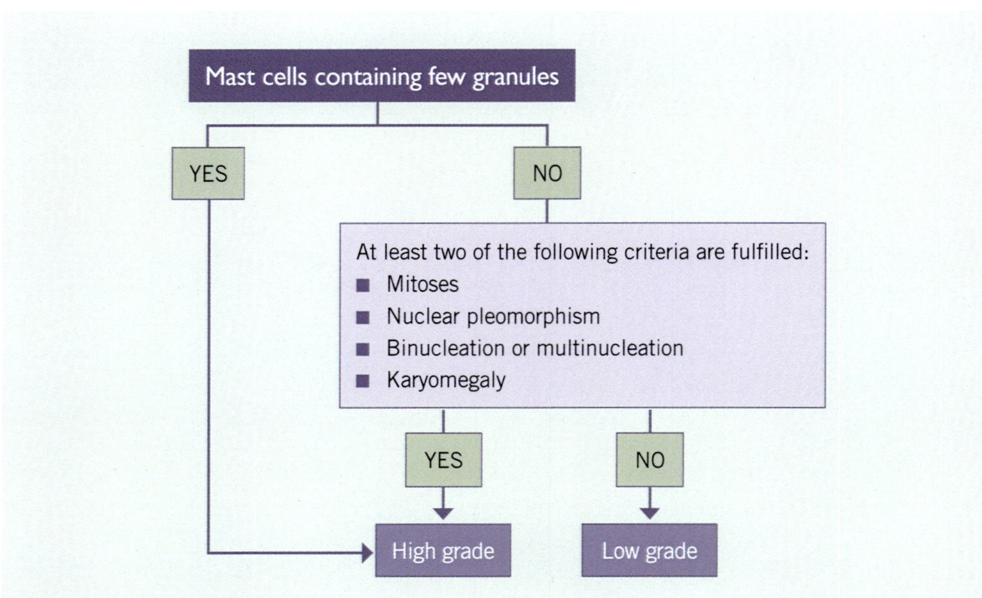


Other studies have proposed that mast cell tumour grade can be estimated based only on nuclear characteristics, according to the criteria of the Kiupel grading system.[5]

From this author's point of view, cytology allows differentiation between two main tumour types:

- Clearly well-differentiated mast cell tumours, in which the majority of mast cells contain so many granules that the nucleus is not visible, but when it is visible (in degranulated cells) it is small, rounded, and homogeneous across cells (Fig. 9–12).
- Clearly undifferentiated mast cell tumours, in which the majority of mast cells contain few granules and/or the nuclear atypia described in the algorithm is evident (Figs. 13–18). The presence of binucleated or multinucleated cells and karyomegaly are the nuclear criteria that best correlate with a decrease in survival time. Mitoses, the presence of which is an important

indicator of undifferentiation, are not usually observed in sufficient numbers. Nuclear pleomorphism is too subjective a criterion and should not be considered as the sole means of determining undifferentiation. In mast cell tumours the granules tend to be located at the opposite pole to the nucleus.

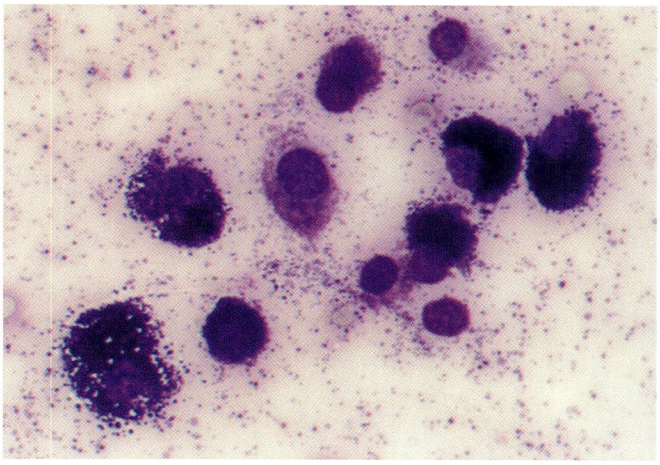
Figure 9.

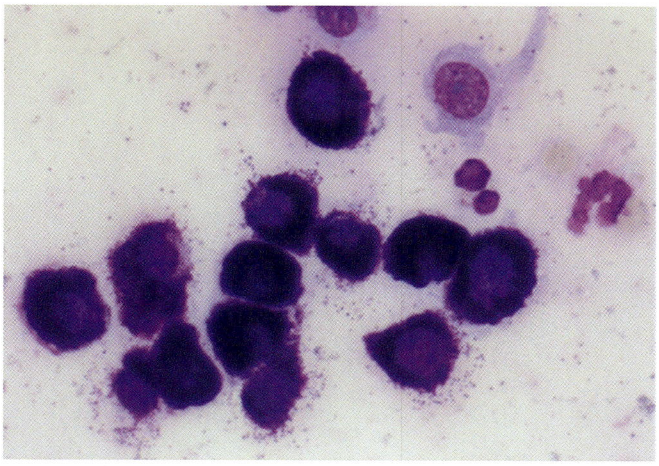
Figure 10.

Figure 11. ▶

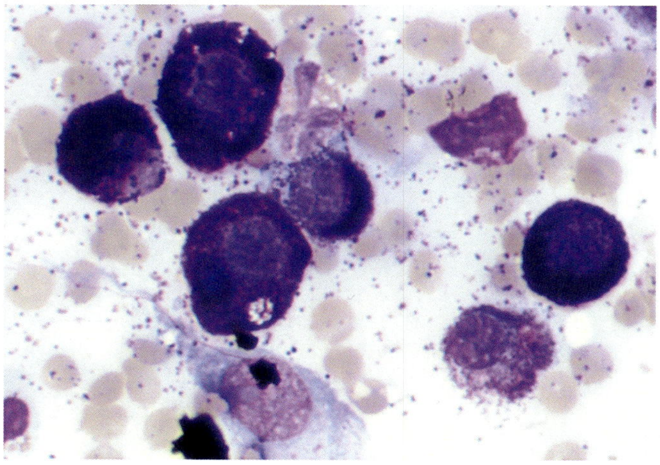

Figures 9–11. Images showing mast cell tumours (estimated grade, well-differentiated). The mast cells contain numerous granules that mask the nucleus.

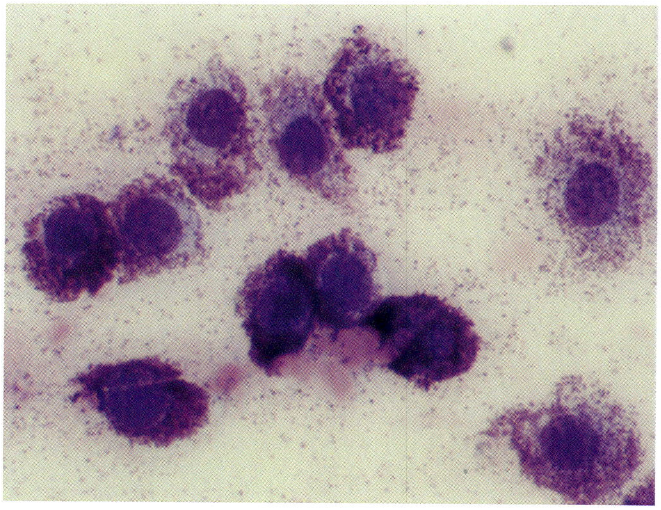

Figure 12. Although the mast cells do not contain many granules (probably due to degranulation), the nuclei are homogeneous, and none of the criteria of the diagnostic algorithm are fulfilled.

Figures 13–17. Images showing mast cell tumours (estimated grade, undifferentiated). In addition to the low level of granulation, marked nuclear atypia (karyomegaly, multinucleation, mitoses) is evident (arrows).

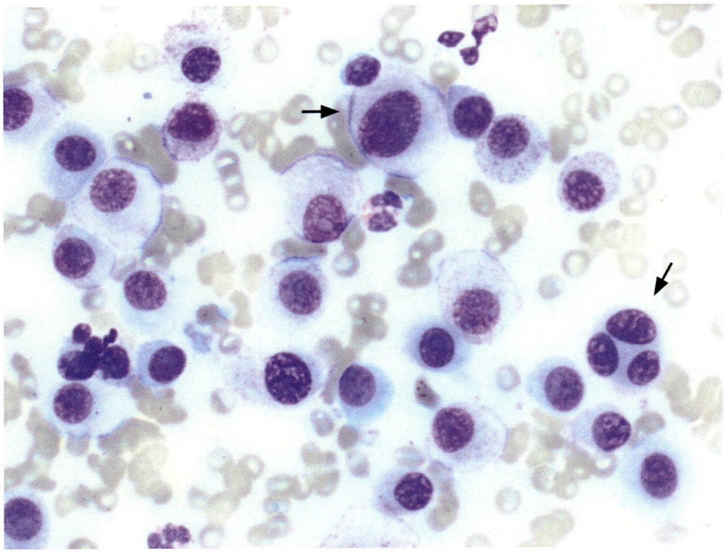

Figure 13.

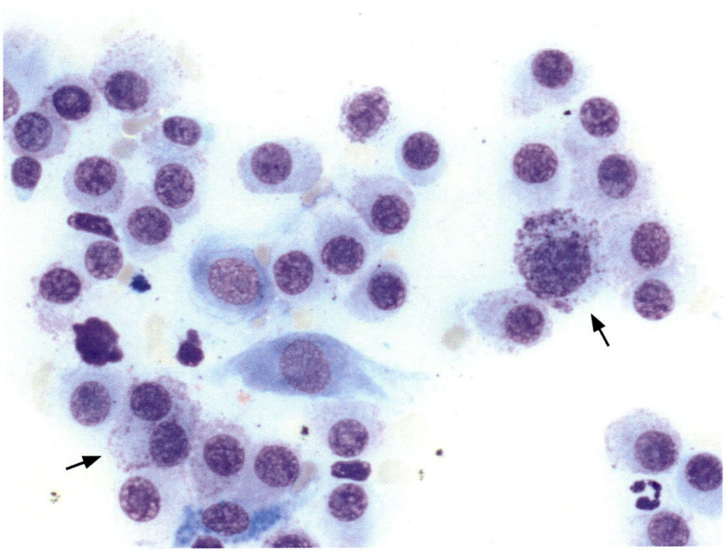

Figure 14.

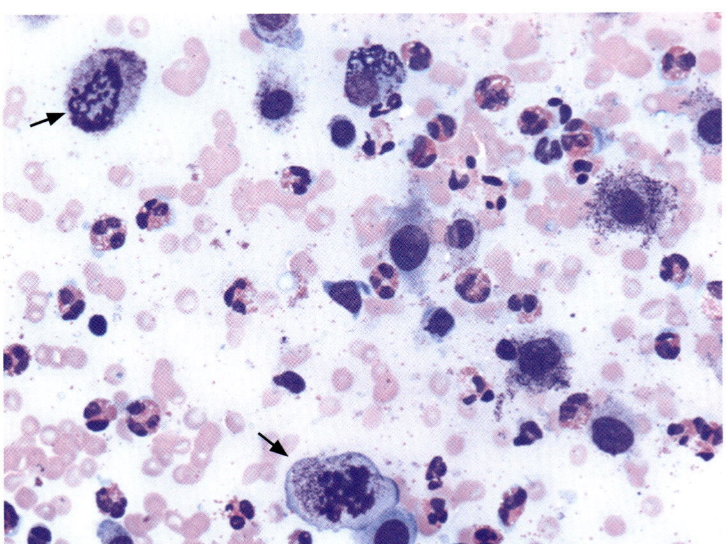

Figure 15.

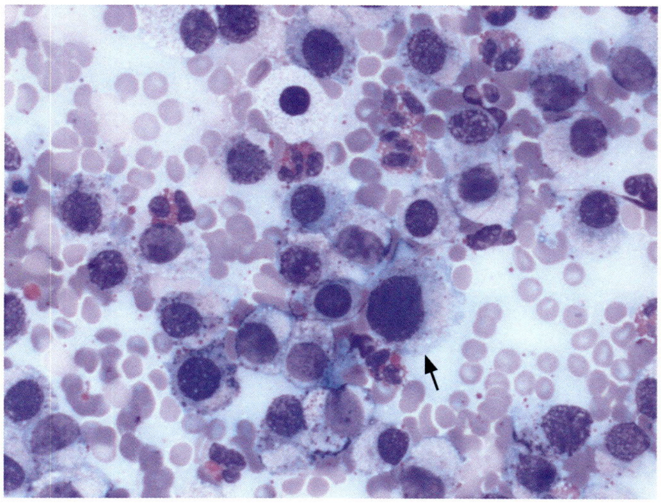

Figure 16.

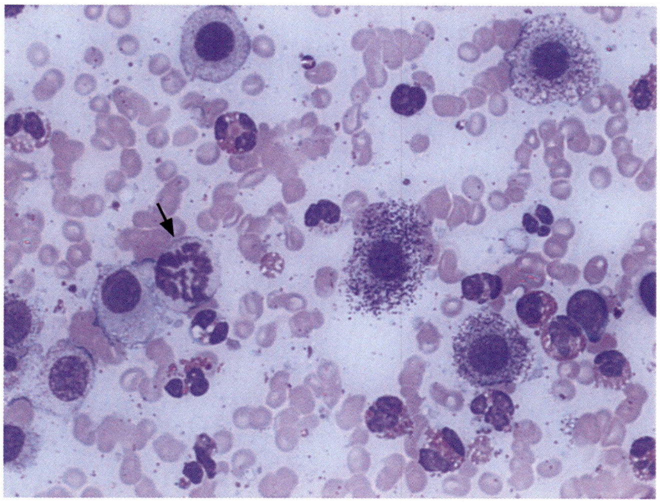

Figure 17.

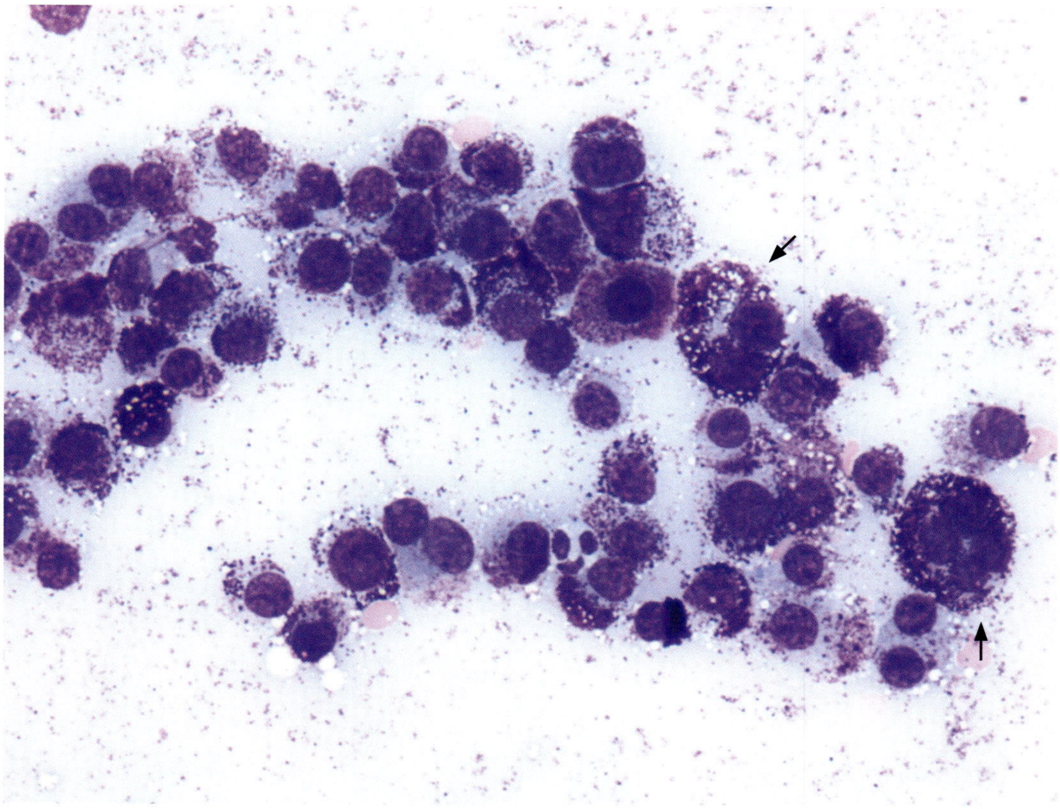

Figure 18. Although the mast cells contain numerous and evident granules, the abundant multinucleation (arrows) is indicative of undifferentiation.

In tumours with the maximum degree of undifferentiation, the characteristic granulation is absent, meaning that the differential diagnosis should include other round cell tumours. Occasionally, the only conclusion that can be reached is that the tumour is an "undifferentiated round cell tumour", and specific stains (toluidine blue) or immunohistochemistry will be required to establish the diagnosis (Figs. 19 and 20).

If the sample does not correspond to one of these two clearly distinct groups, the diagnosis should be limited to a mast cell tumour with an "indeterminate degree of differentiation" (Fig. 19).

Feline mast cell tumours should not be classified according to the degree of differentiation (Fig. 21). Most are derived from cells in which the granules are evident. The cytological interpretation should be limited to defining whether or not the sample corresponds to a mast cell tumour. The presence of few granules and/or nuclear atypia cannot be considered indicative of a more aggressive tumour (Figs. 22 and 23). However, histiocytic mast cell tumours, in which the cells lack granules and closely resemble histiocytes, are also described.

Figures 19 and 20. Images showing a highly undifferentiated mast cell tumour. In most fields, the round cells cannot be identified as mast cells (19).
Cells exhibiting granulation are only occasionally observed (arrow) (20).

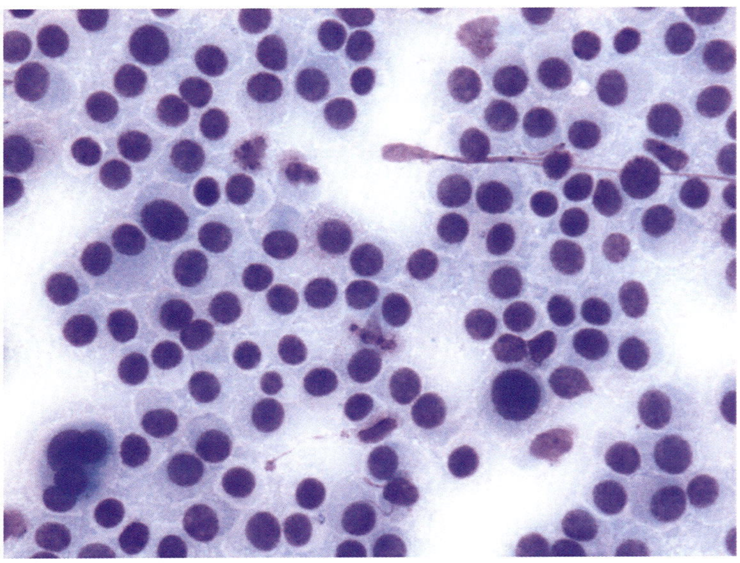

Figure 19.

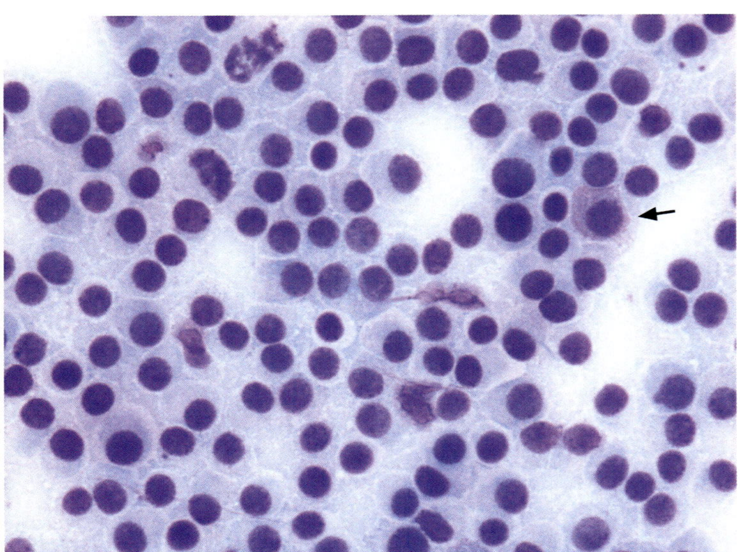

Figure 20.

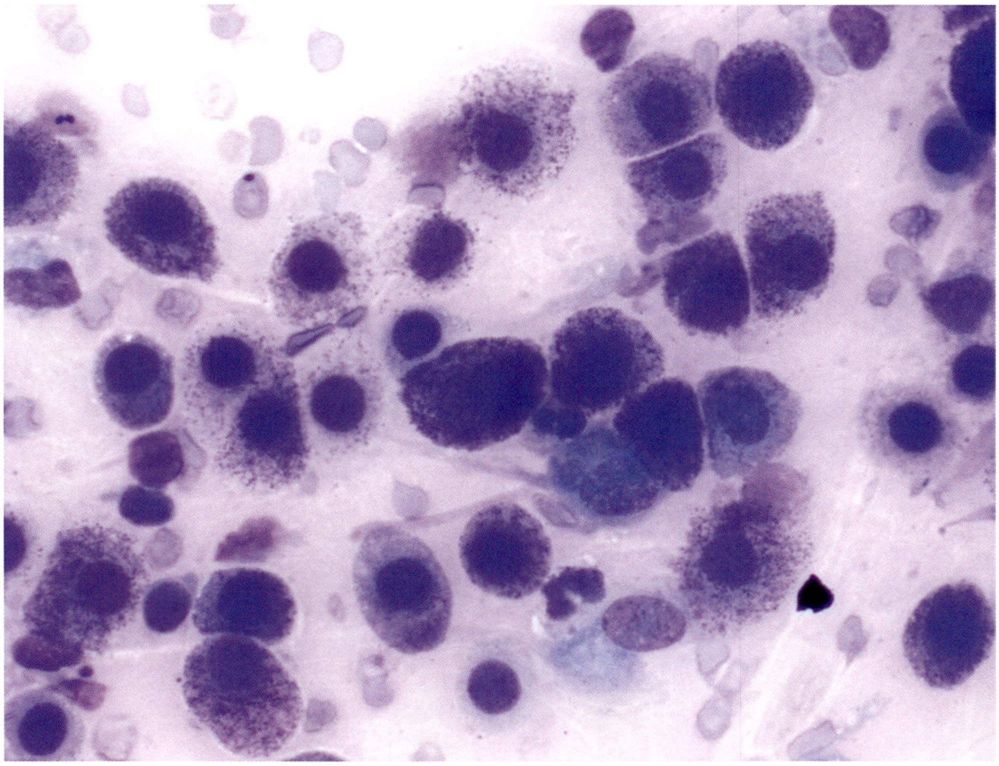

Figure 21. Mast cell tumour of indeterminate grade. The mast cells contain few granules, with no evidence of degranulation, but no other significant atypia is evident.

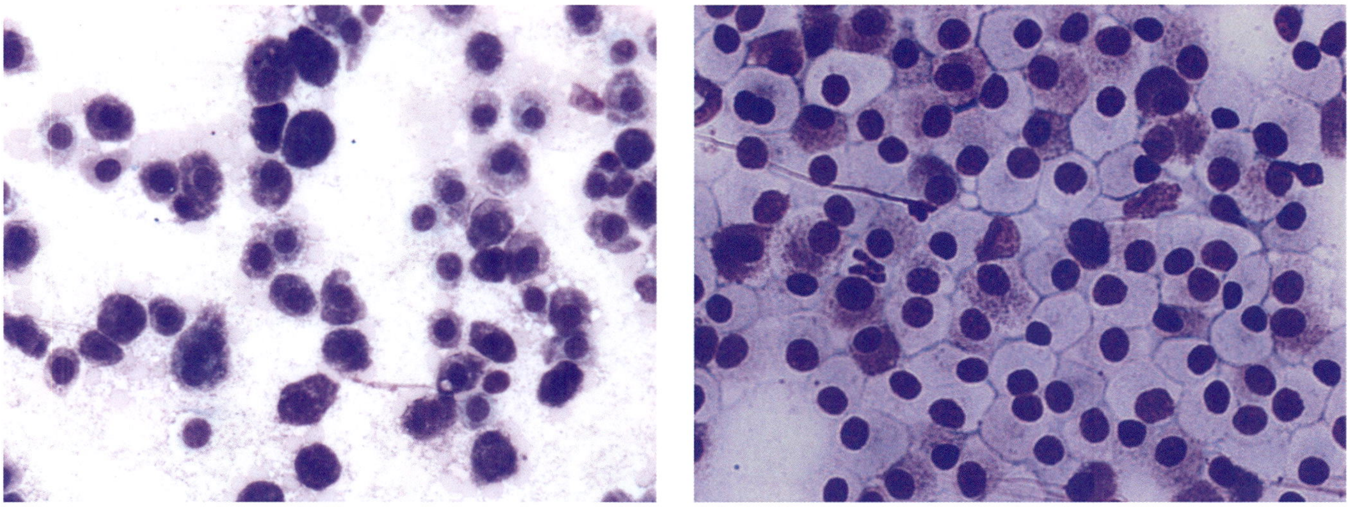

Figures 22 and 23. Feline mast cell tumours. Neither the amount of granules nor the nuclear atypia are indicative of undifferentiation.

## DIAGNOSTIC CRITERIA FOR METASTATIC MAST CELL TUMOUR

In addition to enabling diagnosis of mast cell tumours, cytology is the technique that is usually used to identify metastases in lymph nodes or internal organs.

The criteria used to define lymph node metastasis are somewhat controversial. Mast cells are observed in normal lymph nodes and increase in number in reactive lymph nodes. Normal tissue typically contains solitary mast cells with numerous granules (Fig. 24).

Although there is no single criterion that defines a metastatic lymph node, the most widely accepted include the presence of any of the following characteristics:[6,8]

- Undifferentiated mast cells: the greater the number, the greater the diagnostic accuracy (Figs. 25–29).
- Well-differentiated mast cells: if these are observed, aggregation (more so than cell number) is the most reliable indicator of metastasis. The presence of more than 5 aggregates consisting of more than 3 mast cells is considered diagnostic of metastasis (Figs. 30–33).

Large numbers of mast cells are observed in thymomas. Thymoma cytology is characterised by the presence of numerous mature lymphocytes and, occasionally, groups of epithelial cells. However, infiltrate consisting of well-differentiated mast cells may be observed occasionally (Fig. 34), and in some cases can be so intense as to suggest lymph node metastasis of a mast cell tumour. The presence of these mast cells facilitates differentiation of thymoma from mediastinal small cell lymphoma.

In addition to the lymph nodes, other organs to which mast cell tumours frequently metastasise are the spleen and liver.

Because mast cells can be observed in normal conditions in both organs, caution is required when interpreting cytological findings. In general, metastasis to a given organ can be ruled out if mast cells are absent or are observed as solitary cells (in the liver, the presence of less than one mast cell per 100 hepatocytes is considered normal). By contrast, the presence of abundant and/or grouped undifferentiated or differentiated mast cells is considered indicative of metastasis (Figs. 35 and 36).

Abdominal metastases may be accompanied by ascitic effusion in which mast cells are observed, in some cases accompanied by variable numbers of eosinophils. In poorly differentiated mast cell tumours it may be difficult to distinguish neoplastic mast cells from mesothelial cells (Figs. 37 and 38). The presence of eosinophils alone should not be considered a diagnostic criterion for mast cell tumour, since eosinophilic effusion is characteristic of many other conditions (Fig. 39).

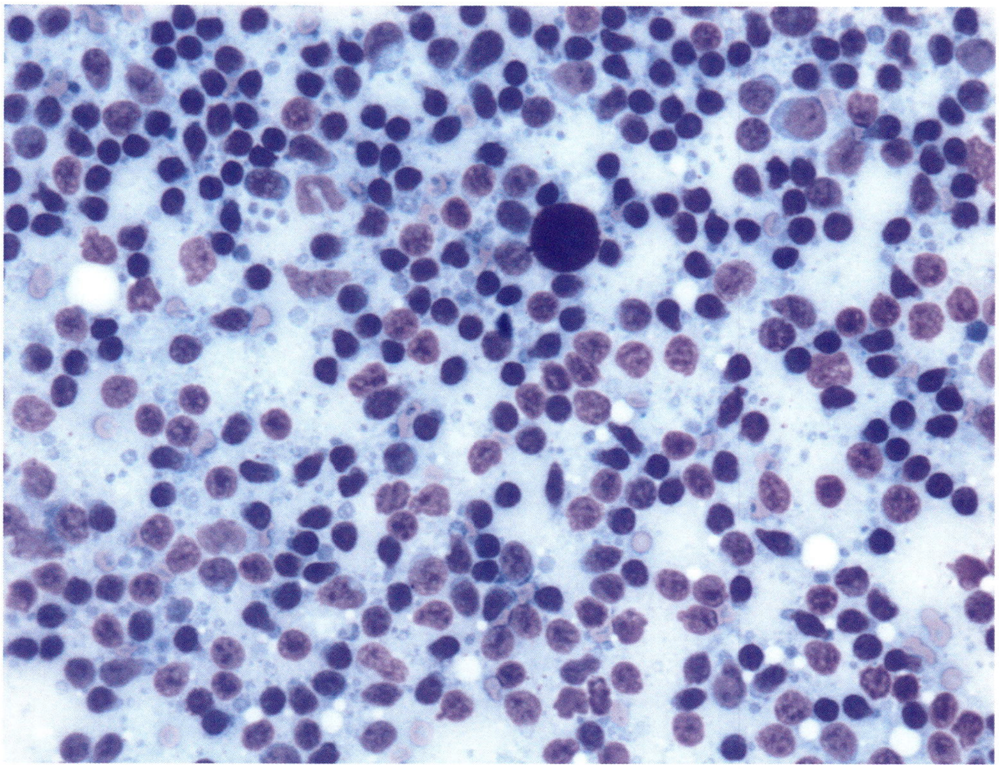

Figure 24. Lymph node cytology. The presence of a solitary, well-differentiated mast cell is not indicative of metastasis.

Figures 25–29. Images show lymph node metastasis of mast cell tumours, with variable numbers of mast cells that are undifferentiated and/or exhibit marked atypia.

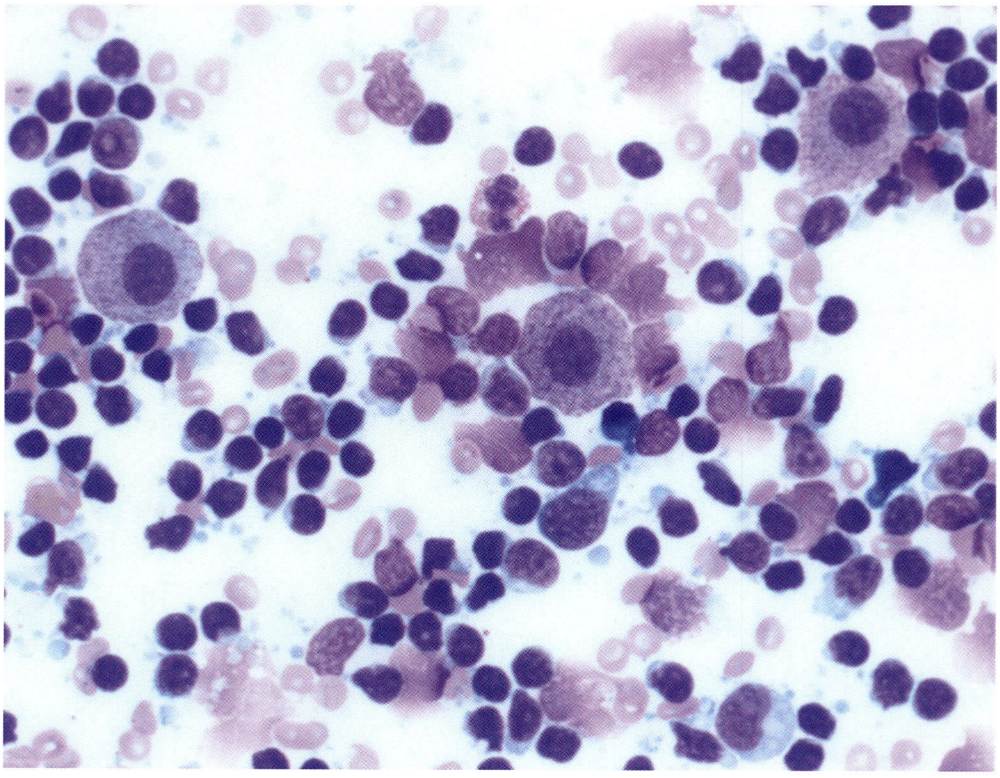

Figure 25.

Figures 25–29. Images showing lymph node metastasis of mast cell tumours, with variable numbers of undifferentiated mast cells and/or marked atypia.

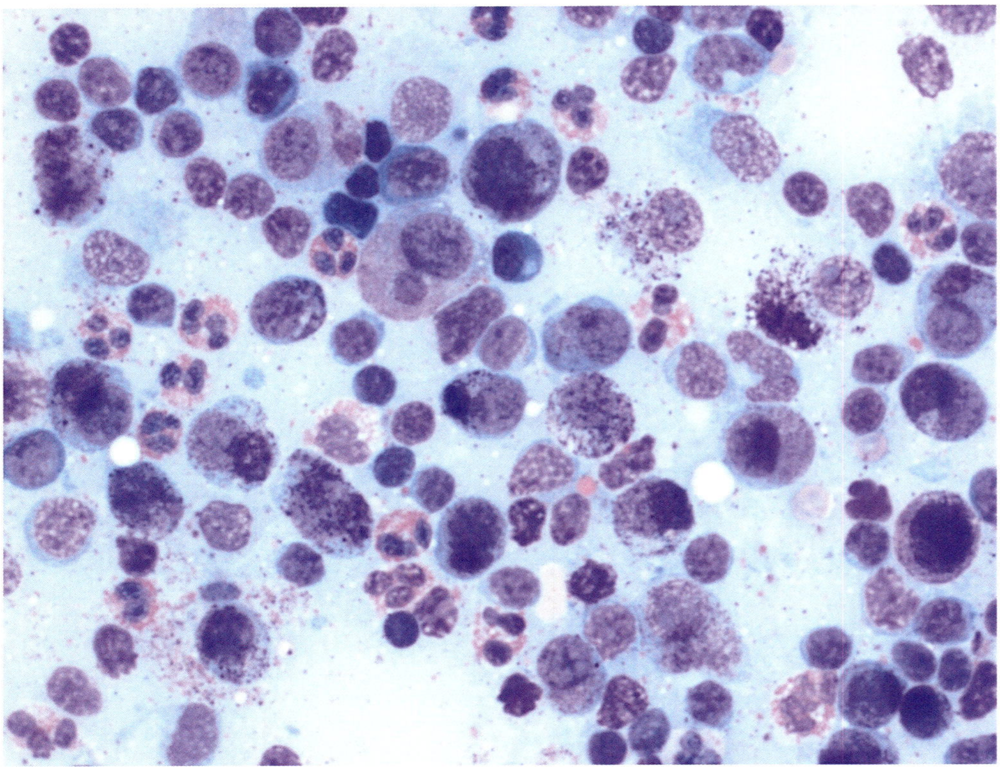

Figure 26.

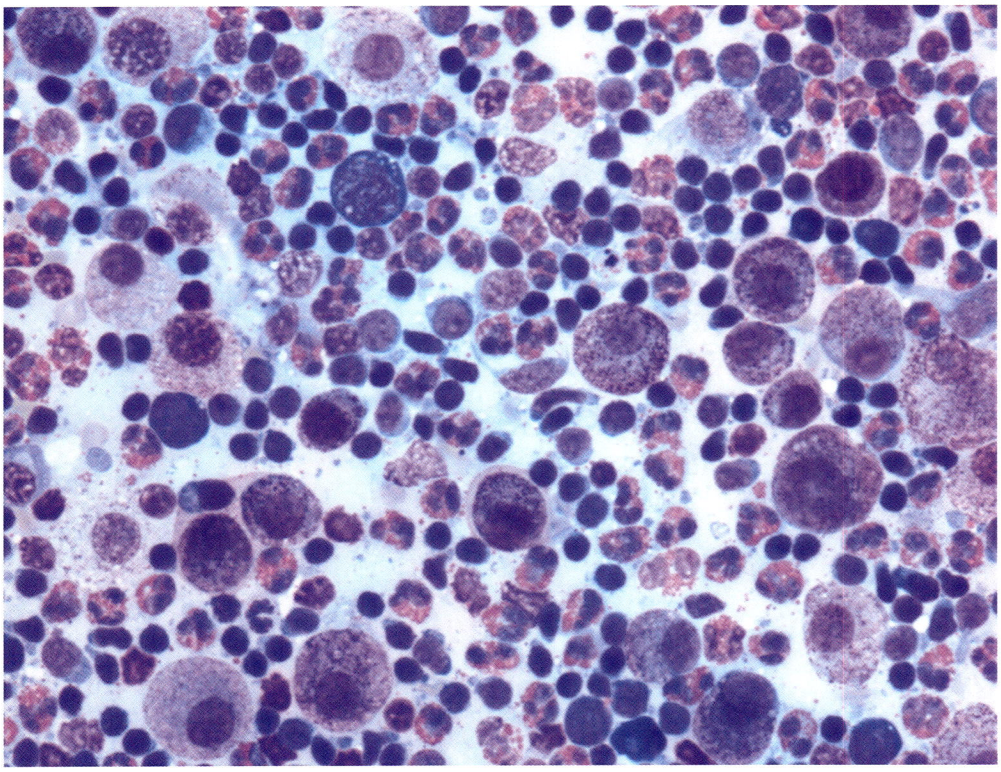

Figure 27.

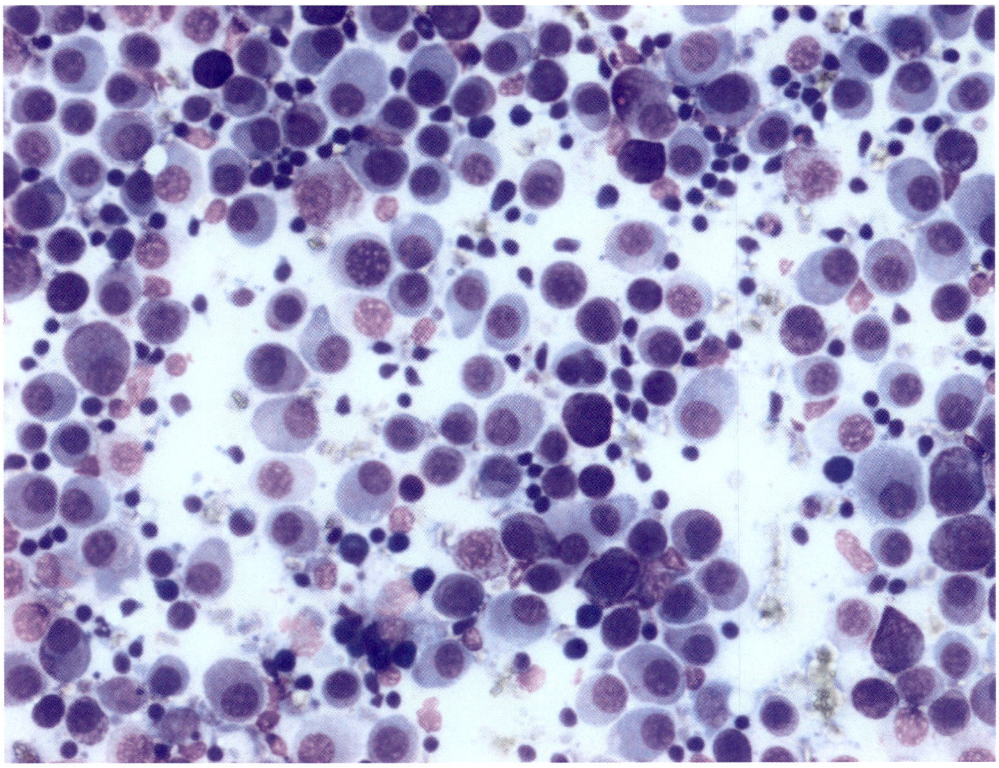

Figure 28.

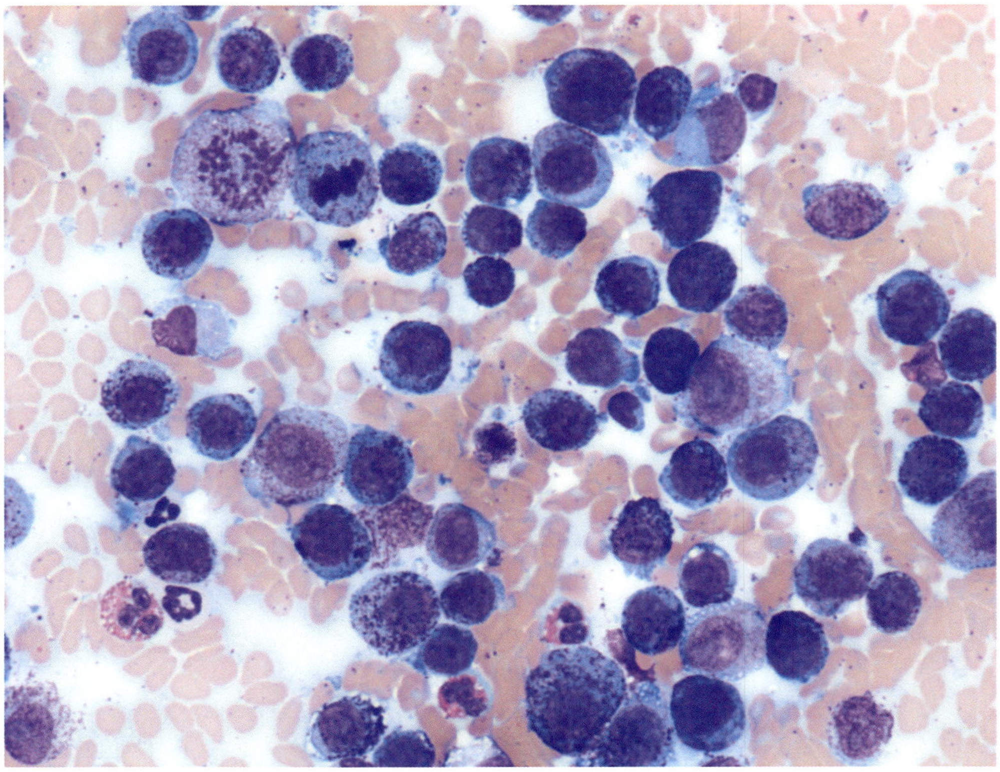

Figure 29.

Figures 30–33. Lymph node cytology. Each of the different fields contains well-differentiated mast cells in large numbers or groups. This criterion is fundamental to define metastasis.

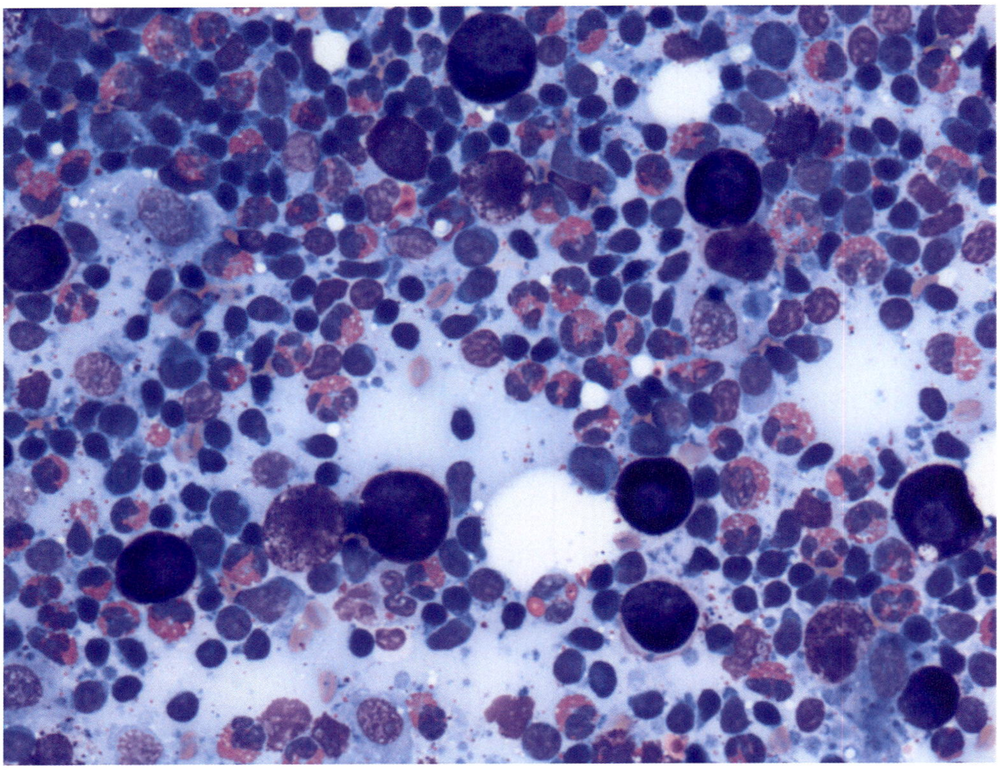

Figure 30.

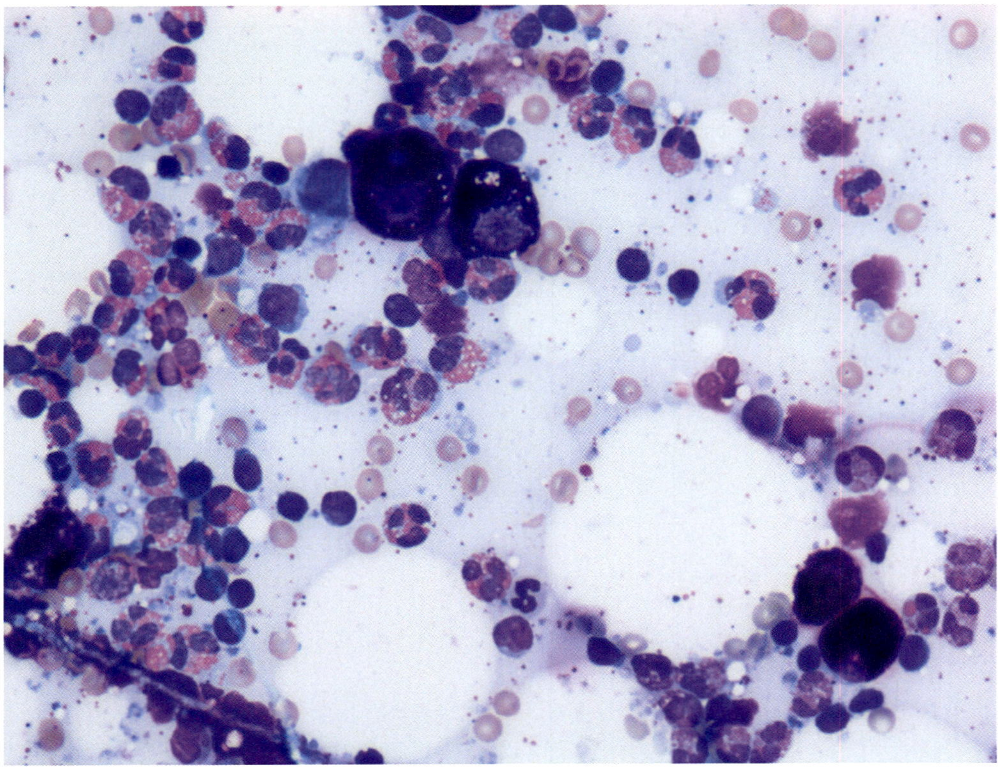

Figure 31.

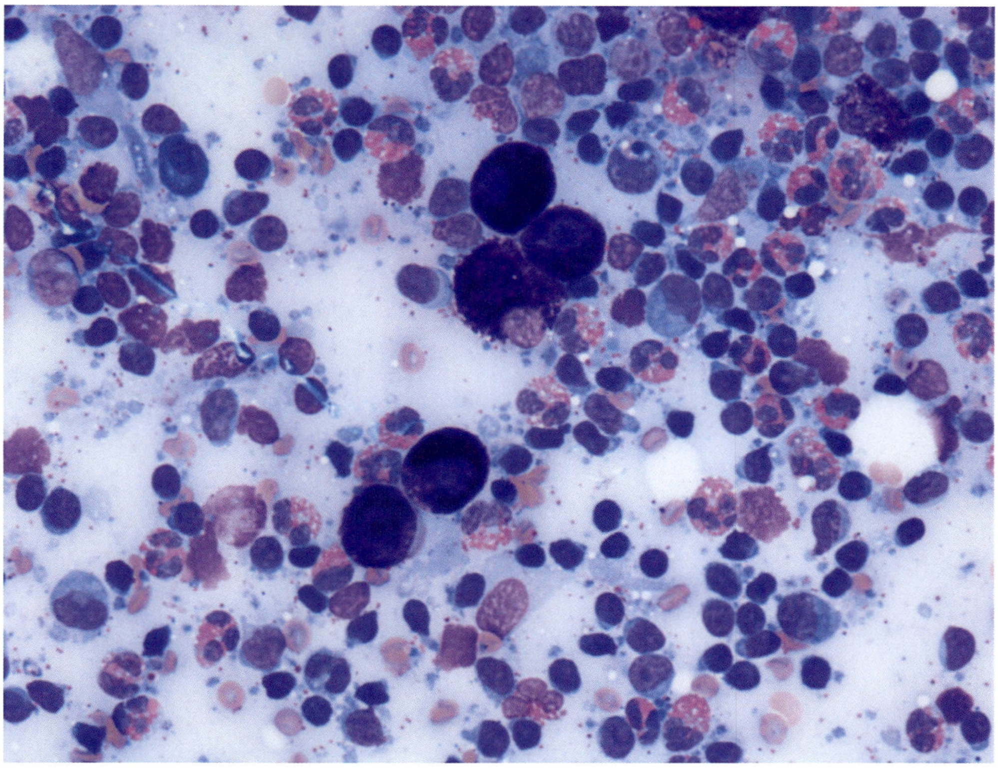

Figure 32.

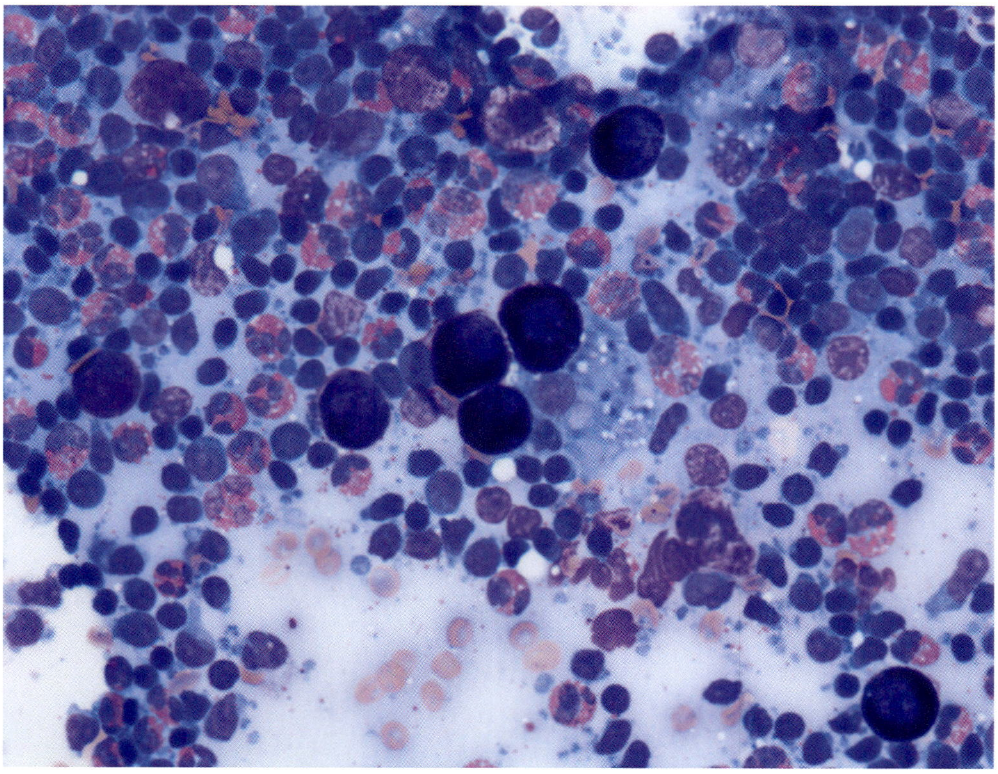

Figure 33.

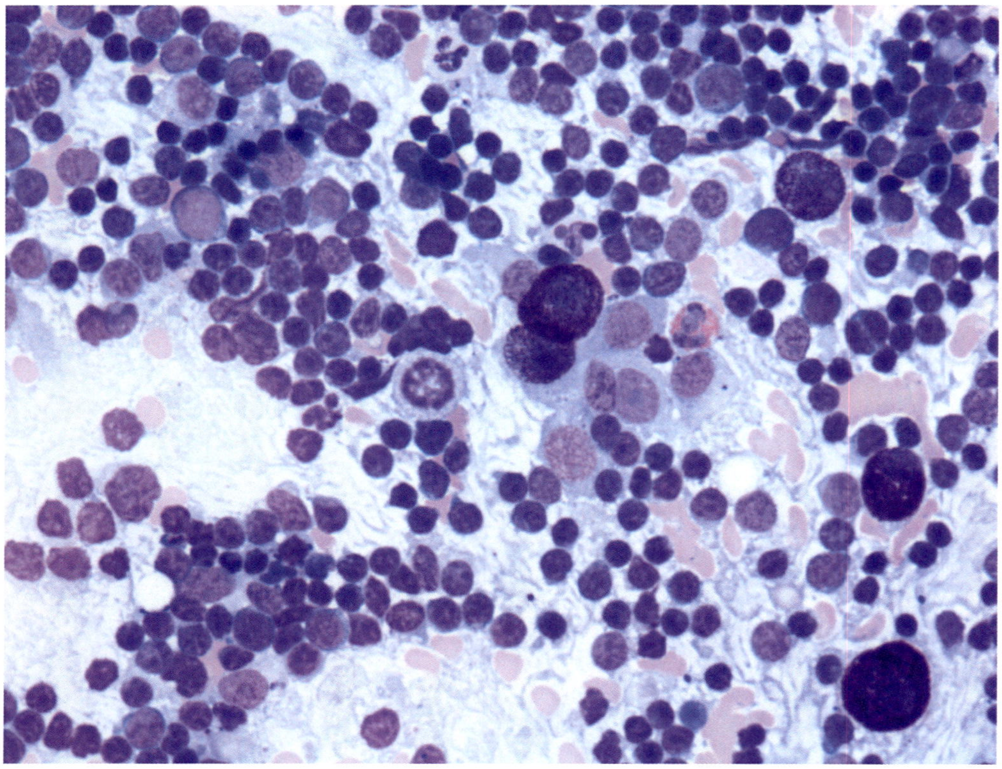

Figure 34. Cytology of a thymoma (mature lymphocytes and epithelial cells) in which well-differentiated mast cells are observed (not to be confused with lymph node metastasis).

Figure 35.

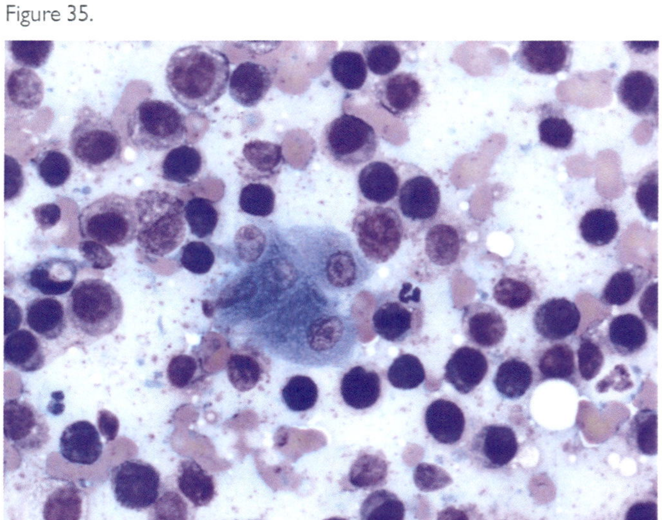

Figure 36.

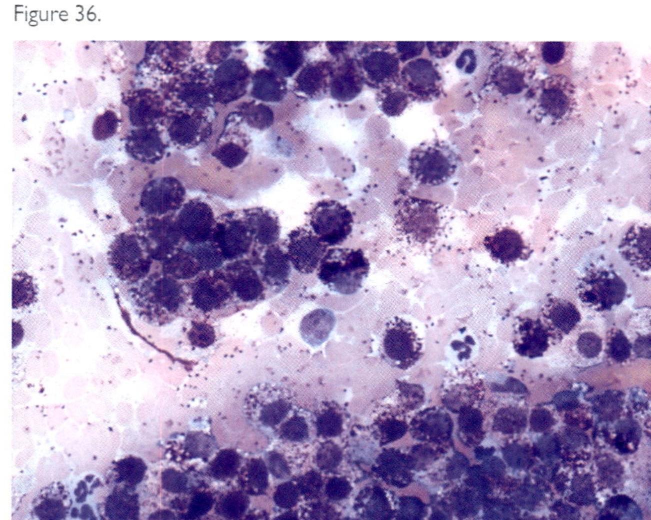

Figures 35 and 36. Liver (35) and splenic (36) metastases of cutaneous mast cell tumours.

Figures 37 and 38. Ascitic fluid cytology, in which numerous eosinophils, undifferentiated mast cells, and few mesothelial cells are observed (arrows).

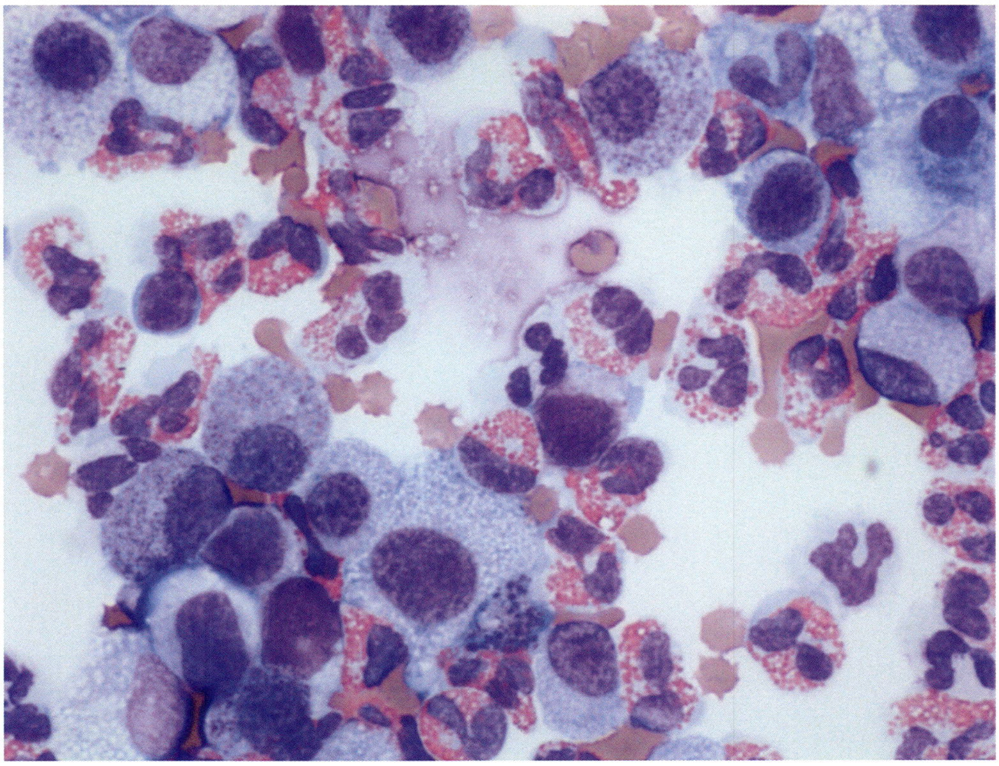

Figure 37.

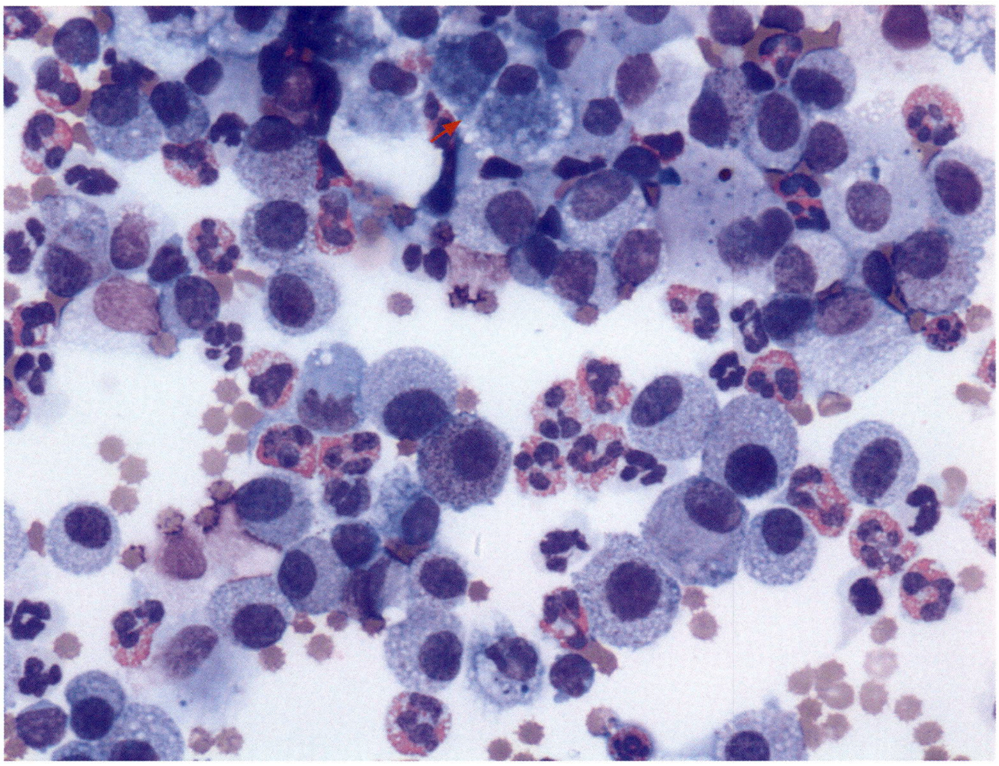

Figure 38.

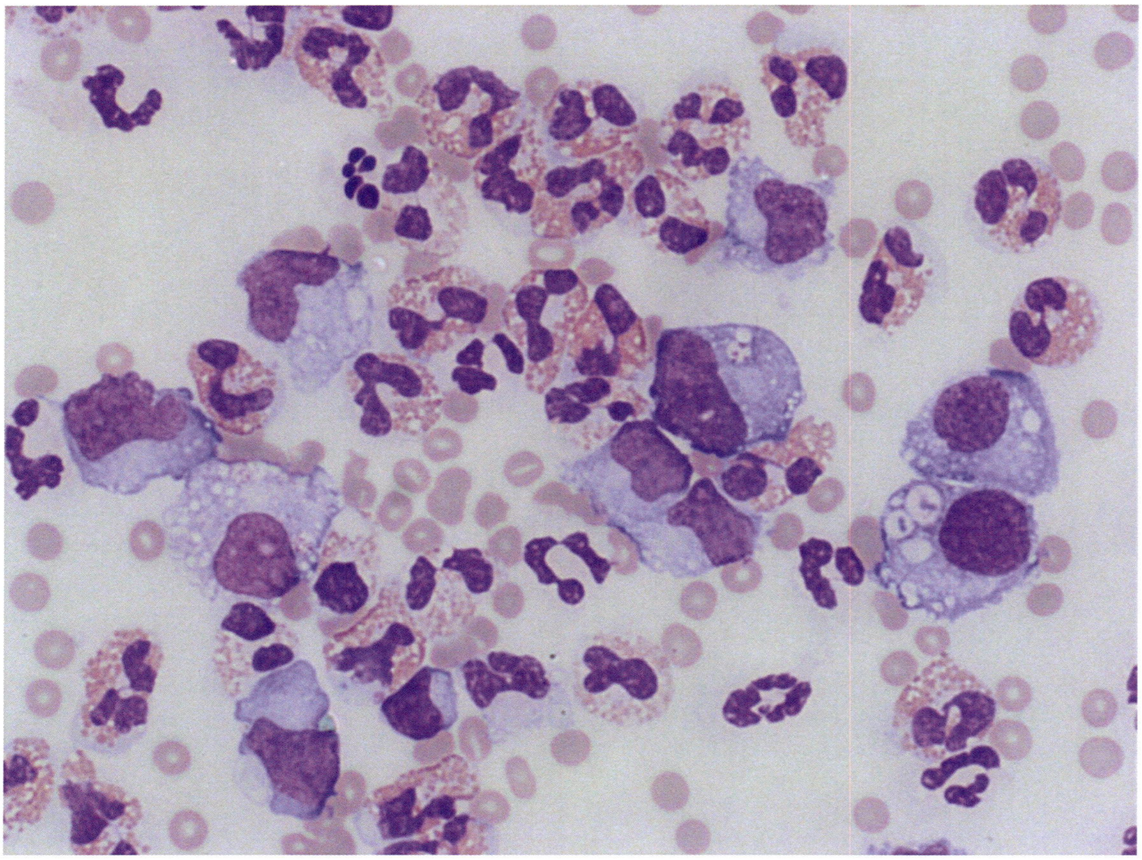

Figure 39. Ascitic fluid cytology, containing numerous eosinophils and activated mesothelial cells (not to be confused with mast cells).

# 04

# Cytology of lymphoma

# Cytology of lymphoma

Cytology is often the first, and in some cases the only, technique used in the diagnosis of lymphoma. While in most cases lymph node cytology is the key to diagnosis, cytology of other structures is usually also performed.

## DIAGNOSIS OF LYMPHOMA BY LYMPH NODE CYTOLOGY

Cytological evaluation of lymph node samples from patients with suspected lymphoma involves the following steps:

1. Determine if the sample is of sufficient diagnostic quality.
2. Diagnose lymphoma.
3. Assess the morphological characteristics of the predominant lymphoid population to estimate the lymphoma subtype.

### ASSESSING THE DIAGNOSTIC QUALITY OF LYMPH NODE SAMPLES

Diagnosis of lymph node lymphoma is strongly influenced by the quality of the sample. Up to 90 % of lymphoma cases in dogs can be diagnosed cytologically. However, this high rate is dependent on the availability of good quality cytological preparations.

Lymph node tissue is very fragile; lymphoblastic cells are the cells most sensitive to rupture. Therefore, if the samples contain a high percentage of ruptured cells, the differential cell count may lack sufficient diagnostic accuracy. As a consequence of cell rupture, it is common to observe numerous naked nuclei (deformed, and less intensely stained) and lymphoglandular bodies (remains of basophilic cytoplasm of varying sizes) (Figs. 1–3).

To classify lymphoid cells according to their size and morphology, it is necessary to view individual cells in a monolayer (i.e. cells that are neither deformed nor compressed). Because lymph node samples contain abundant cells, a common problem is that the preparation is too thick. Therefore, in many cases an adequate differential cell count can only be performed for certain areas of the preparation (Figs. 4–6). If the cytological picture is homogeneous throughout the entire preparation, then the diagnosis can be based on the analysis of several fields. However, in cases in which the differential cell count varies considerably from one area to another, it is not possible to extrapolate the results obtained for several fields. Therefore, the smaller the number of evaluable fields, the lower the diagnostic accuracy.

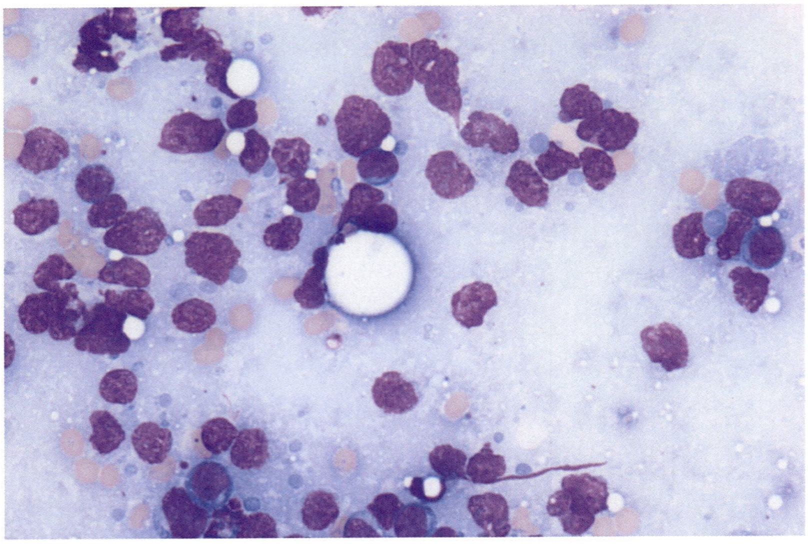

Figures 1–3. Different fields of the same lymph node cytology in a case of lymphoma. Fields 1 and 2 have no diagnostic validity owing to the high proportion of ruptured cells (black arrows indicate naked nuclei; red arrows indicate lymphoglandular bodies). Only field 3, in which intact cells predominate, is valid for interpretation.

Figure 1.

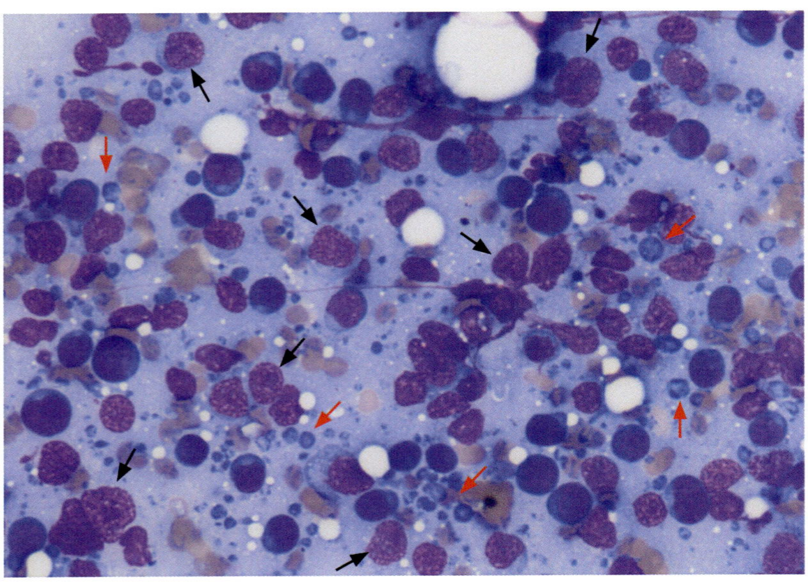

Figure 2.

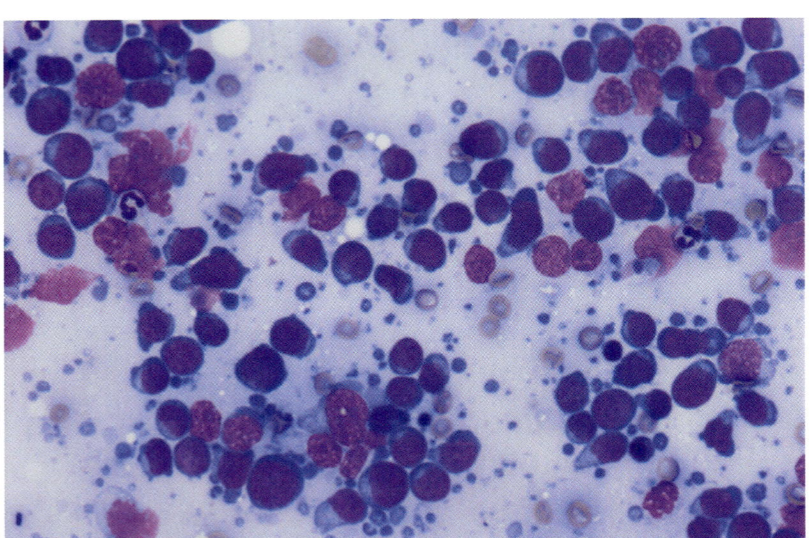

Figure 3.

Figures 4 and 5. Owing to excessive cellularity and deficient staining these fields are of insufficient quality for evaluation for the diagnosis of lymphoma.

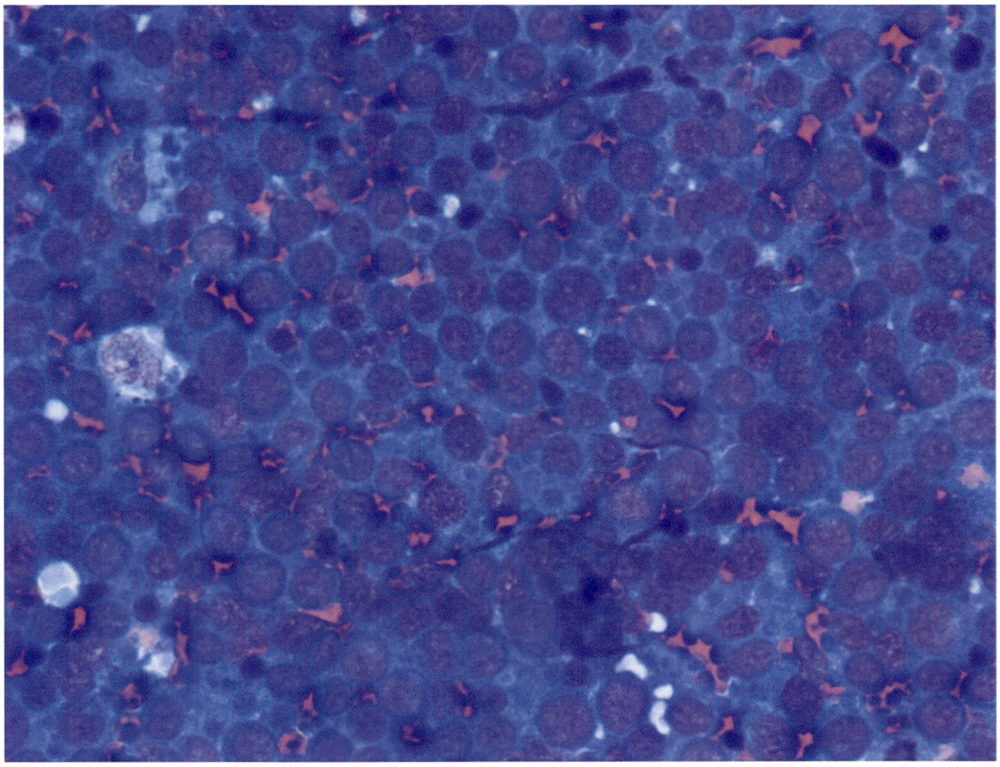

Figure 4.

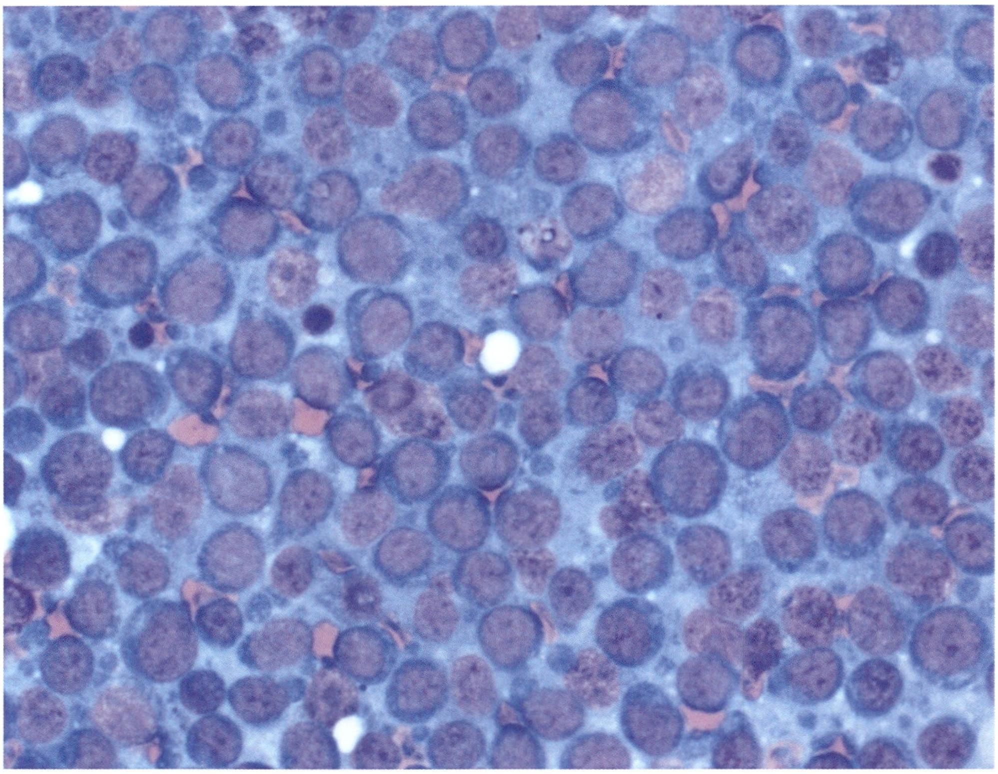

Figure 5.

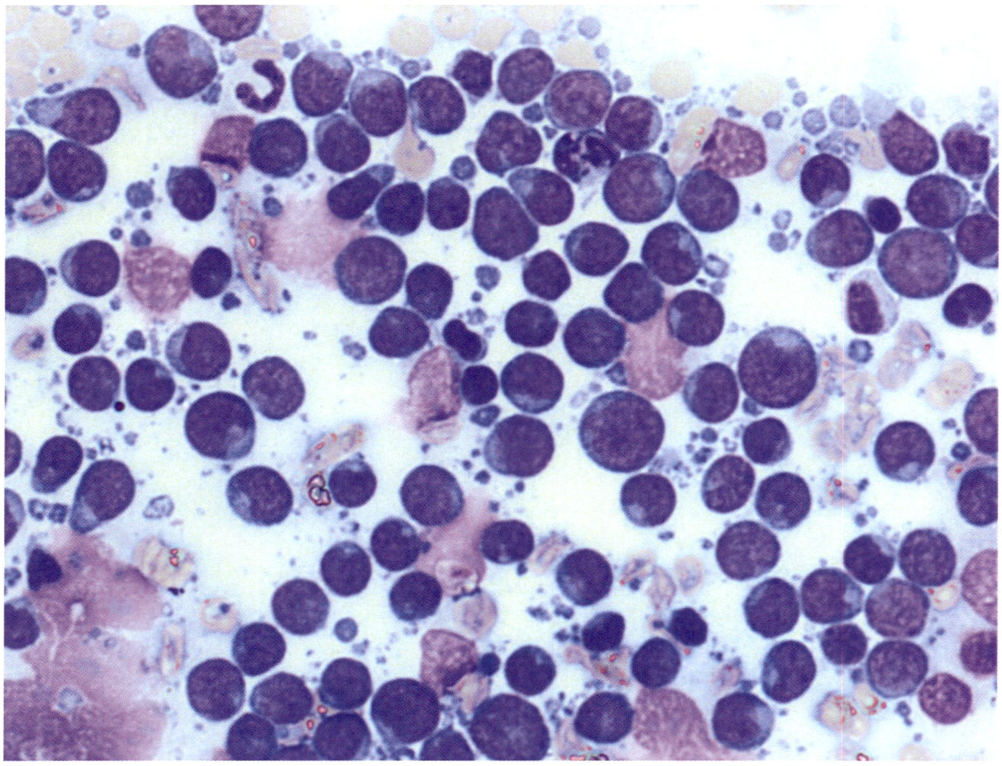

Figure 6. Microscopic field of sufficient quality for evaluation for the diagnosis of lymphoma.

## DIAGNOSIS OF LYMPHOMA

The cytological picture of a normal, hyperplastic, reactive or metastatic lymph node is heterogeneous. Diagnosis of lymphoma is based on observation of a monomorphic population in which a single lymphoid stage predominates. In most cases, this population is lymphoblastic (cells larger than two mature lymphocytes or two erythrocytes).

Lymphoma is suspected if the blast count corresponds to over 50 % of the total population. The higher this percentage, the greater the diagnostic accuracy (Figs. 7–10).

In cases of advanced lymphoma it is relatively easy to establish a diagnosis, even if the increases in blast count are small.

It is important to perform a differential cell count in different areas of the cytological preparation (and in different preparations from the same lymph node). The number of cells counted will vary depending on cellular homogeneity. If the percentages in different areas are very similar, it may be sufficient to count 500–1,000 cells per preparation. However, if there are discrepancies in the percentages, the cell count should be increased proportionally (Figs. 11 and 12). Sometimes, it is impossible to estimate a reliable mean, and only a range of percentages can be established, significantly limiting diagnostic accuracy.

Figure 7.

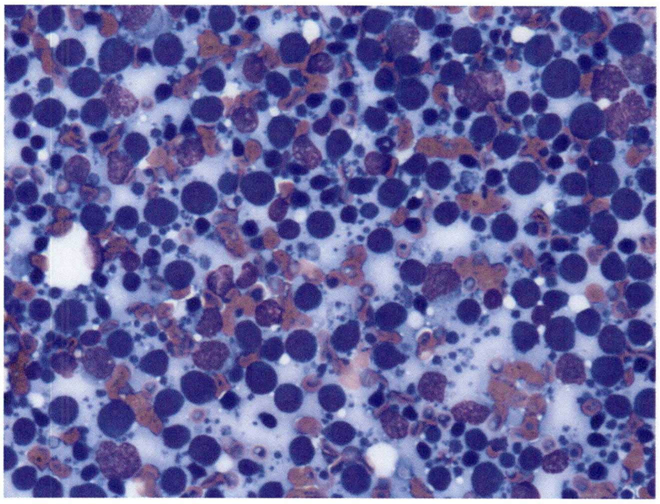

Figure 8.

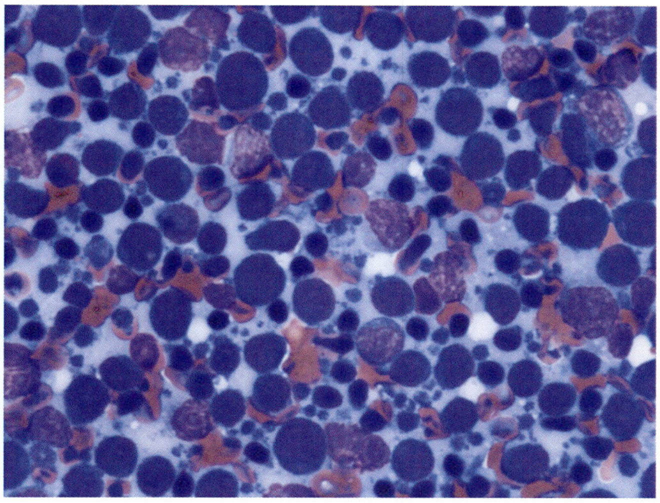

Figure 9.

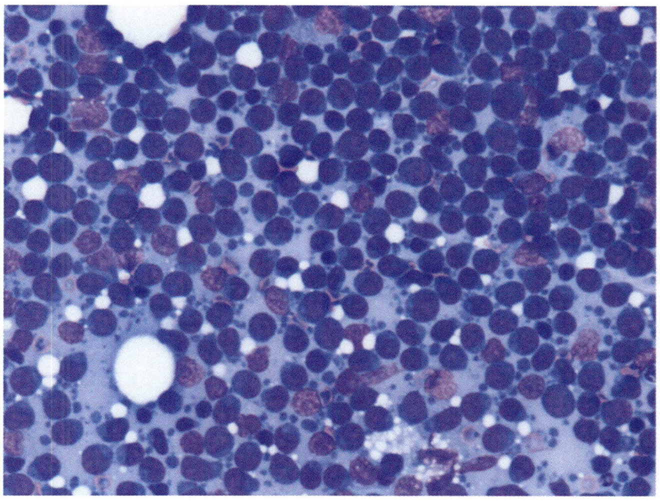

Figure 10.

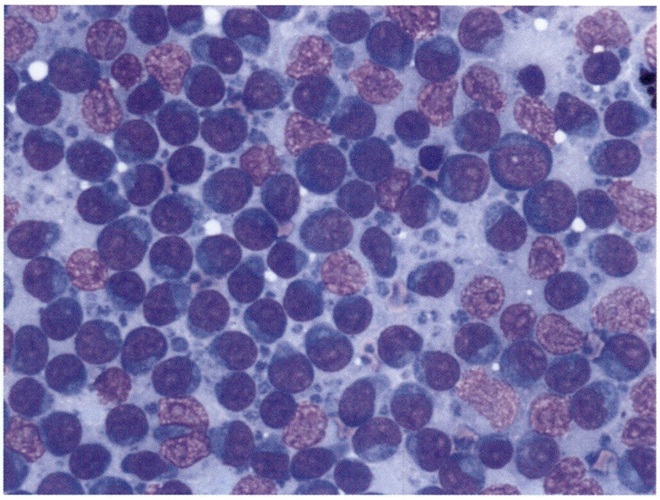

Figures 7–10. Cytological preparations from two patients with lymphoma. Although images 7 and 8 are diagnostic, images 9 and 10 are of greater diagnostic validity, since the proportion of lymphoblasts is much greater than 50 %.

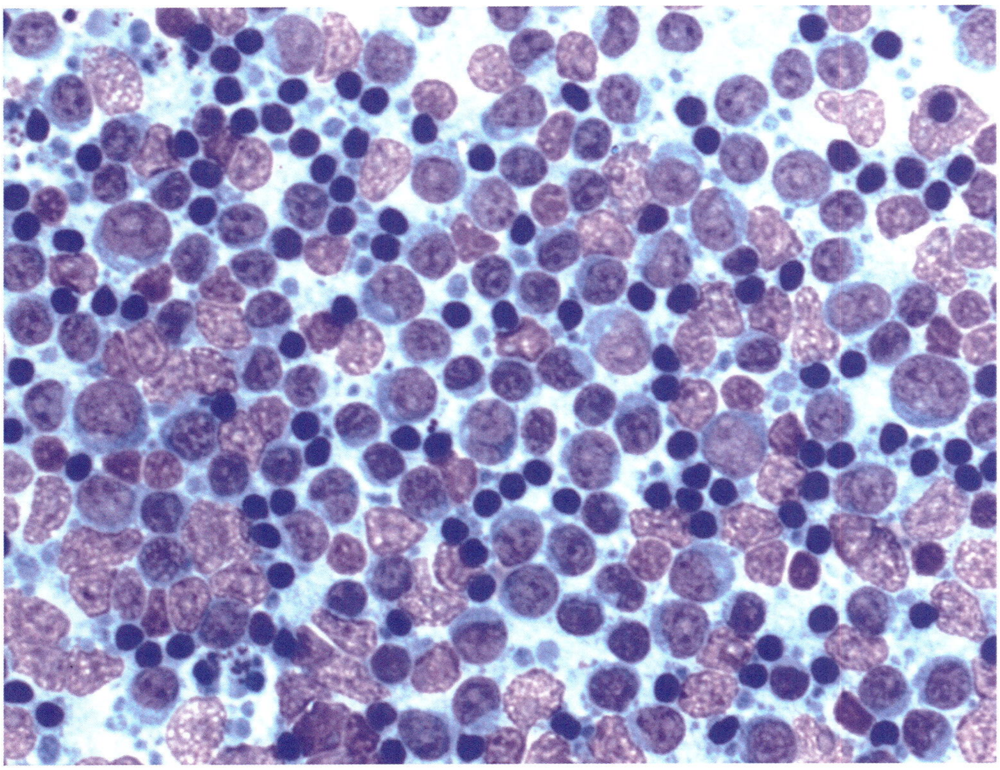

Figures 11 and 12. Two fields from the same cytological preparation. The proportion of lymphoblasts varies markedly between the two fields.

Figure 11.

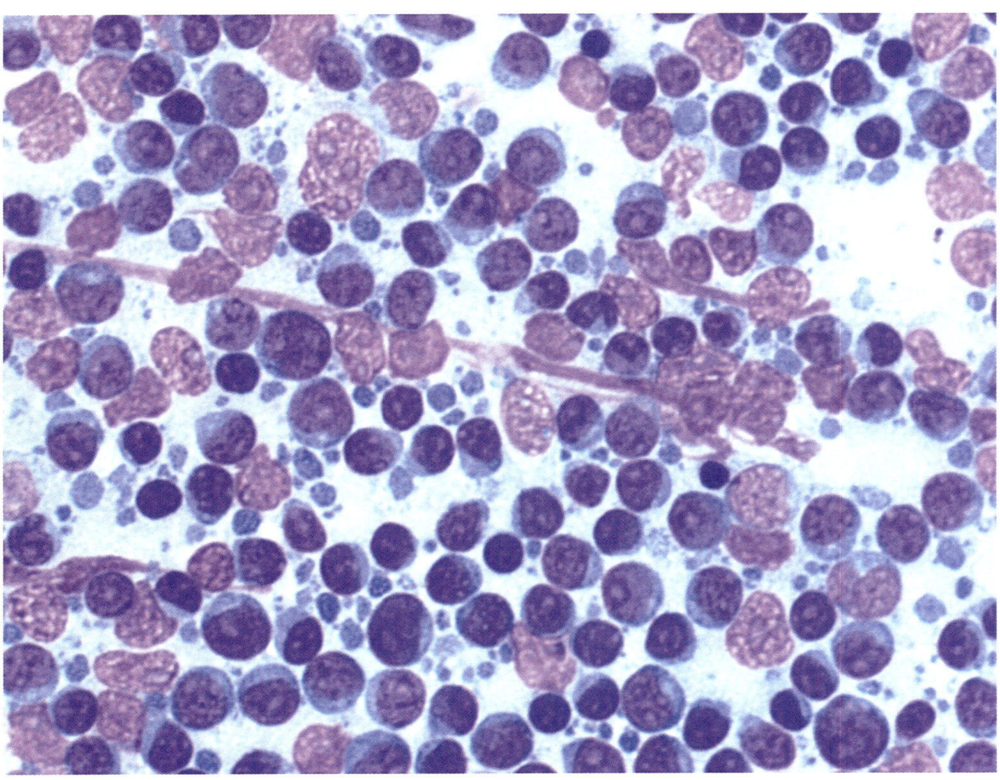

Figure 12.

While the following cytological features are also observed in lymphoma, none constitute a sufficiently valid criterion to allow diagnosis in the absence of a monomorphic cytological picture:

- Increase in the number of atypical mitoses, although it is important to note that mitoses are observed relatively often in normal and reactive lymph nodes (Fig. 13).
- Absence of plasma cells, although plasma cells can be occasionally observed in highly reactive (submandibular) lymph nodes (Fig. 13).
- Increase in the number of macrophages phagocytosing cellular debris (macrophages with tingible bodies), resulting in a so-called "starry sky" pattern at low magnification. Although in humans this cytological picture is associated with Burkitt's lymphoma, in dogs it can be associated with several different types of lymphoma (Fig. 14).
- Presence of numerous lymphoglandular bodies, a consequence of lymphoblast fragility (Fig. 15).

Figure 13.

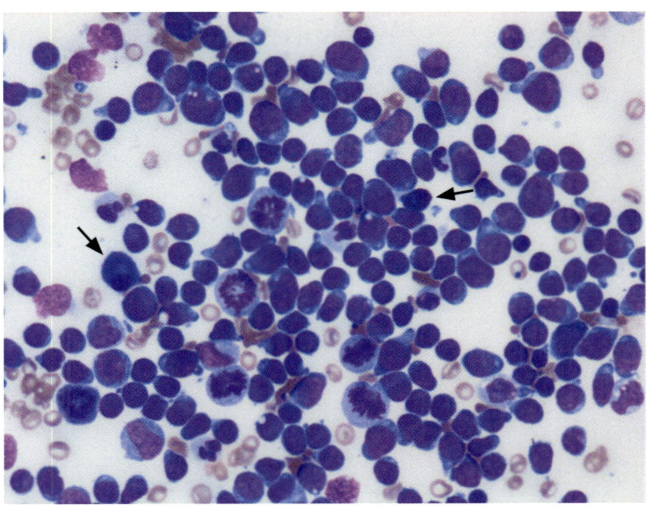

Figure 14.

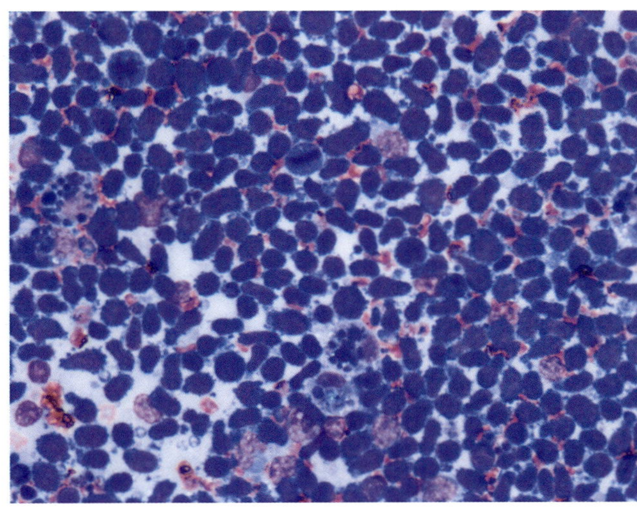

Figure 15.

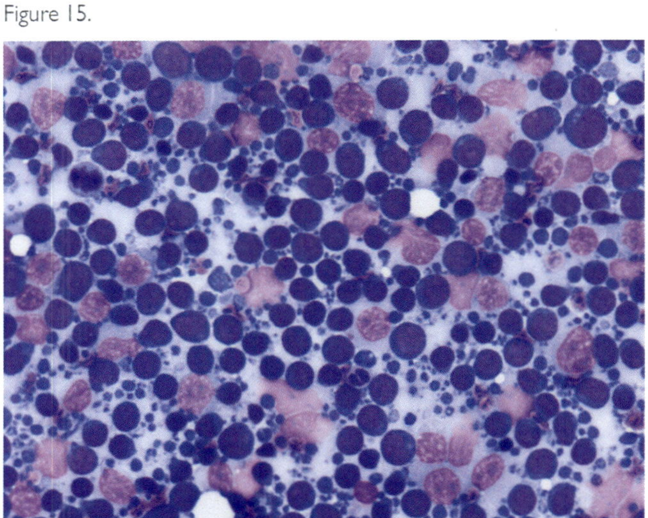

Figure 13. Submandibular lymph node cytology. Although the percentage of large-sized blasts is low, the presence of numerous atypical mitoses supports a diagnosis of (intermediate cell) lymphoma. Plasma cells (arrows) are evident, indicating a reactive component.

Figure 14. Starry sky pattern against a background of lymphoblasts. Macrophages with tingible bodies are evident.

Figure 15. Lymphoma with abundant lymphoglandular bodies.

## CYTOLOGICAL DIAGNOSIS OF LYMPHOMA SUBTYPE

Currently, it is not considered appropriate to apply the same prognostic criteria and therapeutic decisions to all lymphoma patients. In dogs, histological classification of lymphoma subtype has proven to be reliable,[13] and should be combined with immunophenotyping. Certain cytological characteristics can be evaluated to at least enable estimation of the lymphoma subtype with greater prognostic reliability.[14] However, it is not always possible to establish a conclusive classification because the cytological picture can vary depending on the fields evaluated.

Based on cell/nucleus size, the chromatin pattern, and the number, size, and location of the nucleoli, the classification scheme shown in Table 1 can be established (Figs. 16–28).

Cytology is particularly important in the diagnosis of granular lymphoma, since it is difficult to detect the granules in histological preparations or by using rapid stains.

Occasionally, lymphoblasts may exhibit cytoplasmic vacuoles, with a morphology similar to that of Burkitt cells in humans (Fig. 29).

**TABLE 1.** Classification of lymphoma based on nuclear/cell size, chromatin pattern, and the number, size, and location of the nucleoli.

| Degree of malignancy | Type of lymphoma | Nuclear size* | Nucleus | Cytoplasm |
|---|---|---|---|---|
| **Low** | Small cell (lymphocytic) | Small | Round; compact chromatin; without nucleoli | Very scarce. Ends in a cytoplasmic elongation in T-phenotype (hand-mirror lymphocytes) |
| | Marginal zone (B-cell)** | Medium | Round; condensed chromatin; single large nucleolus (macronucleolus) | Scarce, bluish |
| **High** | Diffuse large B-cell | Large | Round; condensed chromatin; single, large and central nucleolus (immunoblasts) or multiple peripheral nucleoli (centroblasts) | Moderate-abundant. Strongly basophilic, sometimes with cytoplasmic clearing |
| | High-grade T-cell | Medium-large | Round (in some cases clefted); finely condensed chromatin; nucleoli usually absent | Scarce to moderate; Slightly basophilic, greyish |
| | Large granular cell | Medium-large | Round; compact or condensed chromatin | Pale with granules*** |

* Small, <1.5 red blood cells; medium, 1.5–2 red blood cells; large, >2–4 red blood cells (in cells with little cytoplasm nuclear and cell size are comparable).

** Can be cytologically identified as high grade; diagnosis requires histopathological confirmation.

*** Magenta granules, sometimes surrounded by a clear, fine halo with a polar distribution (very evident in cats, less so in dogs).

Figures 16 and 17. Small-cell lymphoma. Numerous lymphocytes with "hand-mirror" morphology are observed (T-phenotype).

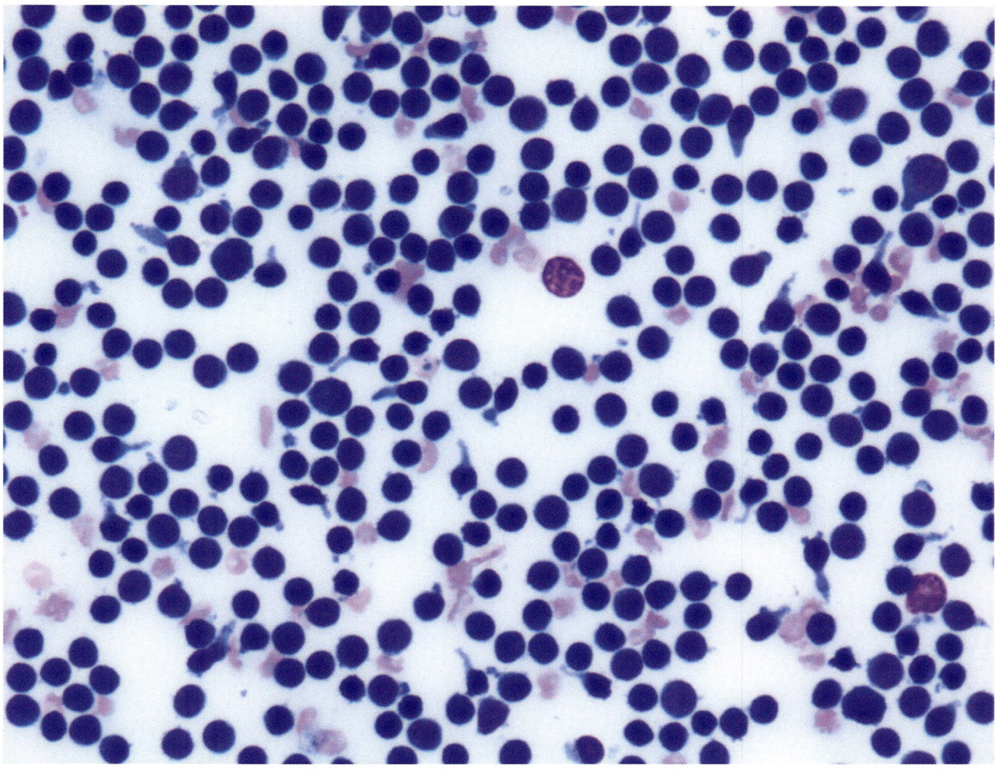

Figure 16.

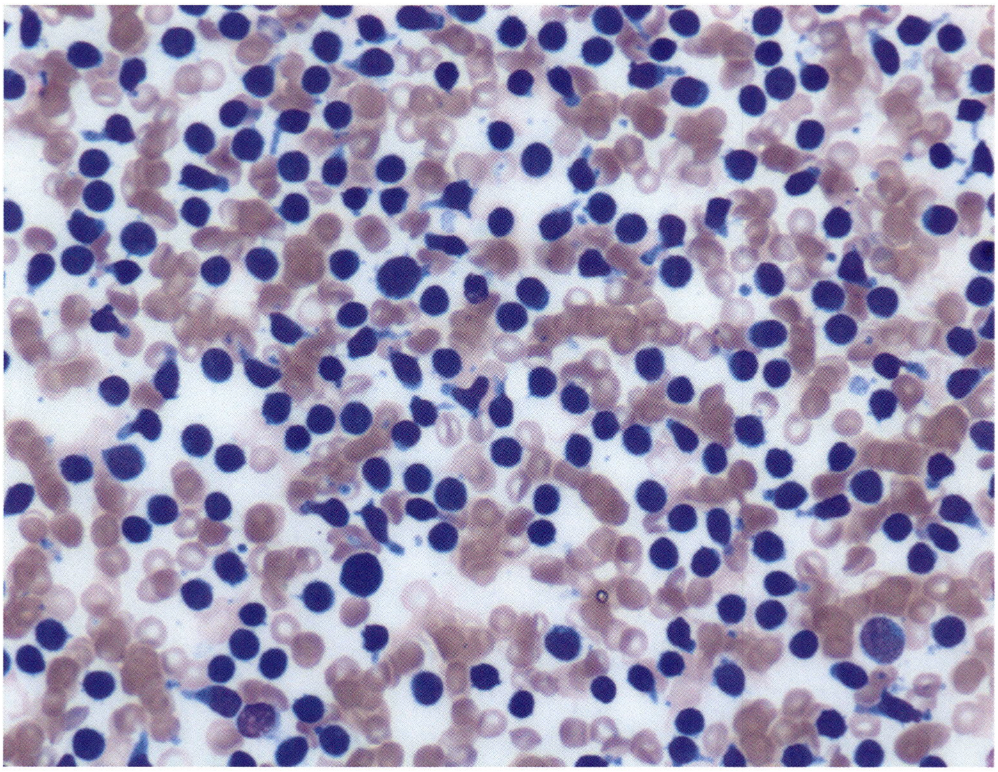

Figure 17.

Figures 18 and 19. Intermediate cell lymphoma with macronucleoli (marginal zone).

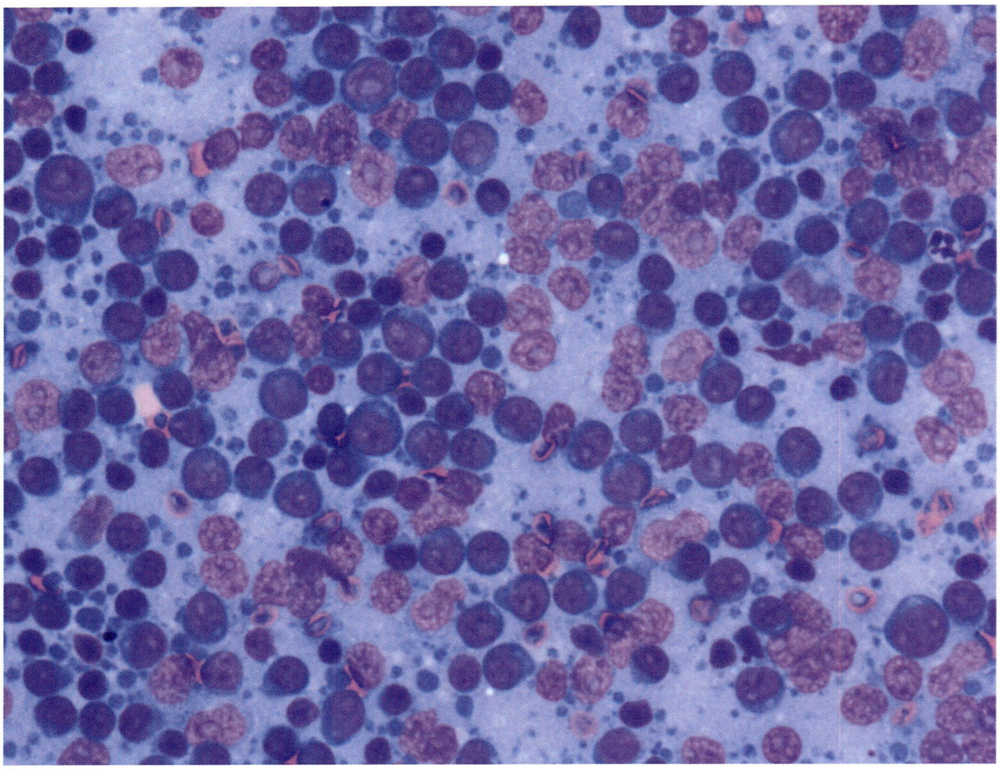

Figure 18.

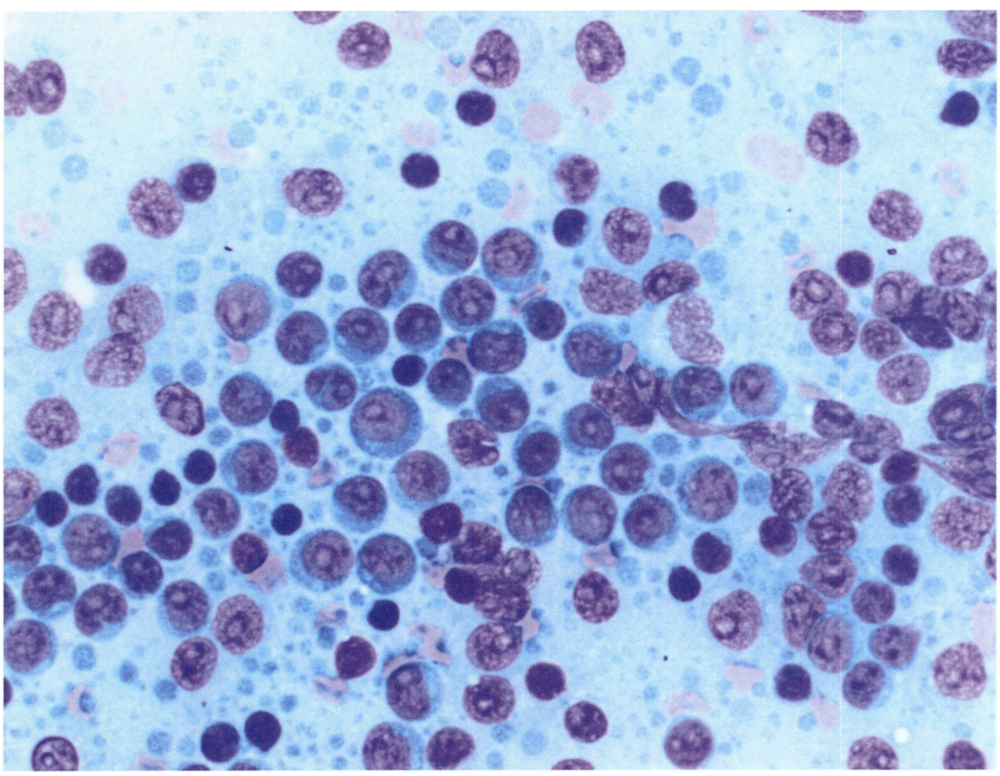

Figure 19.

Figures 20–22. Diffuse B-cell lymphoma. Note the presence of immunoblasts (a single nucleolus) and centroblasts (several nucleoli).

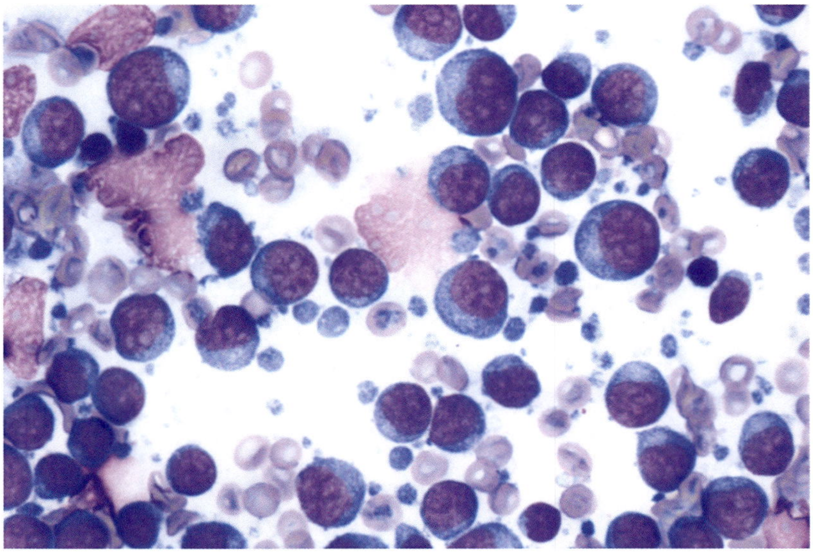

Figure 20.

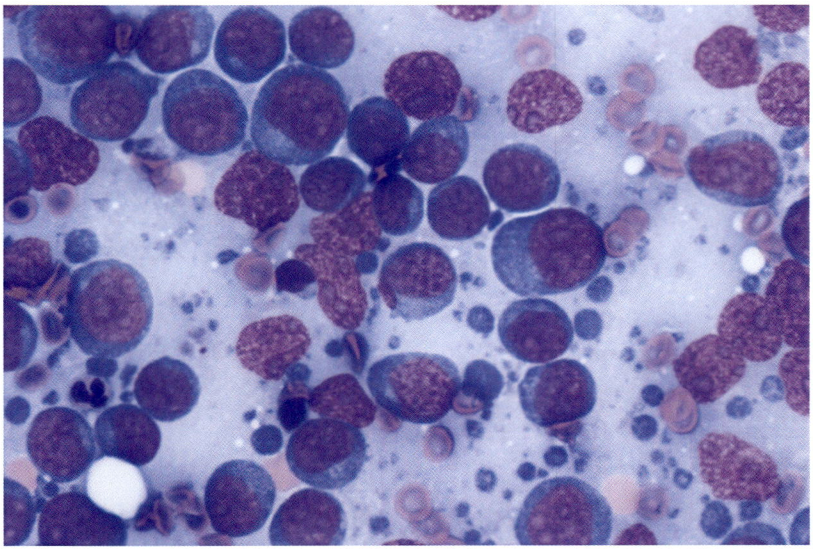

Figure 21.

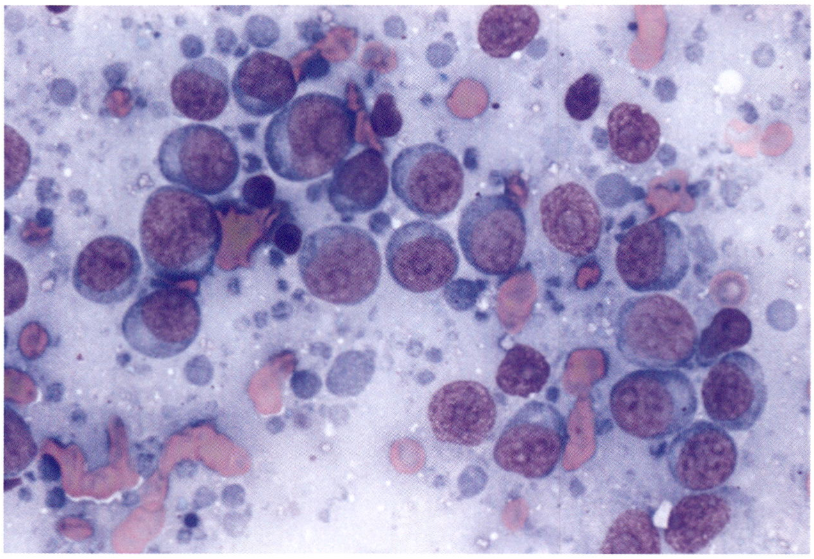

Figure 22.

Figures 23–25. High-grade T-cell lymphoma. The presence of clefted nuclei is common.

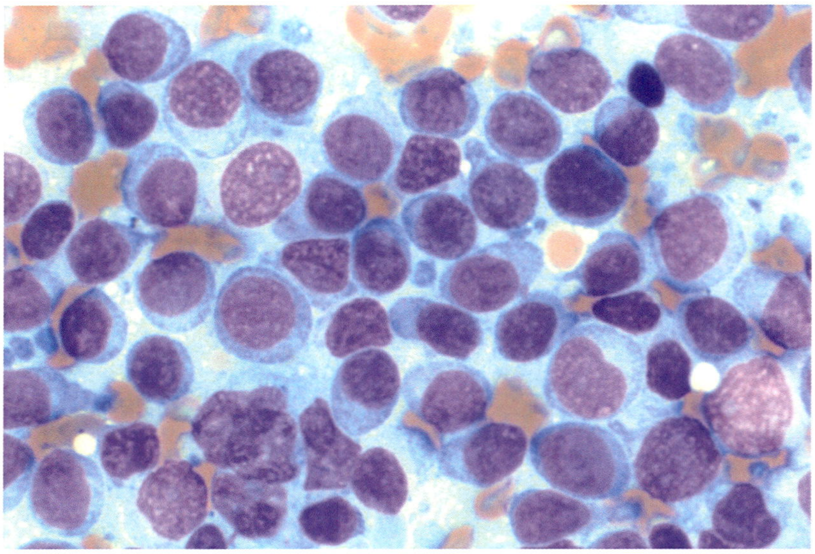

Figure 23.

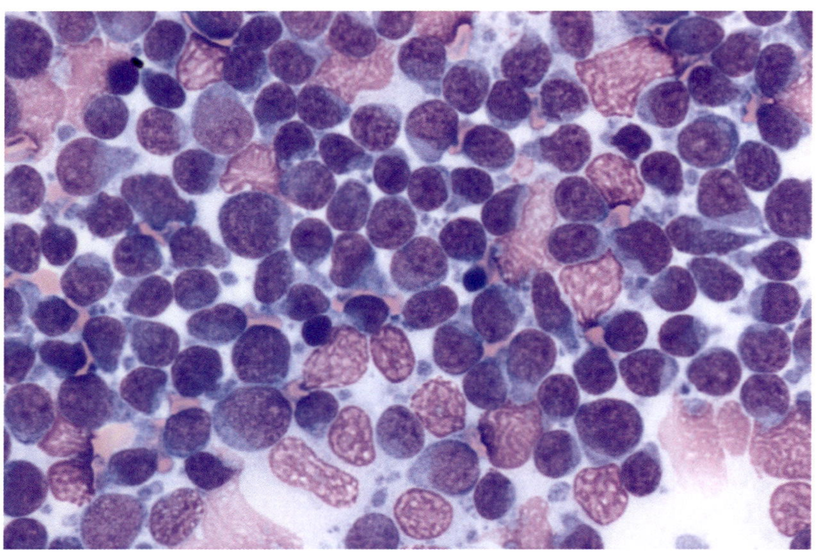

Figure 24.

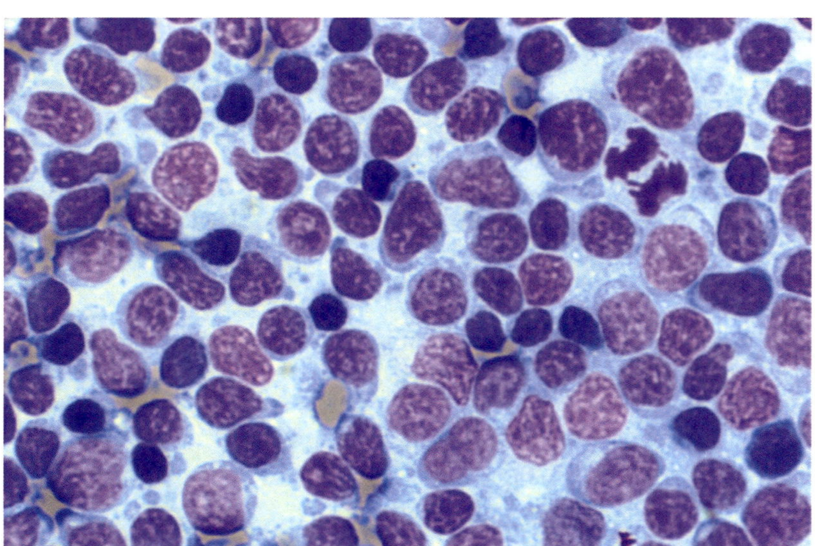

Figure 25.

Figures 26–28. Large granular T-cell lymphoma. The granules are more evident in cats (26 and 27) than in dogs (28).

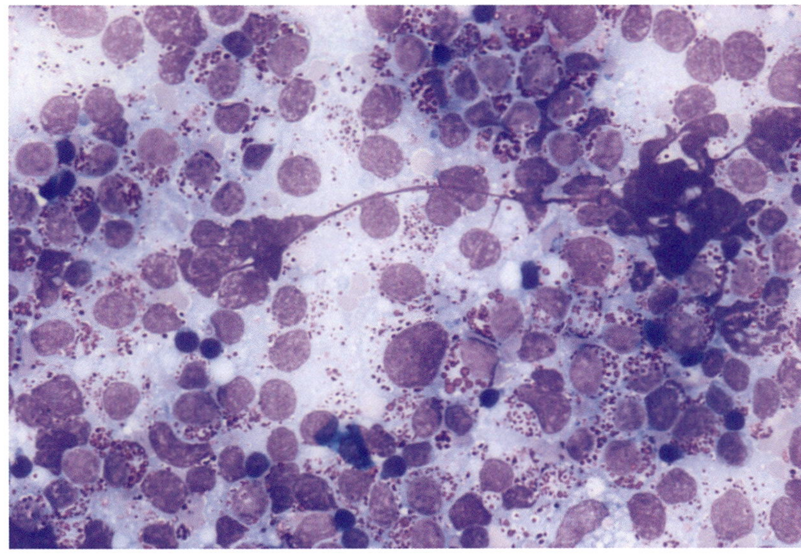

Figure 26.

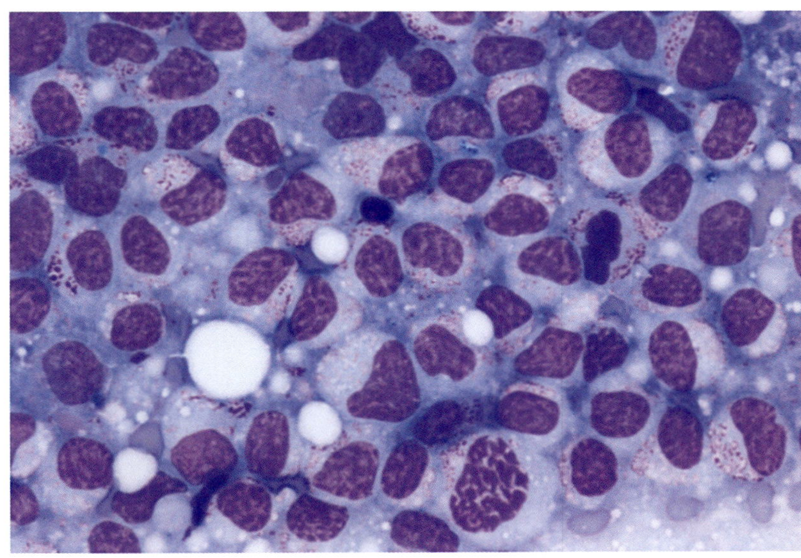

Figure 27.

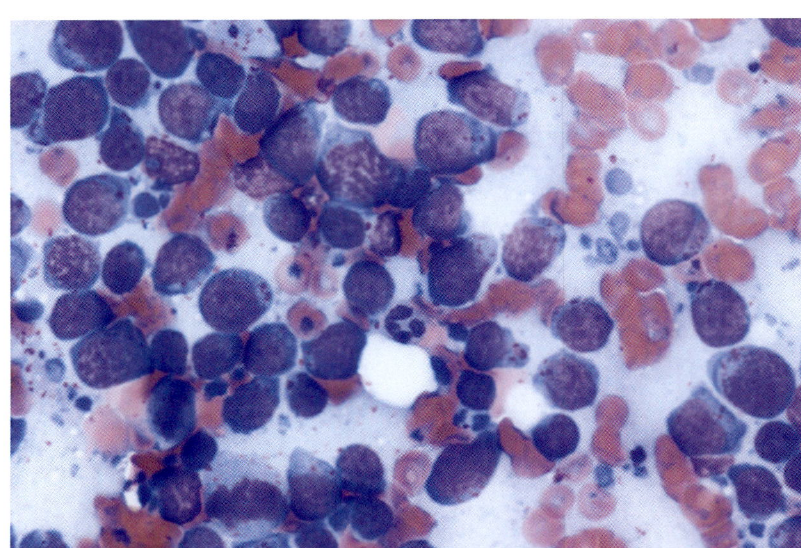

Figure 28.

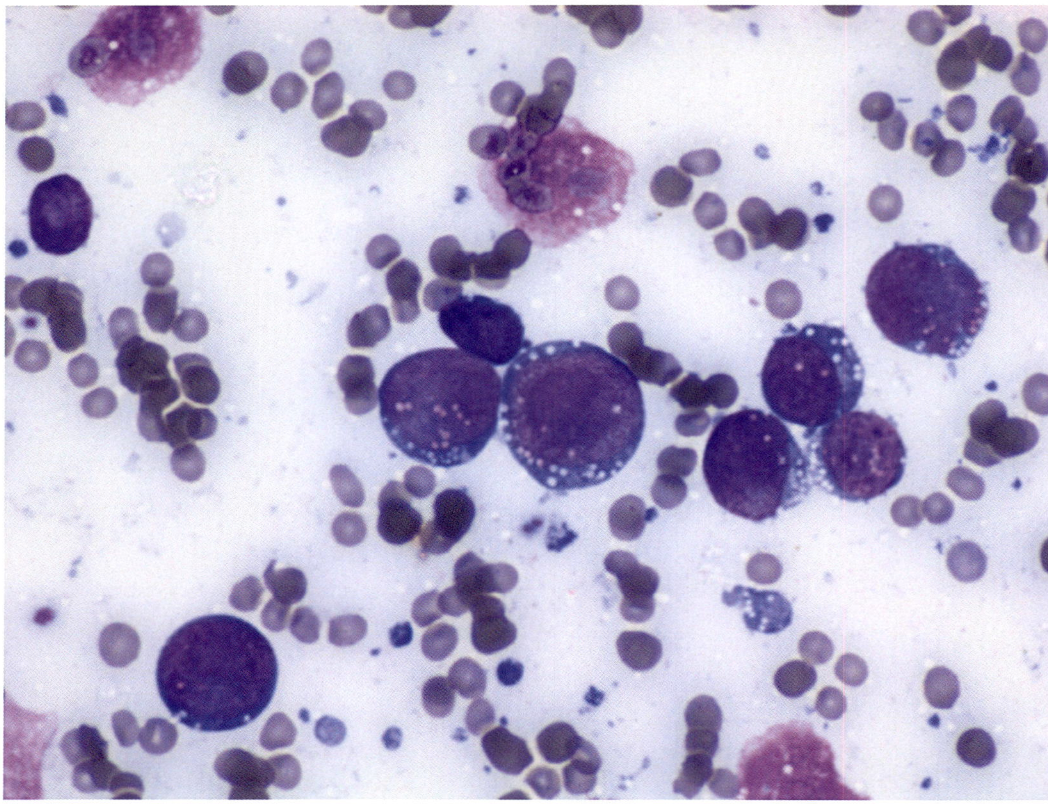

Figure 29. Lymphoma with vacuolated lymphoblasts (cat).

The cytological picture of most large cell lymphomas is highly characteristic. The following are the main differential diagnoses:

- Lymphoid hyperplasia. In dogs it is rare for hyperplasia to be limited to the blast population and to be so intense as to be mistaken for lymphoma. However, in cats this is much more frequent, especially in cases of infectious disease. Therefore, diagnosis of lymphoma at the lymph node level is always more complex and requires great care (see Chapter 2).
- Massive metastasis of other undifferentiated round cell tumours, especially histiocytic sarcoma (Fig. 30). However, in this situation, cells with giant or multinucleated nuclei are common. It is very rare to encounter binucleated lymphoblasts, except for so-called Reed–Sternberg cells (Fig. 31), which are large lymphoblasts characteristic of Hodgkin lymphoma (a rare form of feline lymphoma).

Small cell lymphoma is difficult to differentiate from a normal lymph node, since the predominant cell is the mature lymphocyte (Fig. 32). The absence of lymphoblasts and/or plasma cells is, in this case, an important diagnostic criterion. However, it may be necessary to perform other tests (immunocytochemistry, cytometry, or clonality tests) to confirm the diagnosis.

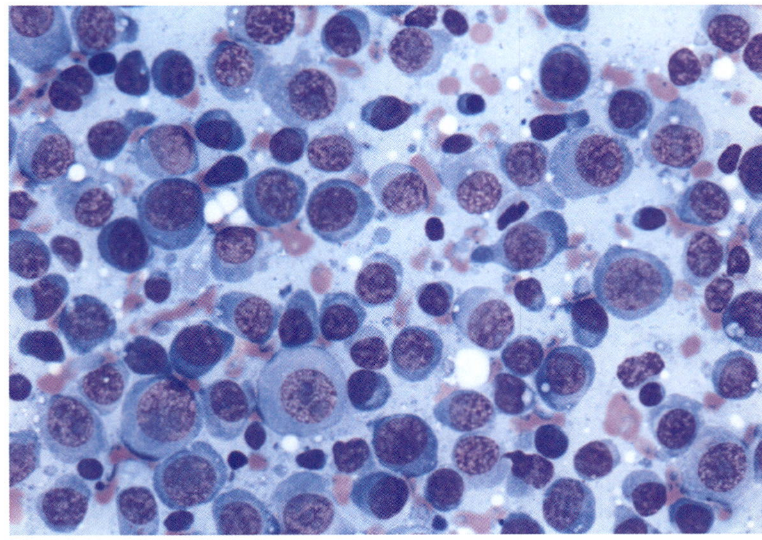

Figure 30. Lymph node cytology. The cytological picture is ambiguous, lying somewhere between histiocytic sarcoma and high-grade T-cell lymphoma.

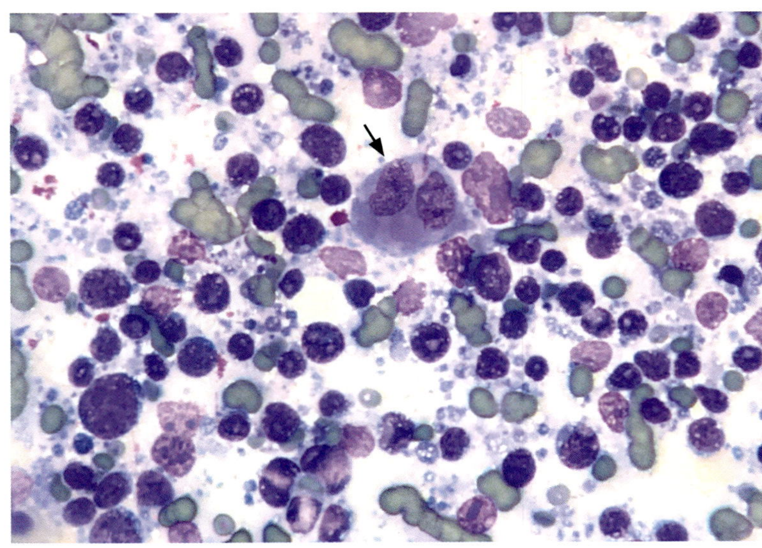

Figure 31. Reed–Sternberg cell (arrow) in a feline lymph node lymphoma. Image courtesy of Dr Víctor Domingo Roa.

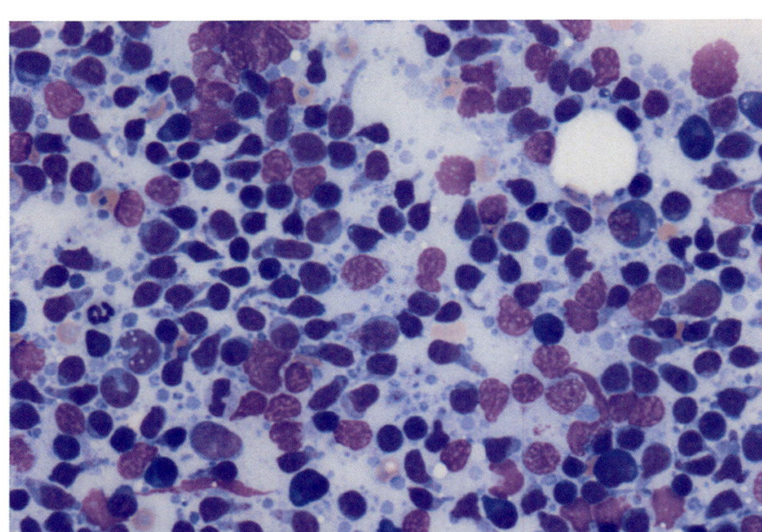

Figure 32. Ambiguous lymph node cytology. A pleomorphic image is observed, but there is a high number of small T cells (higher than usual in hyperplastic lymph nodes).

## DIAGNOSIS OF LYMPHOMA IN OTHER CYTOLOGICAL PREPARATIONS

Although most of the criteria applied to lymph node cytology can be applied to other organs (Figs. 33–37), there are some specific considerations and differential diagnoses that should be borne in mind.

- In the case of the spleen, one important differential diagnosis is extramedullary erythropoiesis, in which the predominant cell population is erythroid precursors, which are morphologically very similar to lymphoblasts. However, other precursors are also frequently observed, enabling differentiation of the two processes (Fig. 38).
- It is impossible to cytologically differentiate lymphoma from infiltration in lymphoblastic leukaemia. It can also be difficult to distinguish lymphoma from acute myeloproliferative leukaemia (Fig. 39). In most cases it is necessary to resort to immunohistochemistry or flow cytometry to establish a diagnosis.
- Small cell lymphomas can be difficult to differentiate from lymphocytic or lymphoplasmacytic inflammation (Figs. 40 and 41).
- In cutaneous lymphoma, the lymphoblasts may contain a greater amount of cytoplasm and clefted nuclei, resembling histiocytes (Fig. 42). If the blast cells are interspersed with fat particles, the picture may be confused with that of panniculitis (panniculitis-like T-cell lymphoma) (Fig. 43).
- Mediastinal lymphoma can be mistaken for thymoma. There is no doubt in cases of large cell lymphoma (Fig. 34), but confusion can arise in cases of small cell lymphoma, since in thymoma mature lymphocytes predominate and the characteristic epithelial cells and dispersed mast cells are not always observed.
- In bodily fluids the nuclear morphology of lymphoblasts can be distorted, causing them to lose their characteristic round shape and adopt a more lobed morphology (clover-shaped or with marked clefts), which can make identification difficult (Figs. 44–46).
- In different forms of meningoencephalitis that present with an increase in the number of lymphocytes in the cerebrospinal fluid, it is common to observe a certain proportion of immature cells that resemble lymphoblasts, although their presence does not imply a diagnosis of lymphoma (Figs. 47 and 48).

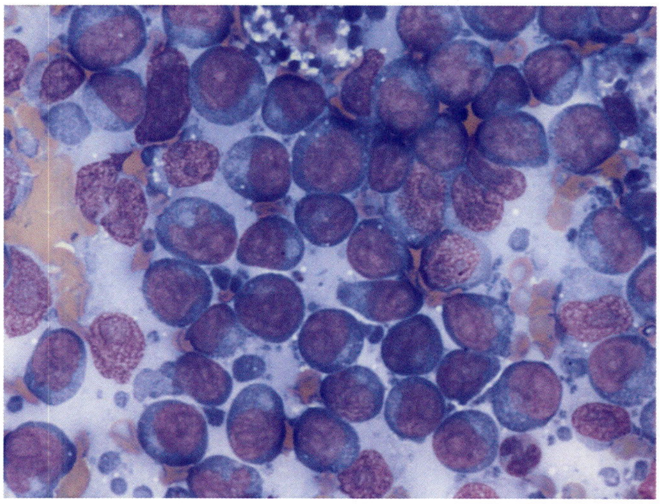
Figure 33.

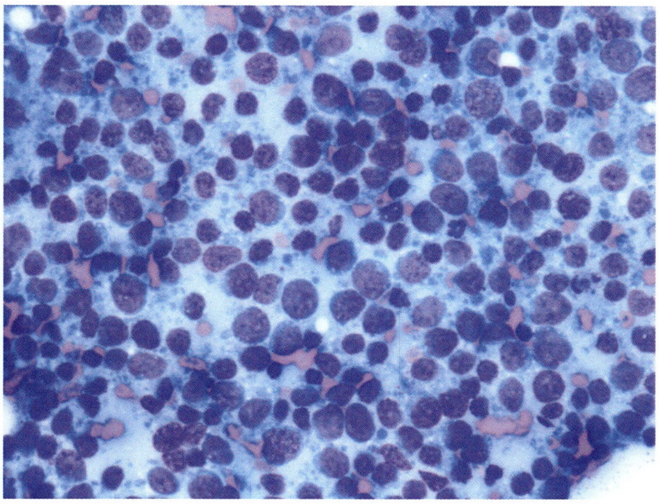
Figure 34.

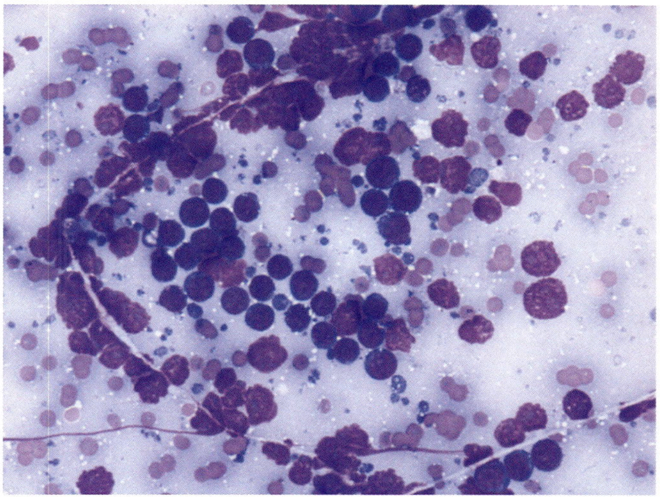
Figure 35.

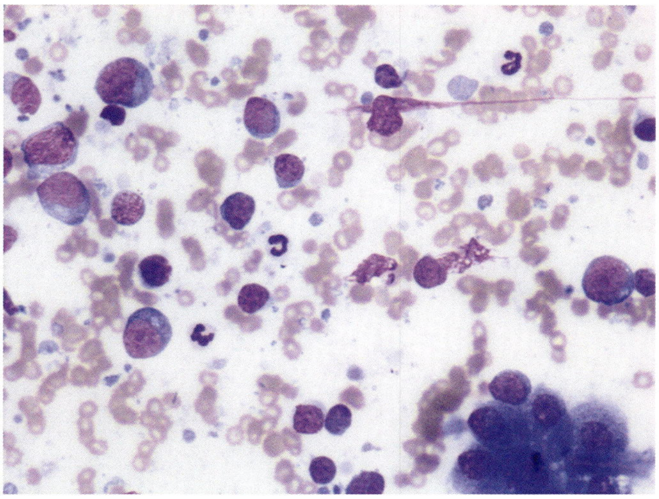
Figure 36.

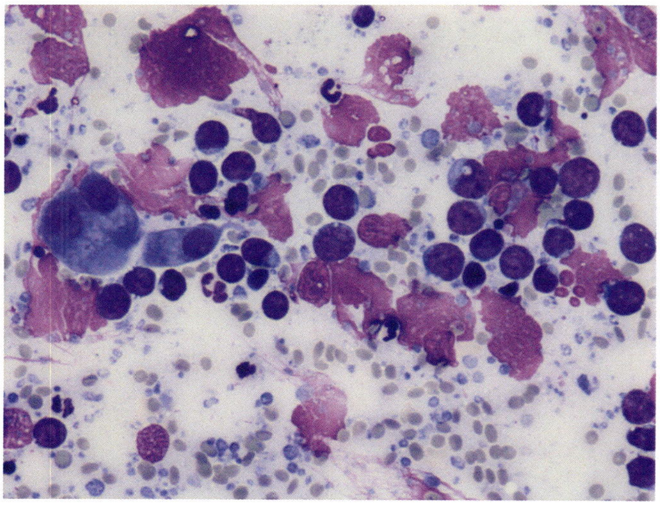
◀ Figure 37.

Figures 33–37. Large cell lymphoma. Samples from the spleen (33), mediastinal mass (34), kidney (35), liver (36), and nasal cavity (37).

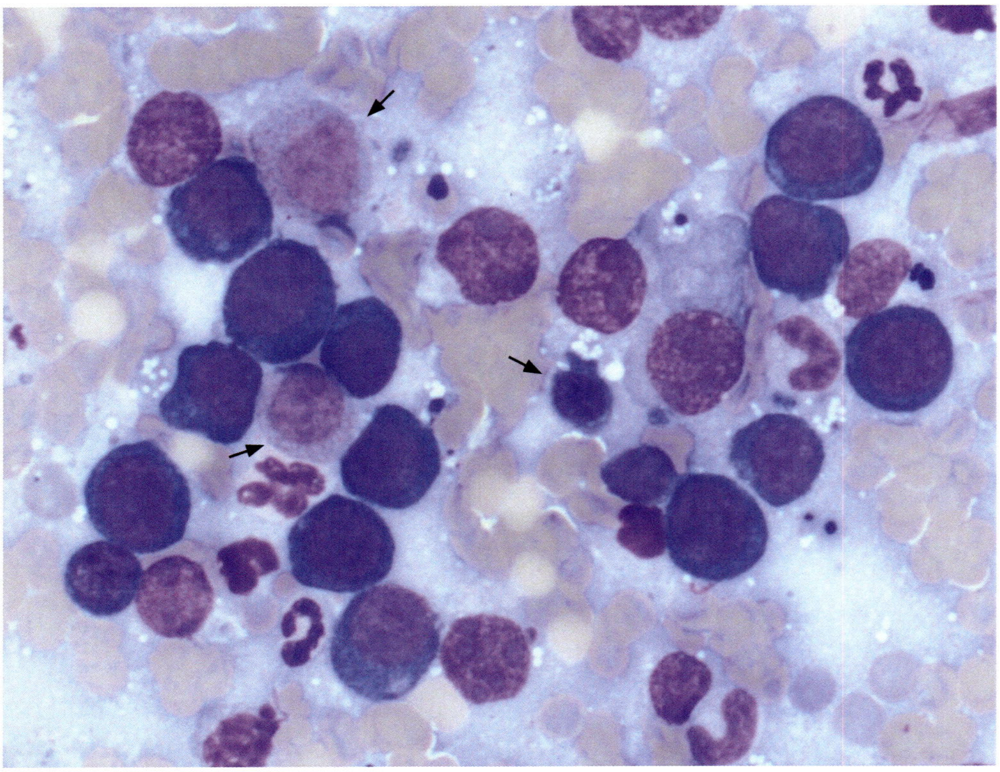

Figure 38. Erythroid precursors exhibiting a lymphoblast-like morphology. Based on the presence of other precursors (arrows), this can be classified as extramedullary haematopoiesis.

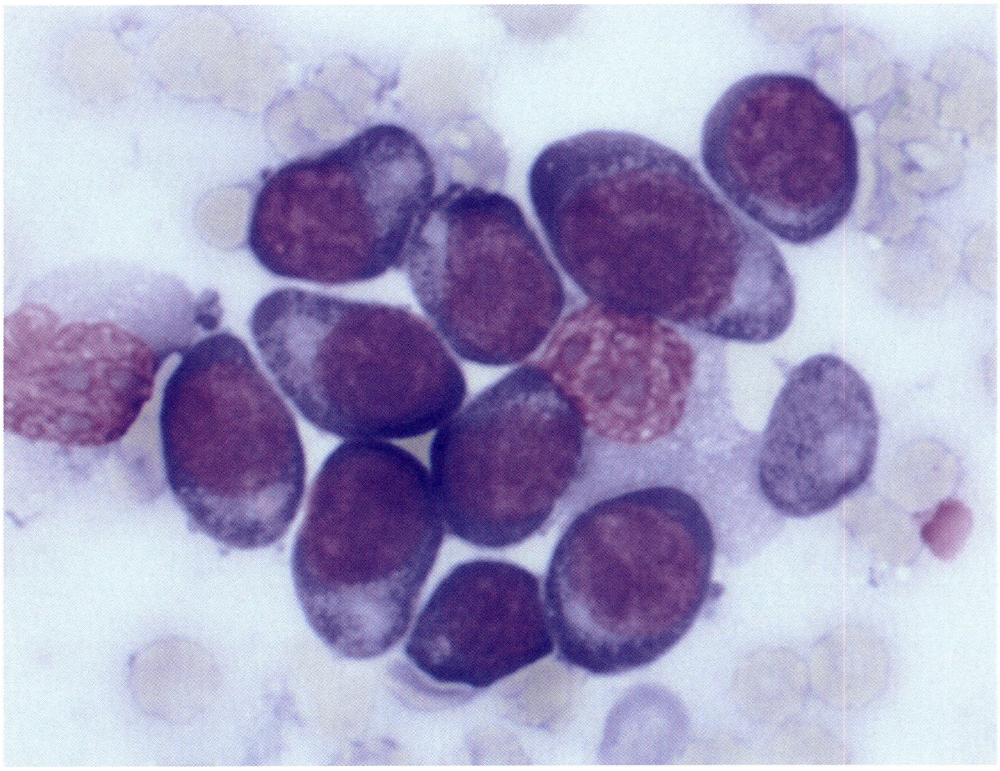

Figure 39. Spleen cytology in a case of myelomonoblastic leukaemia, which is distinguished from lymphoma using other diagnostic techniques.

Figures 40 and 41. Liver (40) and intestinal (41) lymphoma. Differentiation from lymphocytic inflammation can be difficult when small or intermediate cells predominate.

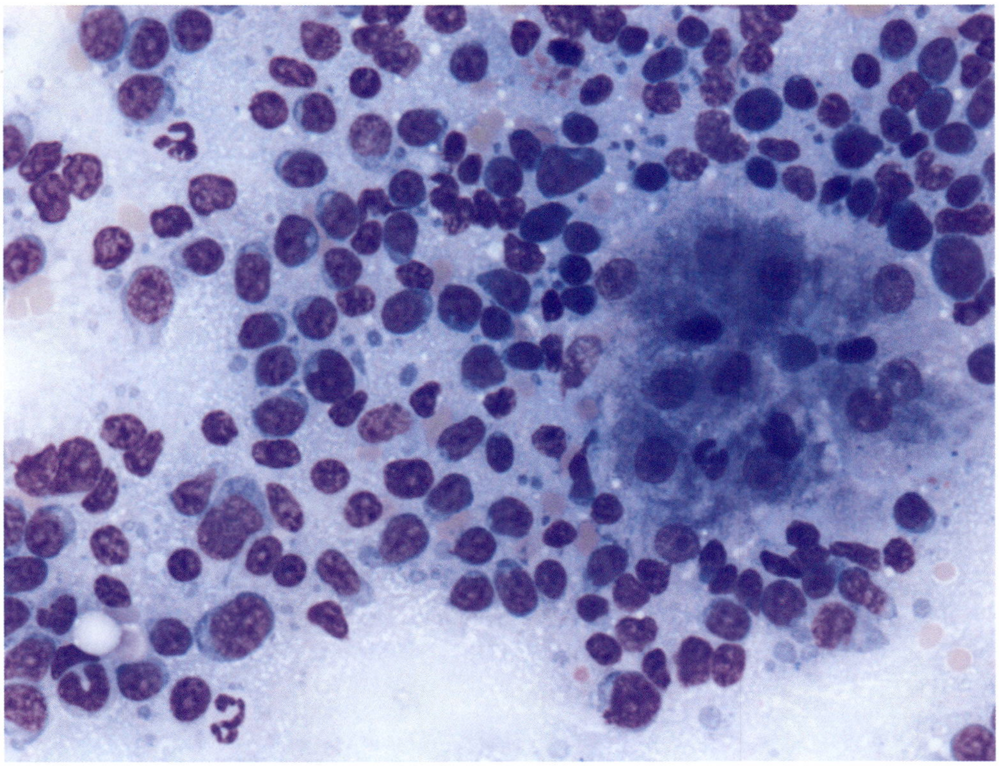

Figure 40.

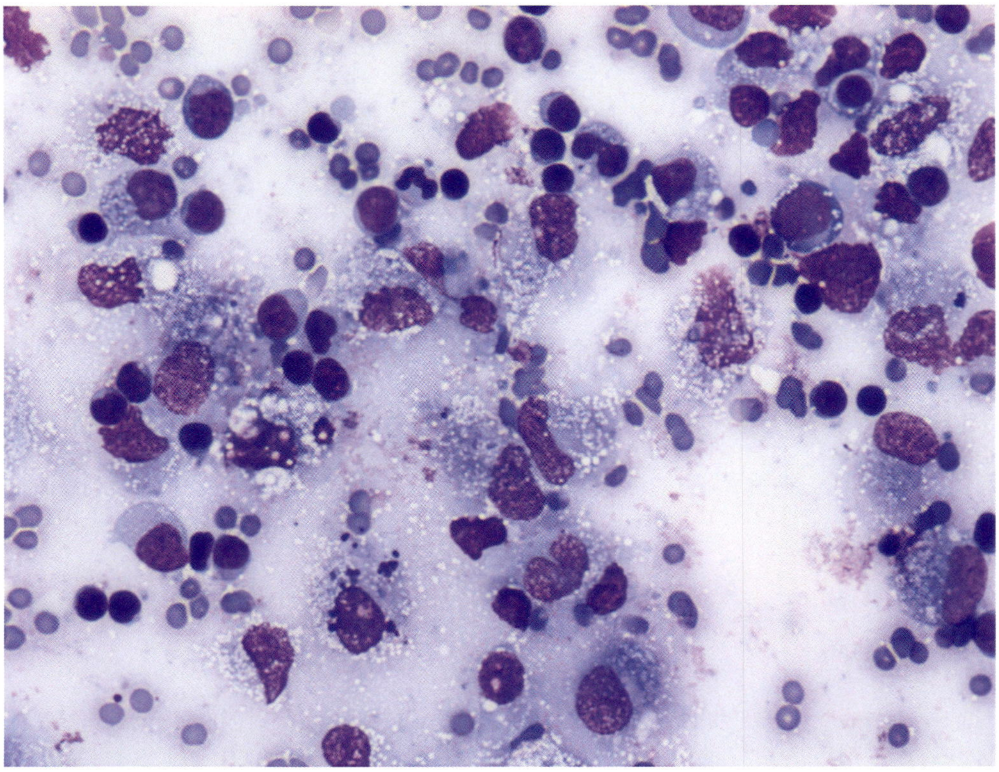

Figure 41.

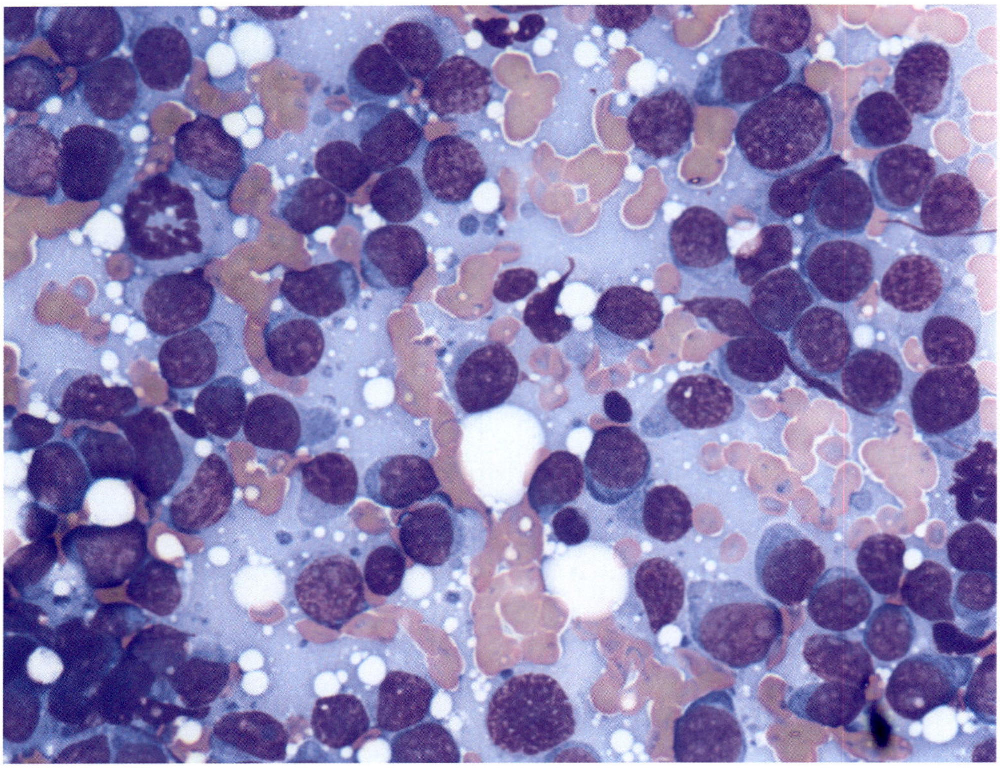

Figure 42. Cutaneous lymphoma in which histiocyte-like lymphoblasts are observed.

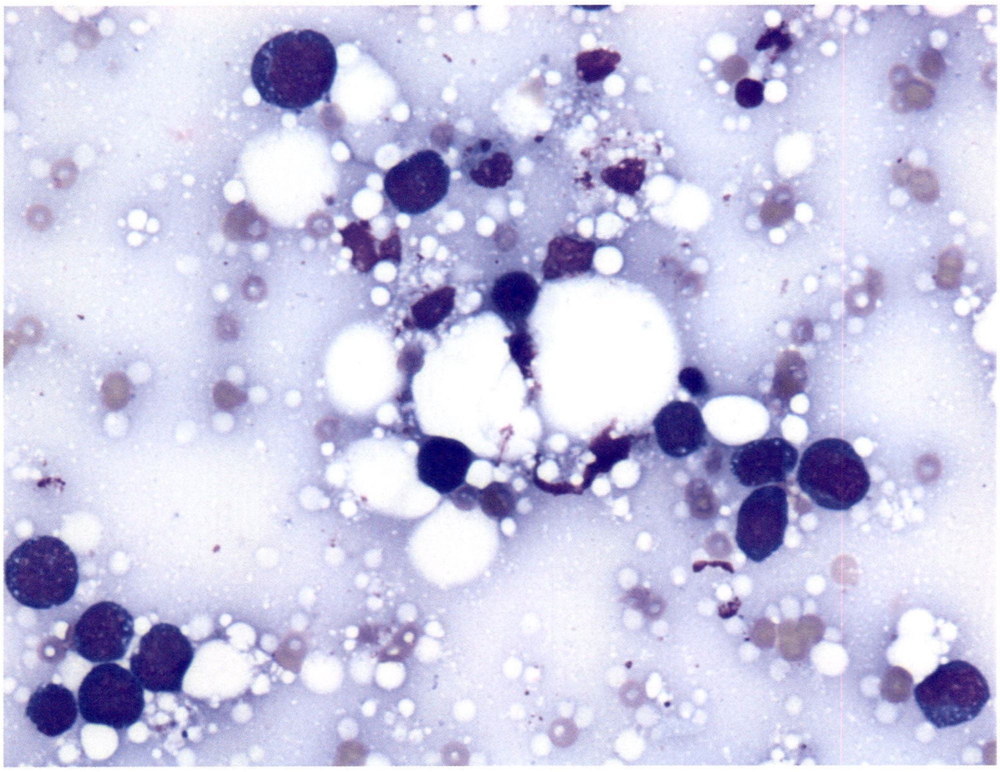

Figure 43. Panniculitis-like T-cell lymphoma.

Figures 44–46. Lymphoma detected in pleural fluid (44), cerebrospinal fluid (45), and peripheral oedema fluid (46). The lymphoblasts are difficult to identify owing to their atypical nuclei.

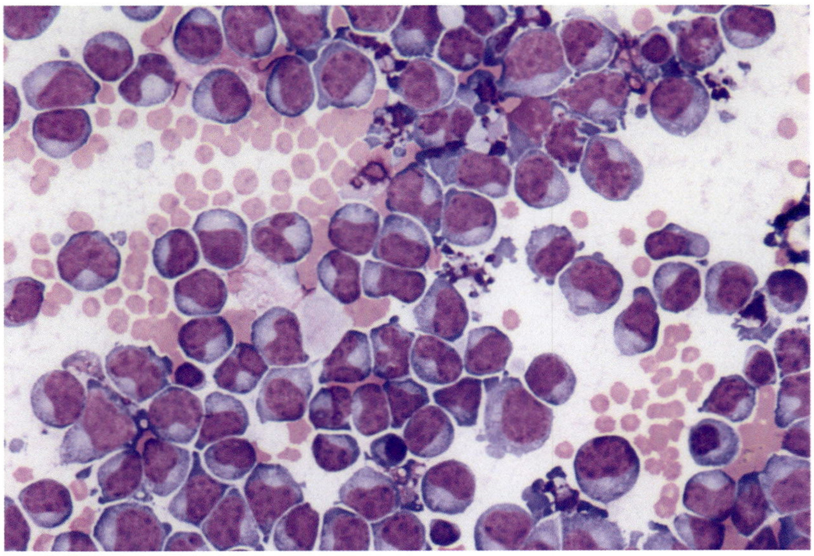

Figure 44.

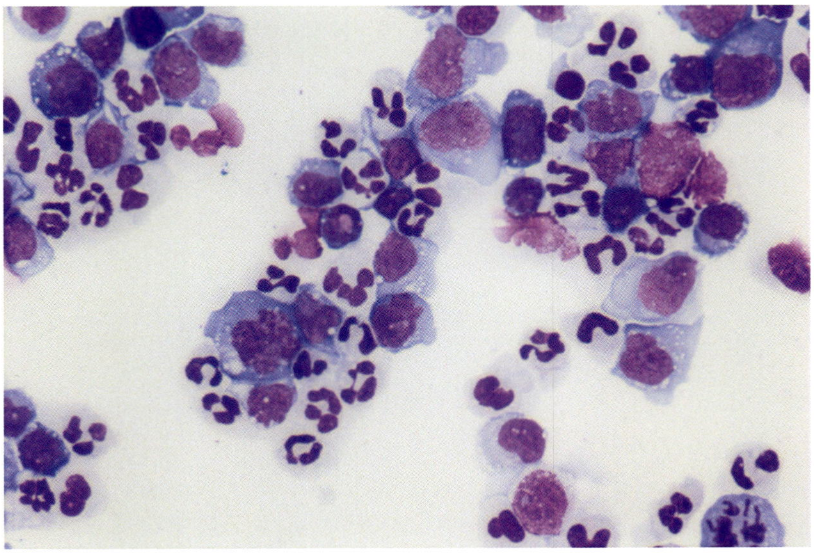

Figure 45.

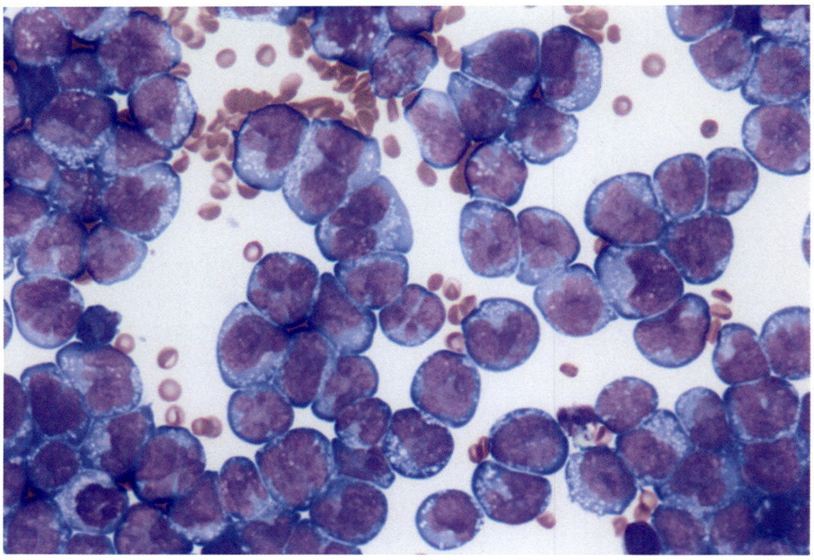

Figure 46.

Figures 47 and 48. Cerebrospinal fluid sample with mixed pleocytosis. The presence of cells that resemble lymphoblasts (arrows) does not imply a diagnosis of lymphoma.

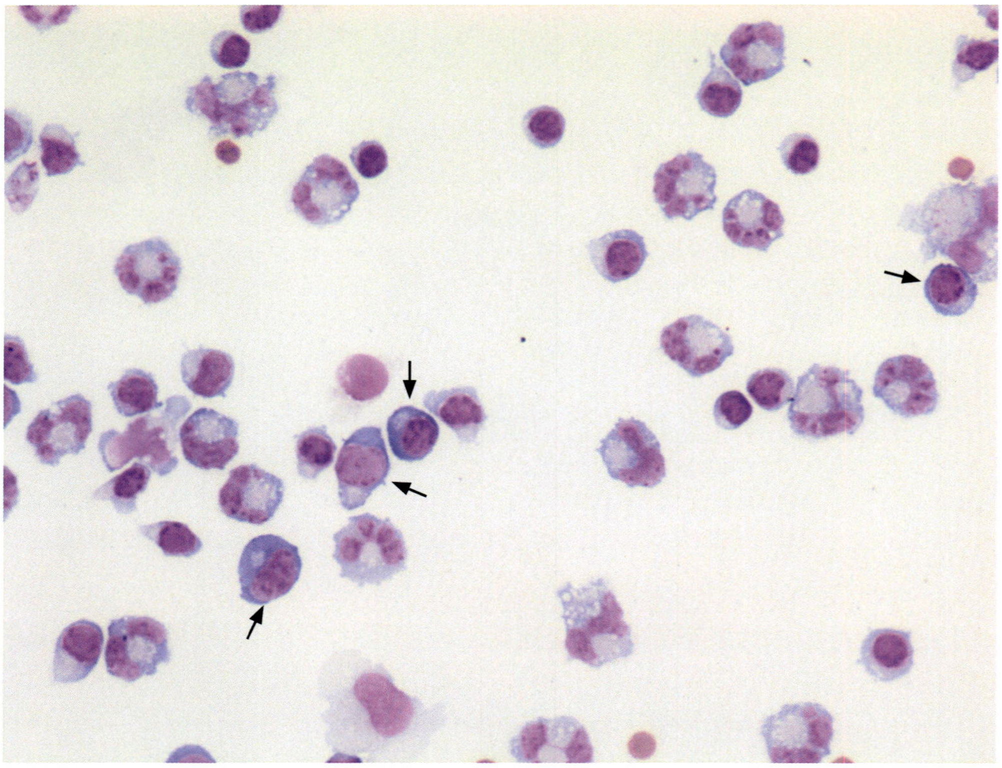

Figure 47.

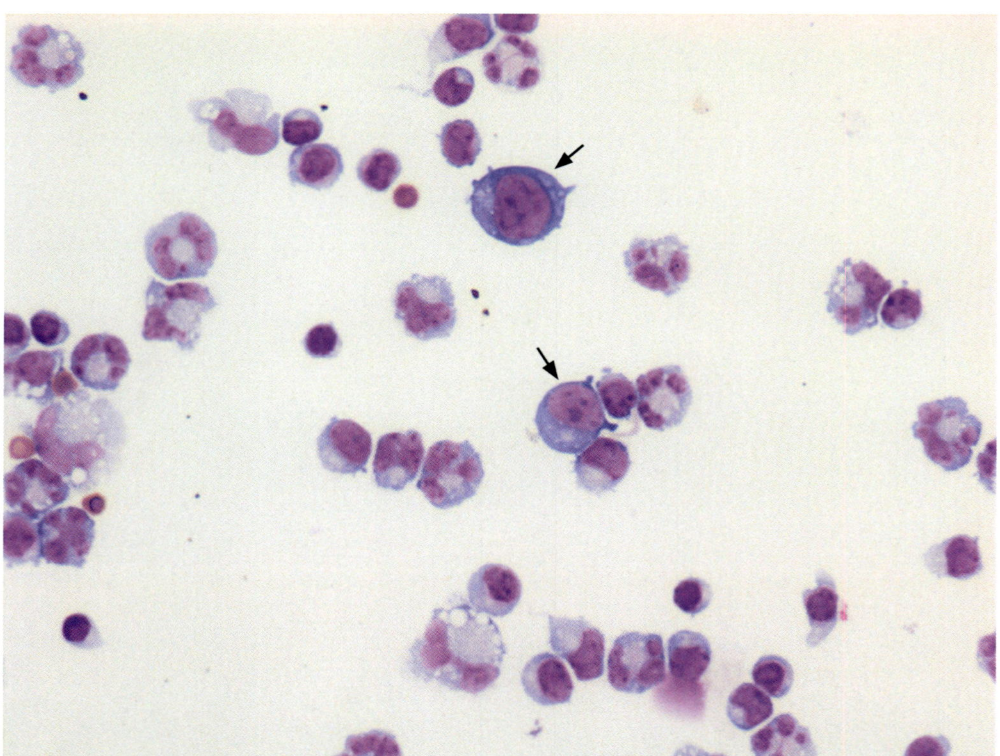

Figure 48.

# 05

# Cytology of histiocytic diseases

# Cytology of histiocytic diseases

Histiocytic diseases are common in dogs, but rare in cats. The most common forms result from neoplastic (histiocytoma and histiocytic sarcoma [HS]) or nonneoplastic (reactive histiocytosis) proliferation of histiocytes. Cytology is widely used to provide preliminary diagnostic clues or even to establish a definitive diagnosis in a significant percentage of patients with histiocytoma or HS.

Histiocytes are $CD34^+$ cells that are derived from pluripotent stem cells of the bone marrow following their differentiation into antigen-presenting cells (dendritic cells) or phagocytes (monocytes/macrophages). Because the majority of histiocytic lesions are derived from dendritic cells, a phagocytic cytological picture is uncommon.

Cytological evaluation of a histiocytic process involves two steps: first, confirming that the process originates with histiocytic cells; and second, assessing the atypia to distinguish benign histiocytoma from HS.

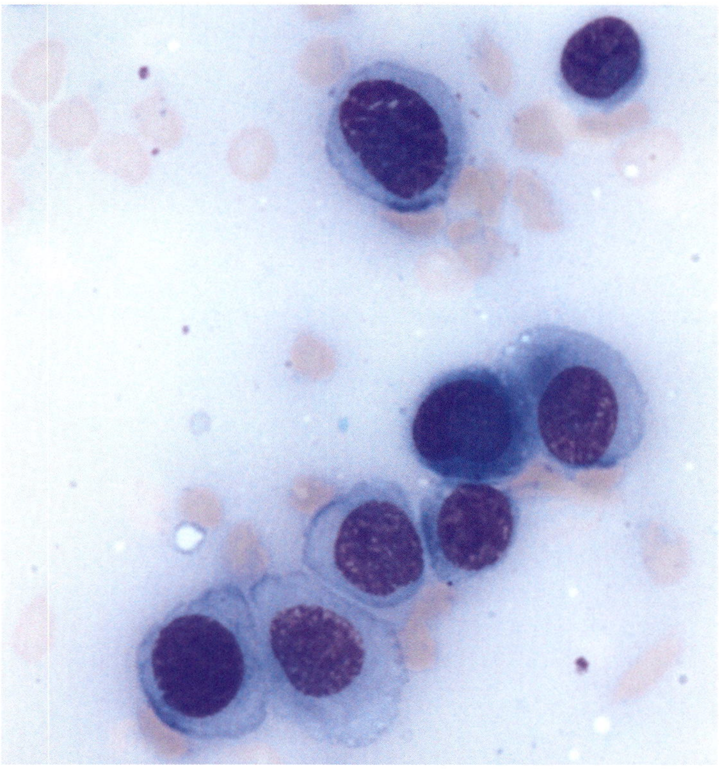

Figure 1. Group of histiocytes exhibiting characteristic morphology.

## IDENTIFICATION OF HISTIOCYTIC CELLS

Cytologically, histiocytes fall within the category of round cells. They are medium-sized (12–30 μm, larger than neutrophils) with a predominantly rounded morphology, although more irregular shapes may be observed. The nucleus, which is often eccentric, is usually rounded or oval shaped, although other morphologies (e.g. kidney shape) are common. Its chromatin pattern is uniform, without evident nucleoli. The cytoplasm is usually moderate to abundant and mildly basophilic, with no evident granules or vacuoles. Unlike most other round cells, the cytoplasmic borders are often poorly defined. Histiocytes are the round cells with the fewest distinguishing cytological features (Fig. 1).

## CYTOLOGICAL CHARACTERISTICS OF HISTIOCYTOMA

Histiocytomas are benign tumours that result from the proliferation of Langerhans cells (dendritic cells of the epidermis). Because these lesions exfoliate many cells, cytology is characterised by a high degree of cellularity, consisting almost exclusively of characteristic histiocytes. Although these are benign tumours, cytology may reveal some degree of cellular pleomorphism (always with a predominance of rounded cells) and nuclear pleomorphism (mild anisokaryosis and the presence of nuclei of varying shapes – rounded, oval, indented, or kidney-shaped). Binucleated cells can be observed. Occasionally, they contain small, poorly-defined cytoplasmic vacuoles. Mitoses are commonly observed. Phagocytic activity is absent (Figs. 2–7).

While cytology of histiocytoma is very characteristic and diagnosis is relatively simple, in some cases, especially in middle-aged patients, it may be necessary to include other round cell tumours in the differential diagnosis.

The main difference between histiocytes and the cells of transmissible venereal tumours is that the latter have homogeneously rounded nuclei, and, most importantly, contain abundant, clear, very well defined cytoplasmic vacuoles that can reach a considerable size. In histiocytes, vacuoles, if present, are usually small and poorly defined (Fig. 8).

It is very easy to distinguish histiocytes from well-differentiated mast cells, but harder to distinguish them from undifferentiated mast cells that lack granules. In these cases, the absence of indented or kidney-shaped nuclei, the presence of evident nuclear atypia, and eosinophilic infiltration (if present) are the main differential criteria (Fig. 9).

The morphology of histiocytes differs to that of mature plasma cells. However, differentiation may not be so marked in plasma cell tumours (Fig. 10).

### Cutaneous lymphoma is the round cell tumour most often confused with histiocytoma.

It is not difficult to distinguish one from the other if the lymphoma cells are typical lymphoblasts. However, occasionally lymphomas can arise from cells that are morphologically very similar to histiocytes, with much more subtle differences (few kidney-shaped nuclei, less cytoplasm, absence of binucleated cells), making it more difficult to establish a clear cytological distinction (Figs. 11–13). In these cases, histology or immunohistochemistry may be required to complete the differential diagnosis.

In histiocytomas in the progression phase, the presence of other cell types is very uncommon. This feature facilitates differentiation of histiocytomas and inflammatory processes (pyogranulomas or granulomas). However, in tumours in the regression phase an increase in the number of mature lymphocytes is observed. Occasionally, activated lymphocytes/lymphoblasts, macrophages, and plasma cells are also observed. It may be necessary to distinguish between this tumour type and reactive histiocytosis, inflammatory lesions, and even lymphoma (Figs. 14 and 15).

Normally, histiocytomas are benign and solitary lesions. "Langerhans cell histiocytosis of skin" has been described in dogs, and is characterised by the presence of multiple lesions. Despite its benign nature, in some cases dissemination to regional lymph nodes can occur. The cells resemble those of solitary histiocytomas, although increased anisokaryosis and a greater abundance of multinucleated cells may be observed. The main entity included in the differential diagnosis is HS, especially if the regional lymph node is affected, but marked cellular and nuclear atypia is absent (Fig. 16).

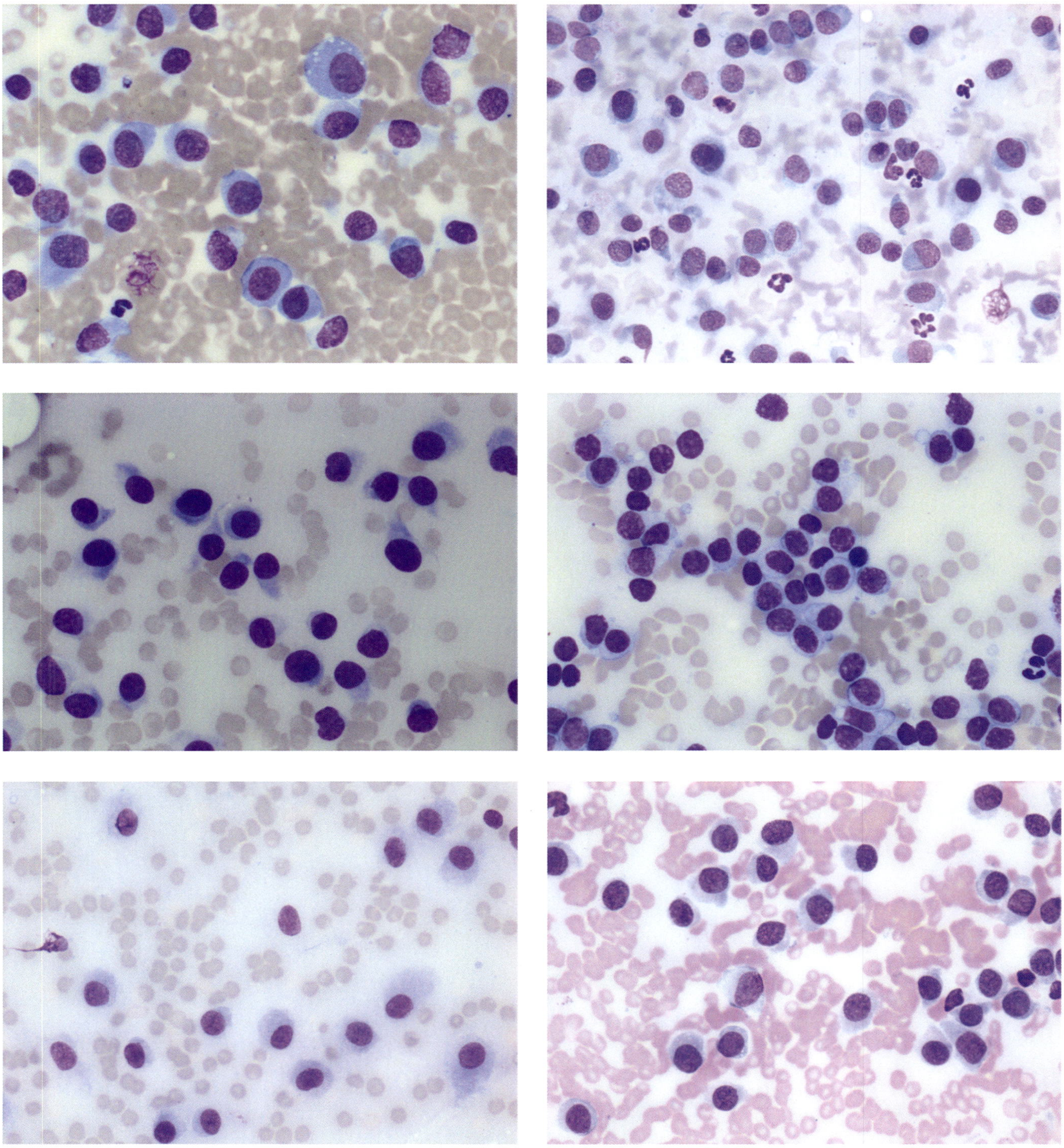

Figures 2–7. Cytological picture of canine cutaneous histiocytoma. Although there is evident variation in the size and shape of the nuclei, all of these images correspond to benign lesions in young dogs.

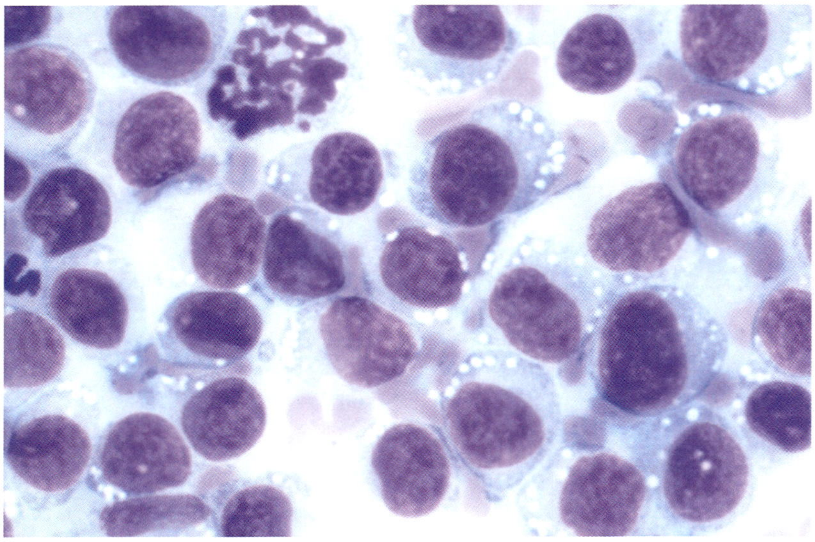

Figure 8. Transmissible venereal tumour. Although in this image the nuclei are not as round as usual, the type and number of cytoplasmic vacuoles enable differentiation from histiocytoma.

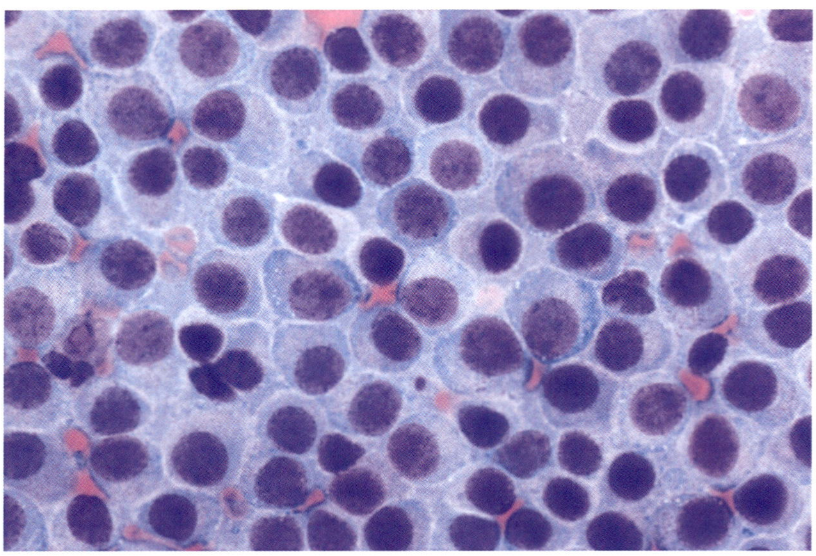

Figure 9. Undifferentiated mast cell tumour. Owing to the almost complete absence of cytoplasmic granules, the mast cells closely resemble histiocytes. The fact that the nuclei are very round can facilitate differentiation.

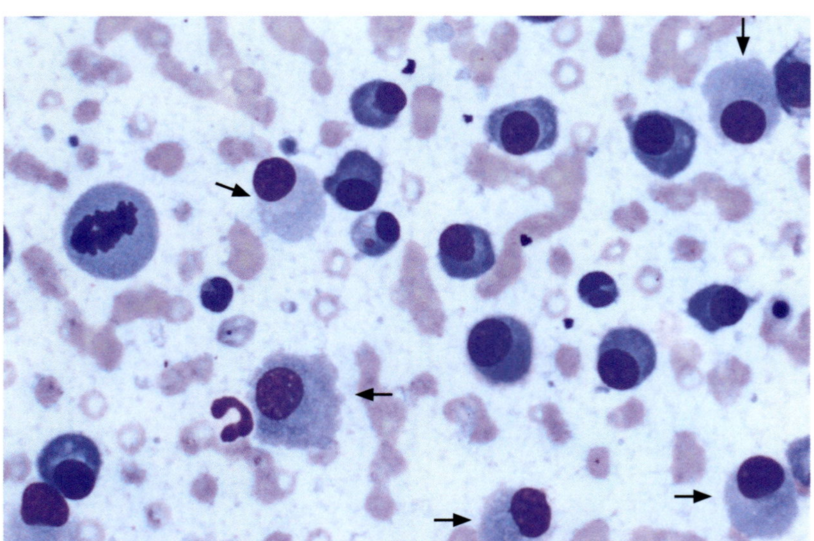

Figure 10. Plasmacytoma. The cells are small and oval, with an intensely basophilic cytoplasm. The most immature cells (arrows) could be confused with histiocytes.

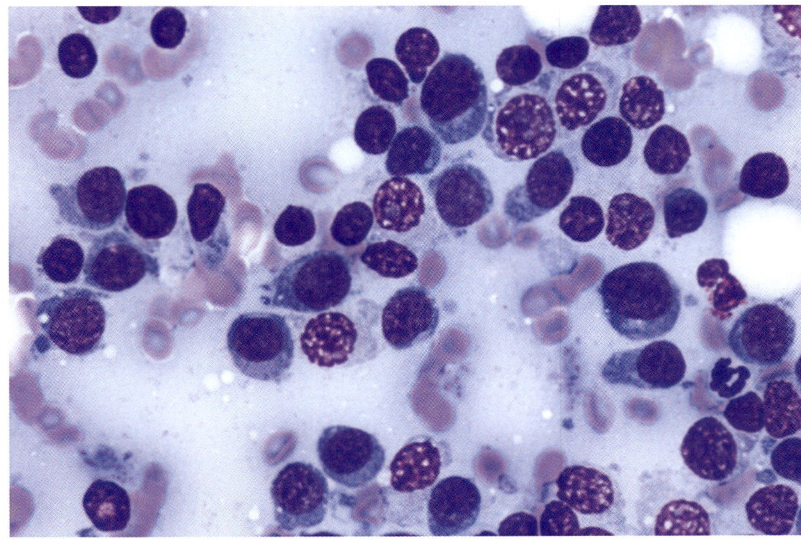

Figure 11. Cutaneous lymphoma. The cells do not exhibit the typical lymphoblast morphology. Histology was required to differentiate this lymphoma from a histiocytoma.

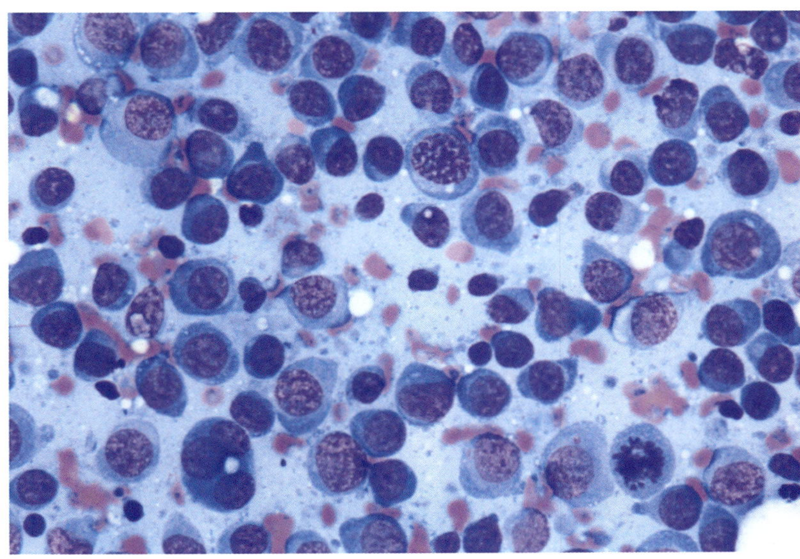

Figure 12. Lymph node cytology. Ambiguous cytological picture showing signs of both lymphoma and metastasis of histiocytic disease. In general, the cell morphology is more compatible with histiocytes than with lymphoblasts. The presence of a trinucleated cell is highly suggestive of histiocytic disease.

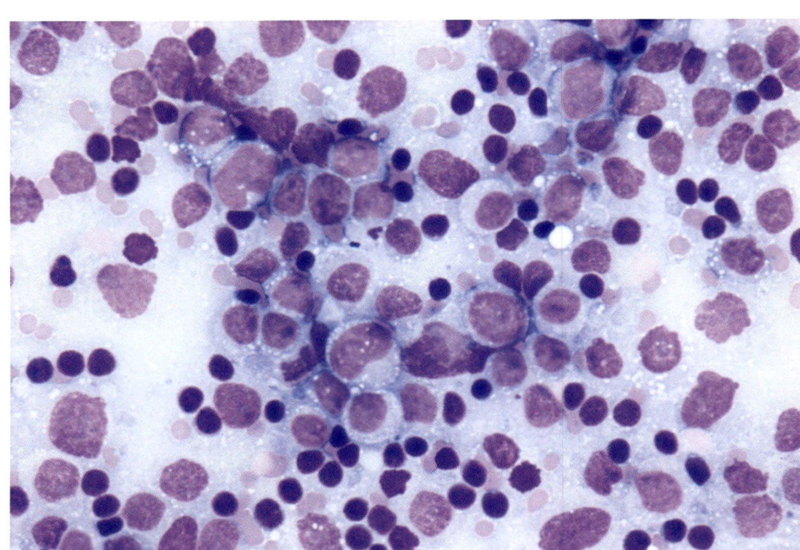

Figure 13. Lymph node cytology (cat). There are abundant mature lymphocytes and a population of cells with histiocytic morphology. However, a diagnosis of lymphoma was established based on histology and immunohistochemistry.

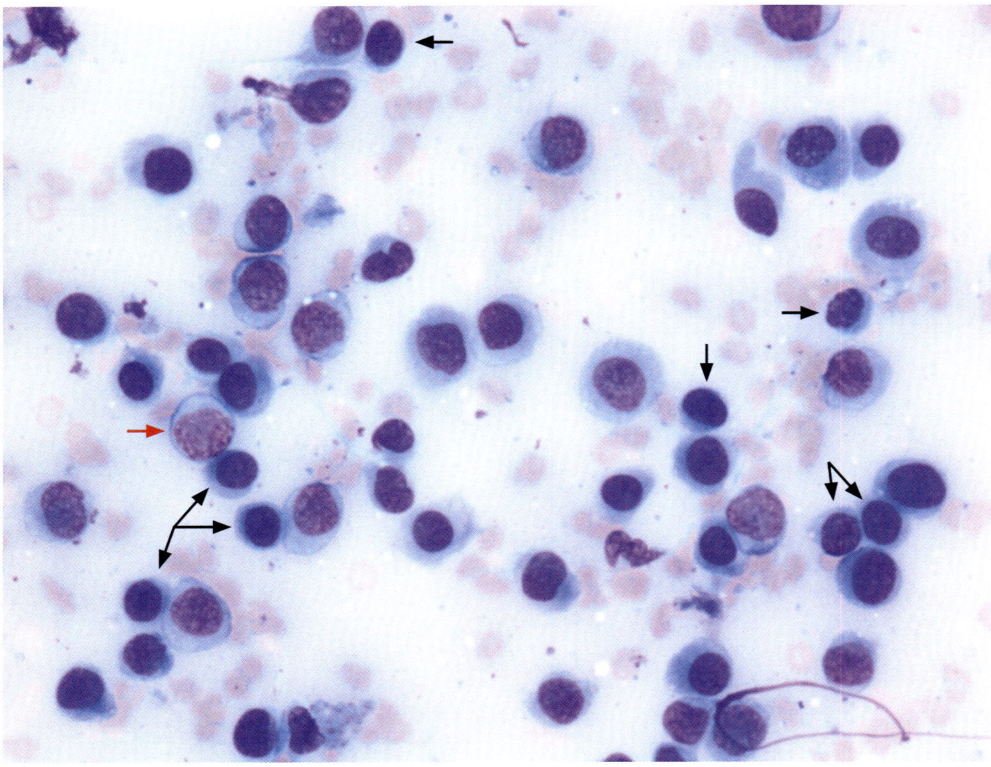

Figures 14 and 15. Histiocytomas in regression. In addition to histiocytes, there are abundant lymphocytes (mostly mature or reactive, indicated with black arrows, and some lymphoblasts, indicated with a red arrow).

Figure 14.

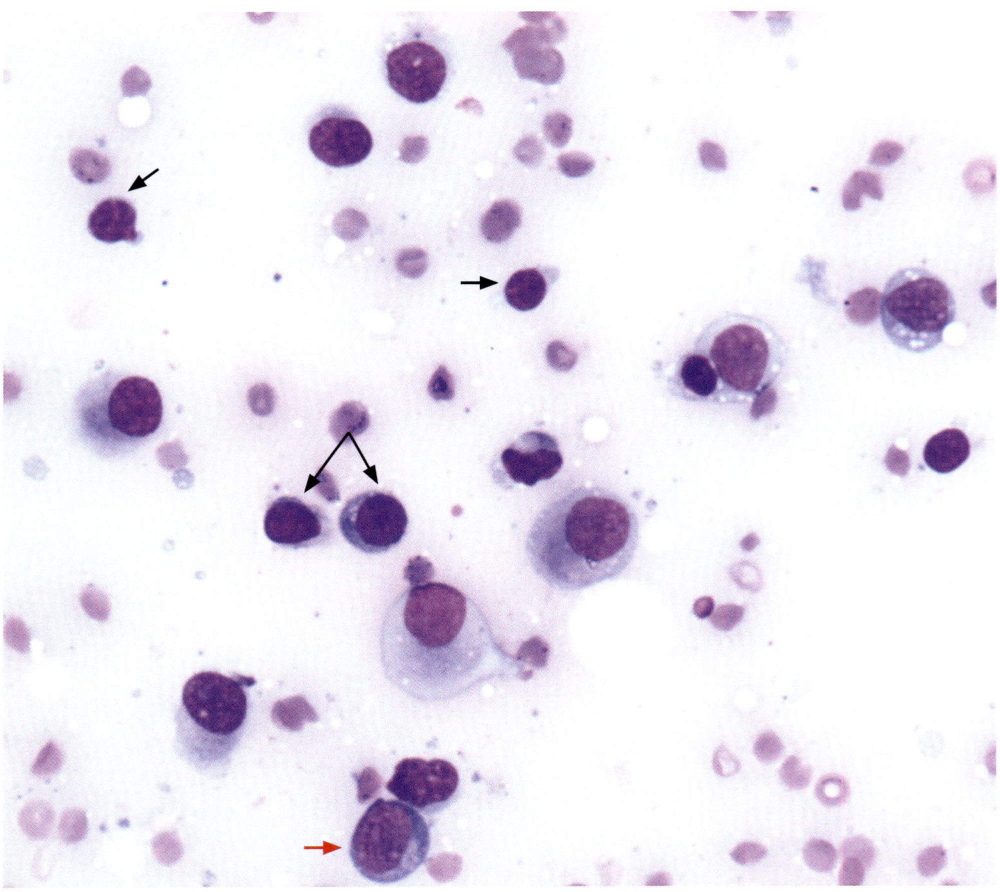

Figure 15.

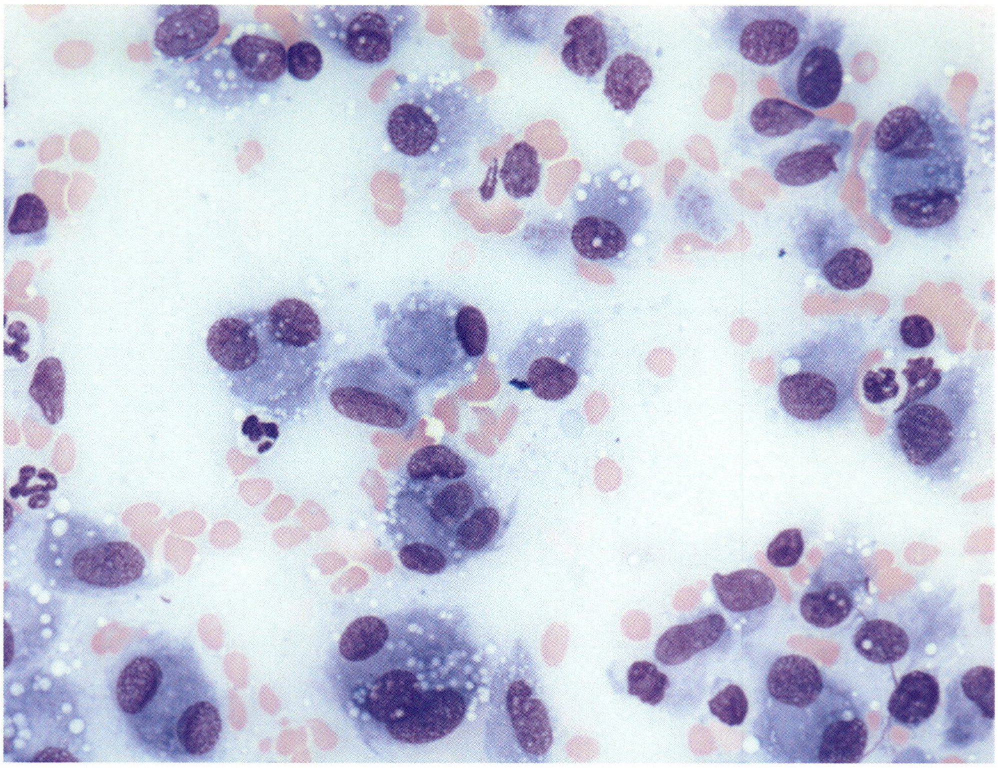

Figure 16. Langerhans cell histiocytosis of skin. Cytologically, the image is ambiguous. It does not resemble the cytological picture typical of solitary cutaneous histiocytoma, but the degree of atypia is not sufficient to consider histiocytic sarcoma.

## CYTOLOGICAL CHARACTERISTICS OF HISTIOCYTIC SARCOMA

Despite its denomination (sarcoma), HS (formerly known as malignant histiocytosis) is a malignant neoplasm of histiocytic cells.

Most cases are derived from dendritic cells. Regardless of its origin (cutaneous or affecting different organs, including the lymph nodes, spleen, liver, lung, nervous system, bone marrow, and joints), the cytological findings are similar and highly characteristic. The large cells are very pleomorphic, with abundant granular cytoplasm, which is usually vacuolated. Although rounded cells predominate, fusiform cells may also be present. The cytological picture clearly indicates malignancy, as evidenced by marked nuclear atypia, including anisokaryosis with the presence of giant nuclei; numerous multinucleated cells with intracellular anisokaryosis; irregular nuclear forms (lobulated morphology in some cases); and very prominent and atypical nucleoli and a condensed chromatin pattern. Atypical mitoses are very common (Figs. 17–26).

The high proportion of multinucleated giant cells can confer an appearance similar to that of giant cell sarcoma. The differential diagnosis should also include highly undifferentiated mast cell tumours (the main differential criterion is the degree of nuclear pleomorphism, and in mast cell tumours rounded nuclei predominate) (Fig. 27) and amelanotic melanoma.

Haemophagocytic HS is the only histiocytic tumour derived from macrophages. It is characterised by the presence of erythrophagocytosis in addition to the characteristic cytological findings of HS (although the cell morphology does not correspond to activated macrophages). Although less frequent, leukophagocytosis may also be observed (Figs. 28 and 29).

Figures 17–24. Images of histiocytic sarcoma in samples of skin (17, 18), lymph node (19), spleen (20), lung (21), and liver (22–24), with very atypical histiocytes and numerous giant and multinucleated cells.

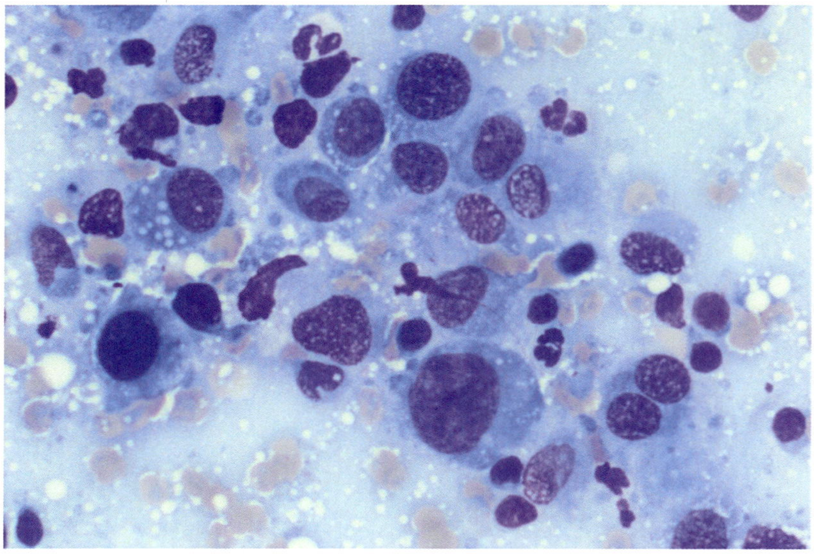

Figure 17.

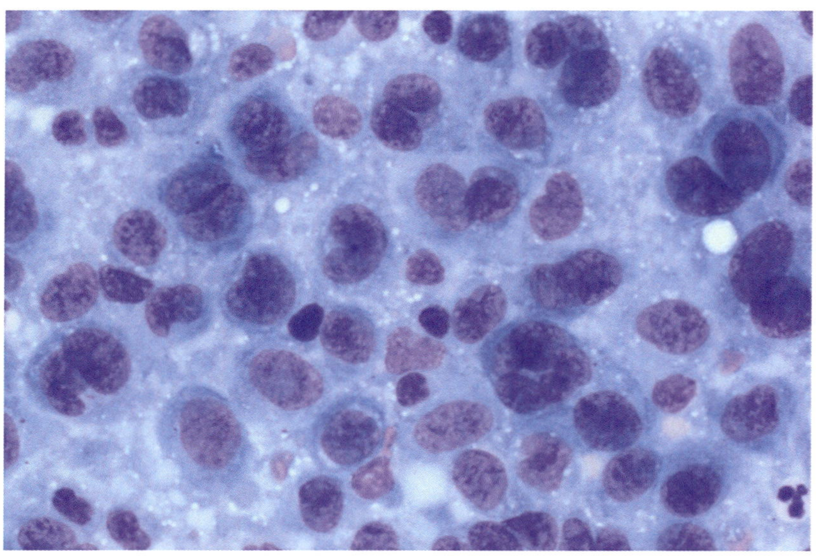

Figure 18.

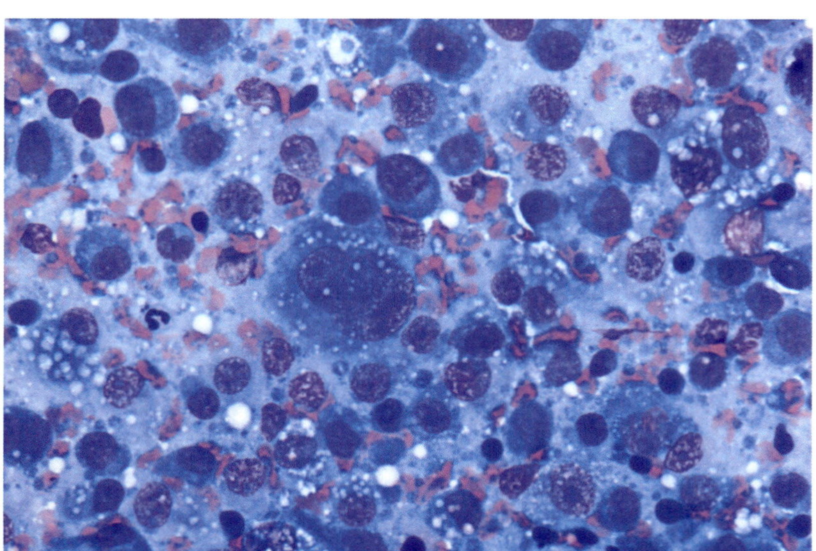

Figure 19.

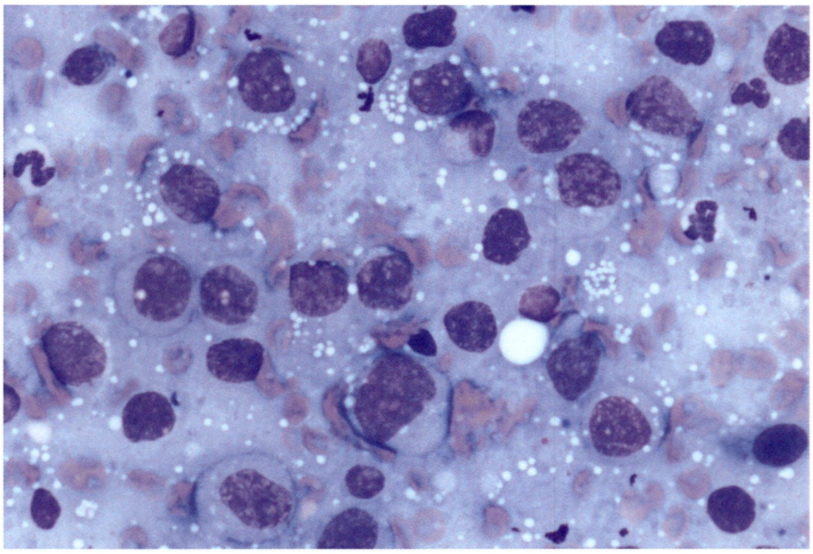

Figure 20.

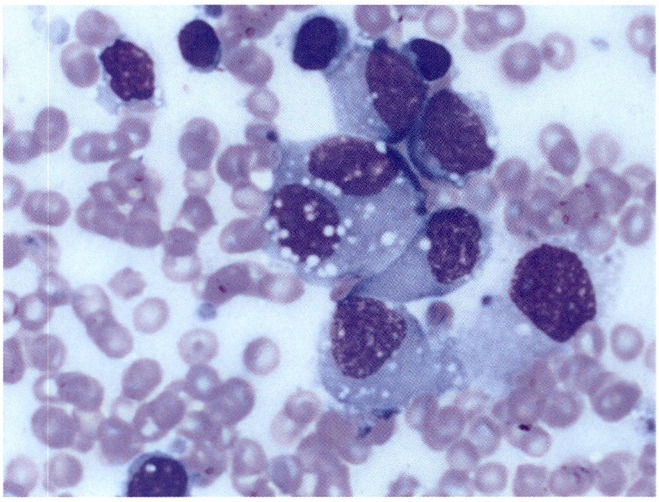

Figure 21.

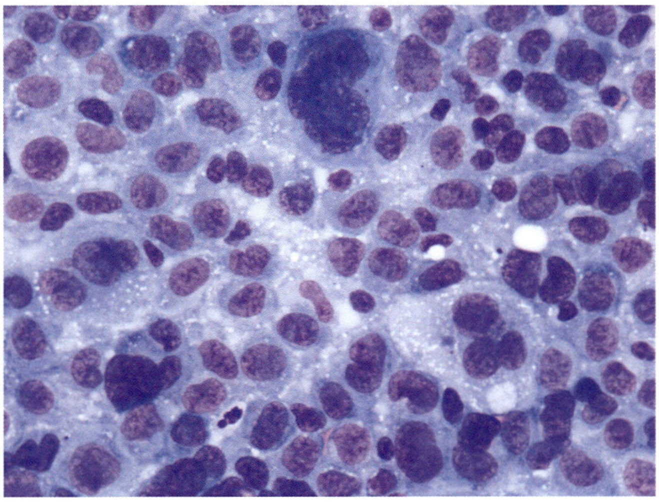

Figure 22.

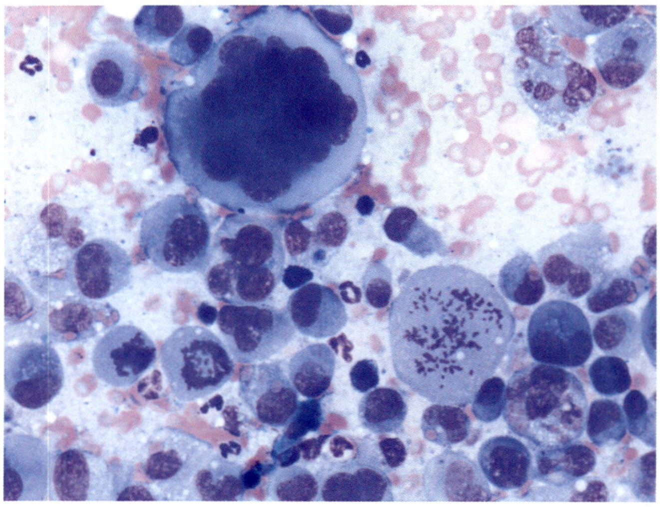

Figure 23.

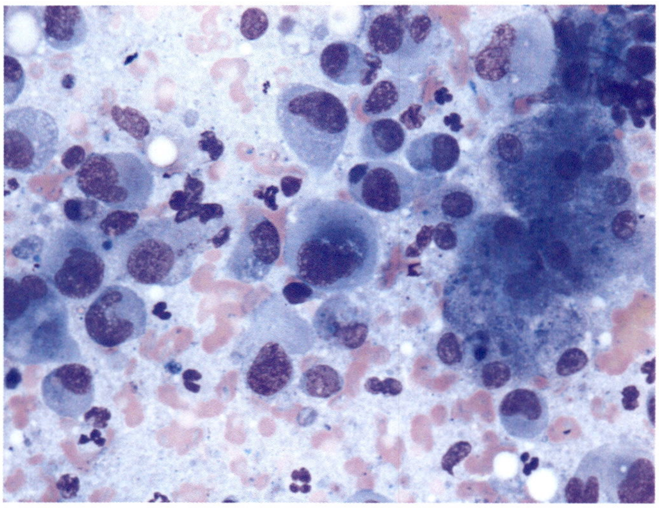

Figure 24.

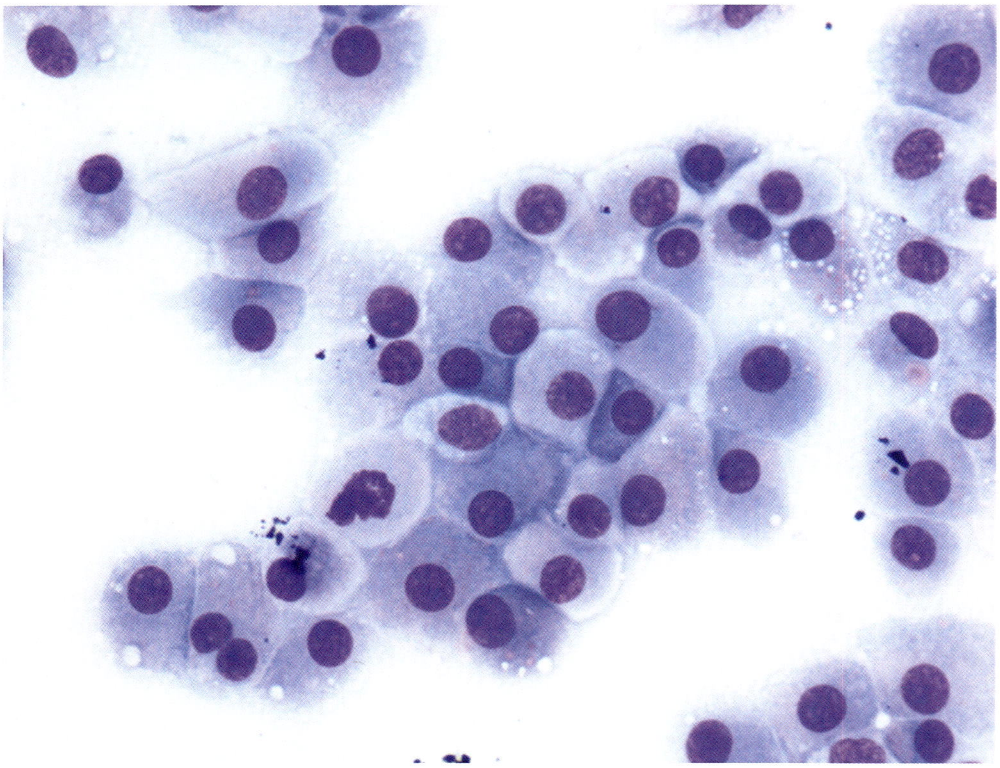

Figure 25. Histiocytic sarcoma (HS) of the skin. This cytological picture is very unusual. The cells appear more polygonal than rounded and the nuclei do not exhibit marked atypia. The cytological diagnosis was malignant tumour of indeterminate origin. A diagnosis of HS was established based on histology and immunohistochemistry findings.

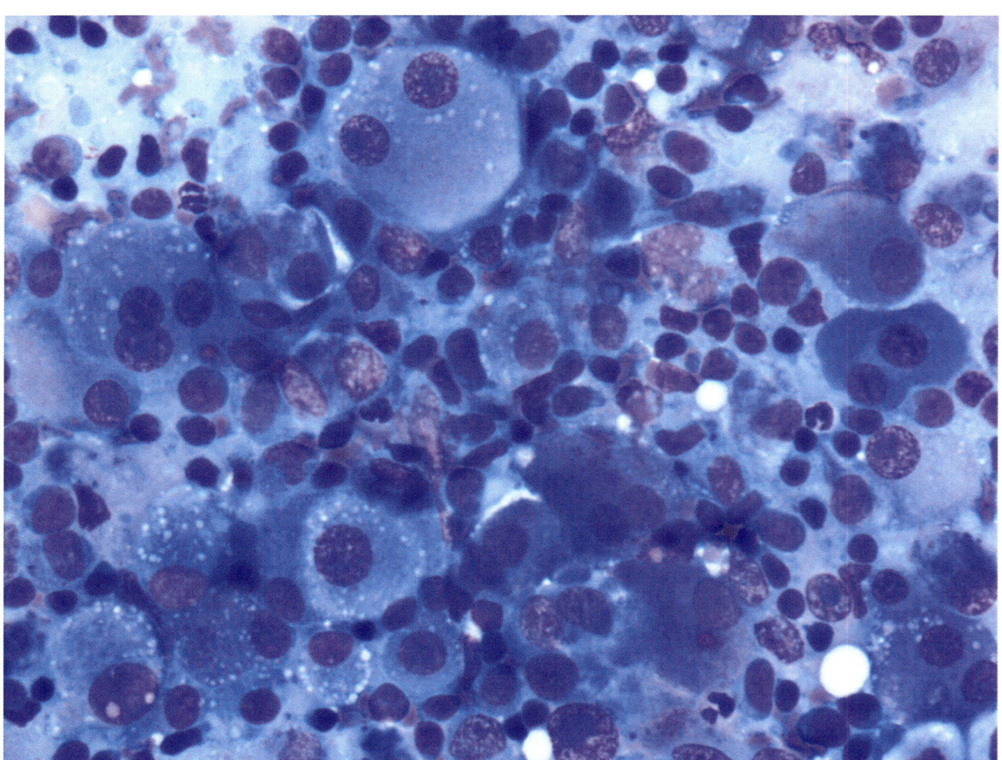

Figure 26. Lymph node metastasis of histiocytic sarcoma (same case as shown in Figure 25). The cell morphology is more characteristic than that of the primary tumour.

Figure 27. Cutaneous sample obtained from a Shar Pei patient with a history of undifferentiated mast cell tumour. The cytological diagnosis was an undifferentiated round cell tumour. The liver samples (Figs. 23 and 24) clearly indicate its histiocytic origin.

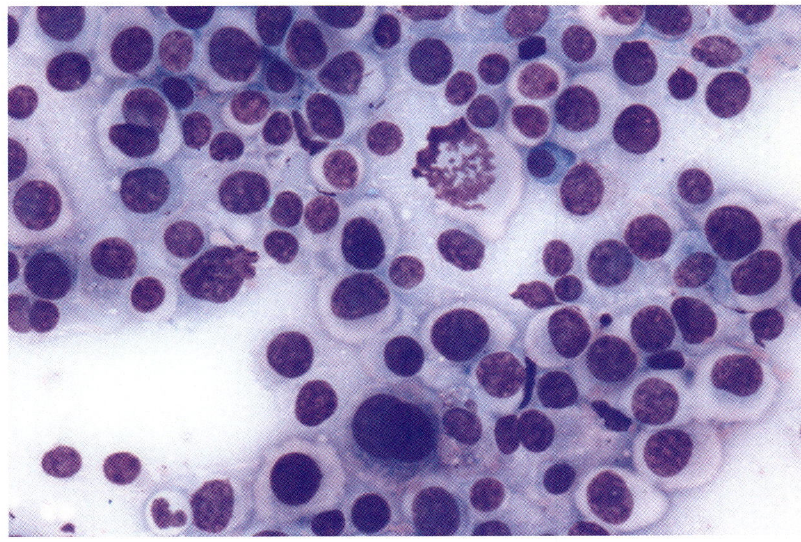

Figures 28 and 29. Haemophagocytic histiocytic sarcoma. Two fields of a liver cytology preparation showing malignant histiocytes and erythrophagocytosis (arrow in Figure 29 indicates a hepatocyte).

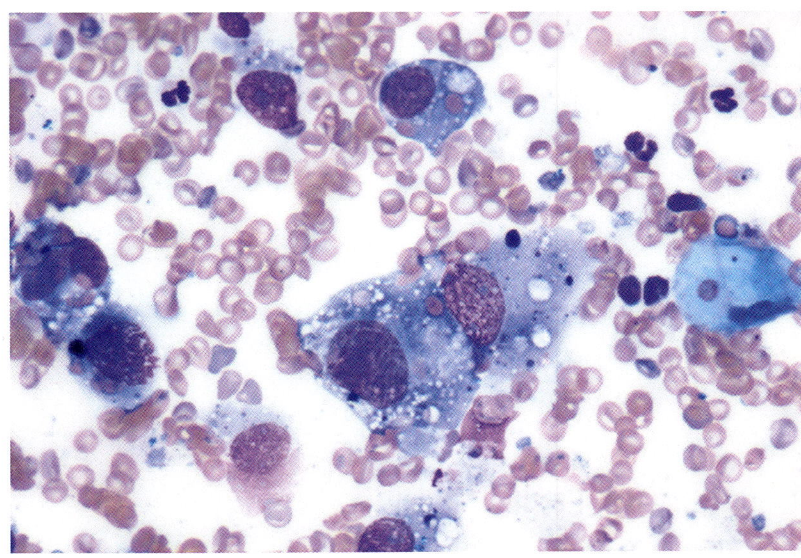

Figure 28.

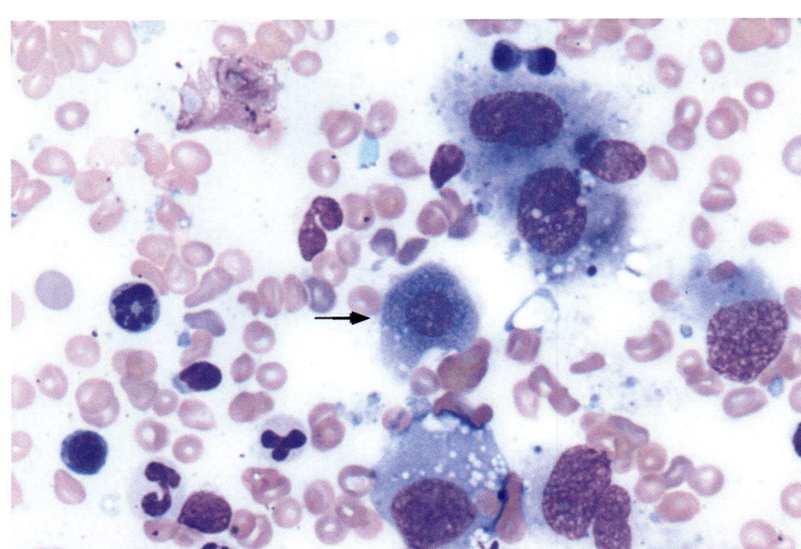

Figure 29.

## CANINE REACTIVE HISTIOCYTOSIS/FELINE PROGRESSIVE HISTIOCYTOSIS

Histiocytosis is caused by dysregulation of the immune system, and is therefore an immune-mediated process. In most cases, cytology is nonspecific or ambiguous, and is therefore not considered appropriate for the diagnosis of these processes.

Unlike histiocytoma, it is uncommon to only observe histiocytes in cases of reactive histiocytosis, since polymorphic lymphocytes can account for 50 % of the total cell population. A small percentage of nondegenerate neutrophils and occasional macrophages may also be observed. The mixture of cells may be mistaken for granulomatous or pyogranulomatous inflammatory reactions. The main difference is that in histiocytosis most cells are dendritic, and therefore do not evolve into macrophages. Consequently, neither giant multinucleated macrophage cells nor signs of phagocytosis are usually observed (Fig. 30).

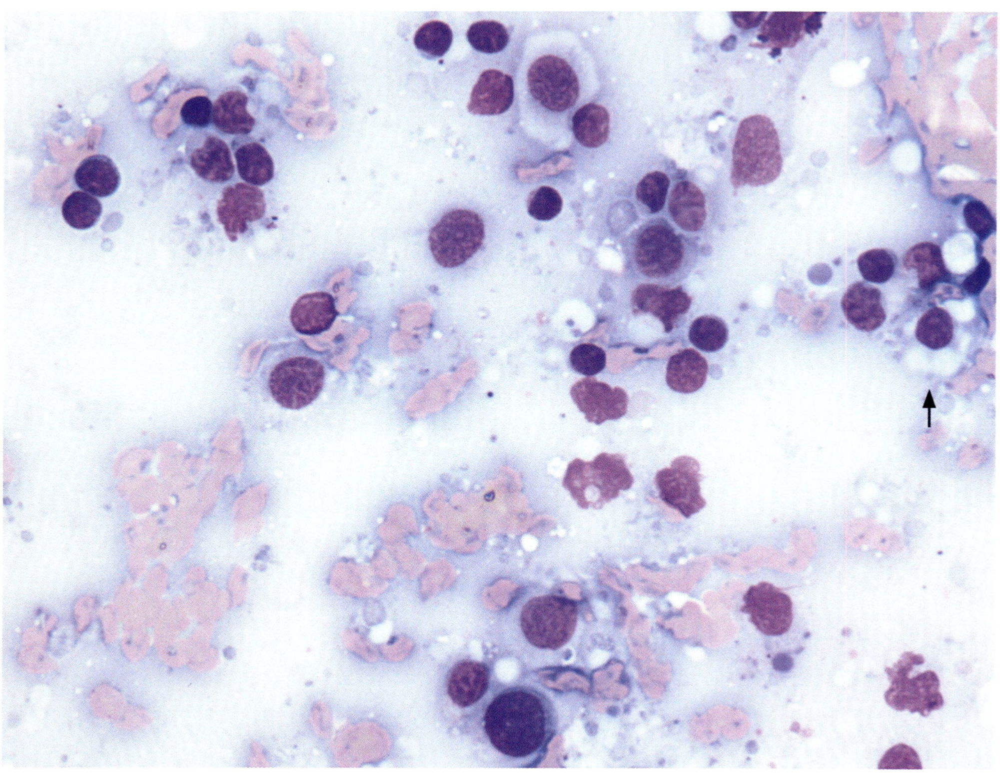

Figure 30. Cytology with abundant lymphoid cells, fewer histiocytes, and a macrophage (arrow). This cell mixture is compatible with reactive histiocytosis (unconfirmed diagnosis).

# 06

# Cytology of sarcoma

# Cytology of sarcoma

Sarcomas are malignant tumours of mesenchymal origin and can develop from different conjunctive structures, including fibrous, nervous, myxoid, adipose, muscle, bone, and endothelial tissue. Owing to the wide distribution of these tissues in the body, sarcomas are very common tumours in both dogs and cats.

Cytology is a common first-line approach for the diagnosis of sarcoma, but is not without diagnostic limitations, mainly due to the difficulty in determining the specific tissue of origin or the histological grade of malignancy. Published studies have shown that cytology offers high sensitivity, specificity, and diagnostic accuracy for the determination of malignancy (84 %, 98 %, and 93 %, respectively), but that these values decrease when histological type is also evaluated (77 %, 98 %, and 89 %, respectively).[3,11]

Despite these limitations, evaluation of good quality cytological preparations provides useful information for prognosis and treatment. This evaluation involves the following steps:

1. Identification of the cell lineage.
2. Estimation of the degree of malignancy.
3. Identification of any specific characteristics that would allow determination of cellular origin.

## IDENTIFICATION OF THE CELL LINEAGE

The mesenchymal lineage is characterised by exfoliation of few individual cells that tend to be fusiform, with poorly-defined cytoplasmic borders and rounded or oval nuclei (Fig. 1). The more differentiated the sarcoma is, the closer it approaches these characteristics, but as the degree of undifferentiation progresses the cells become more atypical (Fig. 2). In the case of anaplasia, it can be difficult to identify the lineage and only a diagnosis of "malignant tumour of indeterminate lineage" can be reached.

When conducting a cytological analysis of lesions in internal organs, normal stromal cells or cells indicative of fibrosis should not be mistaken for metastatic sarcoma cells. The former are usually scarce (or absent), and exhibit no atypia (Fig. 3).

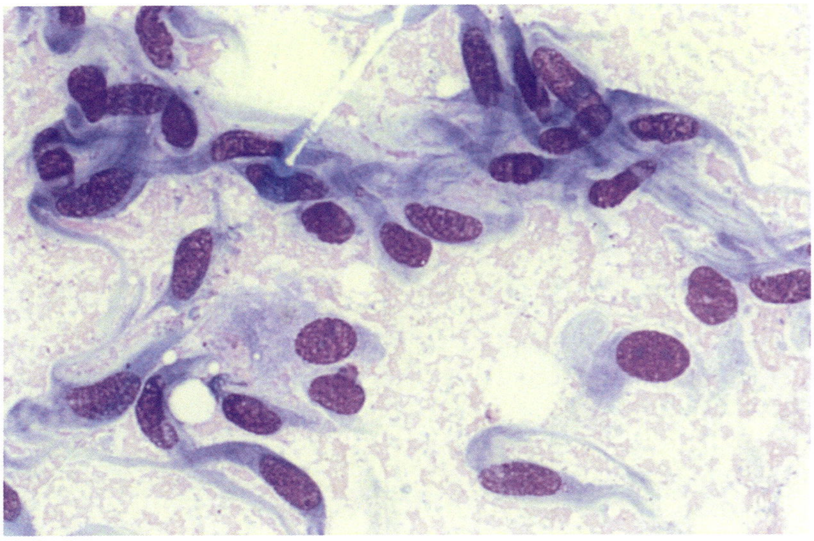

Figure 1. Conjunctive cells displaying typical characteristics.

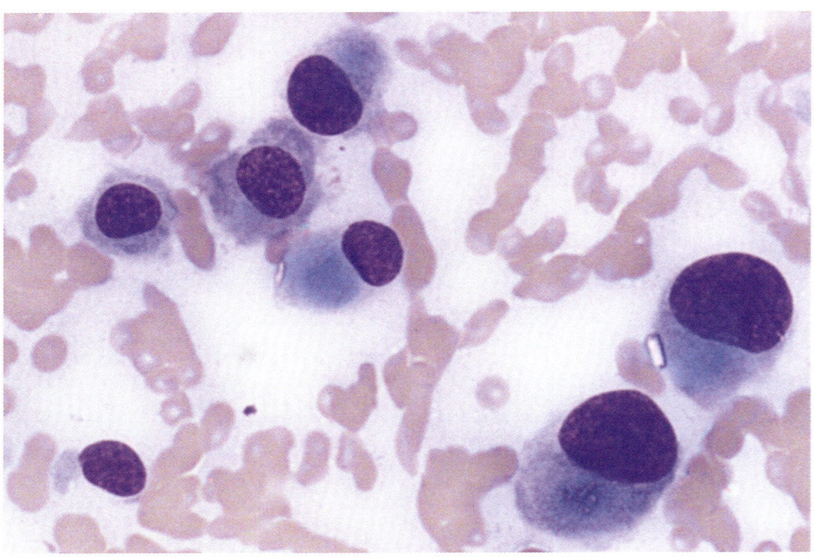

Figure 2. Undifferentiated sarcoma. The cells do not exhibit the morphology typical of conjunctive cells.

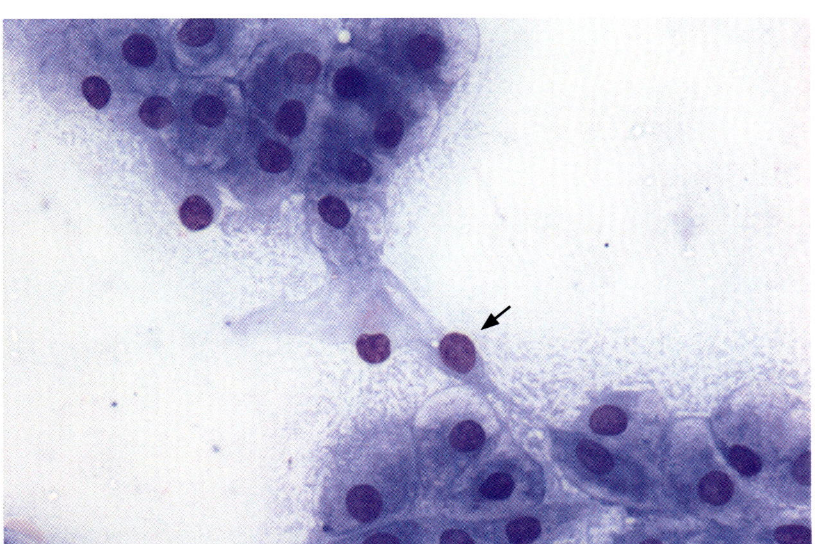

Figure 3. Liver cytology. Non-neoplastic conjunctive cells of stromal origin (arrow) are observed among the hepatocytes.

# ESTIMATION OF THE DEGREE OF MALIGNANCY

If the sample is of sufficient cellularity, it may be possible to estimate the degree of malignancy. However, although an approximation can be made based on the cytological picture, only histopathological evaluation can determine the definitive histological grade.

## LOW-GRADE SARCOMA

Cytology of low-grade sarcoma usually reveals a high degree of cellularity. It is easy to identify the conjunctive origin since fusiform cells predominate, although some pleomorphism is evident.

It is common to observe cellular accumulations, which form as a consequence of high cellularity or cell distribution within the tumour. If these accumulations are abundant, the sample may appear epithelial at low magnifications (Figs. 4 and 5). The cells of the accumulations may be interlaced with a pink extracellular matrix of collagen (Fig. 6).

The key to identifying low-grade sarcoma lies in the evaluation of the cytological characteristics of malignancy. It is possible that no more than three nuclear criteria of malignancy are fulfilled, in which case the lesion is identified as a conjunctive lesion of doubtful malignancy. In most cases, the minimum number of nuclear atypia indicative of malignancy is present, but the atypia is either mild or does not affect a large proportion of cells.

Mitoses are scarce, or absent.

The cytological picture suggests benignity: cells similar to one other, with no evident nuclear atypia, mild anisokaryosis, occasional nucleoli, condensed chromatin (but homogeneous throughout the population), and occasional binucleated or multinucleated cells (Figs. 7–12).

Due to the scarcity of malignant characteristics, the main differential diagnoses are benign lesions.

Cytological preparations of hyperplasia/mesenchymal proliferations or benign tumours are usually of low cellularity, although a poorly exfoliative sarcoma can never be ruled out (Fig. 13).

In an inflammatory context, the tissue cells can be activated and acquire evident atypia. Generally, in cases of low-grade sarcoma no significant inflammatory component is observed. Therefore, if inflammatory cells predominate, the activation of the conjunctive cells is most likely due to dysplasia (Fig. 14). However, the diagnostic accuracy is reduced in this scenario.

Figures 4 and 5. Cell accumulations in a low-grade sarcoma. At low magnification this tumour can be mistaken for an epithelial tumour. At higher magnifications, the characteristics of the conjunctive cells can be distinguished.

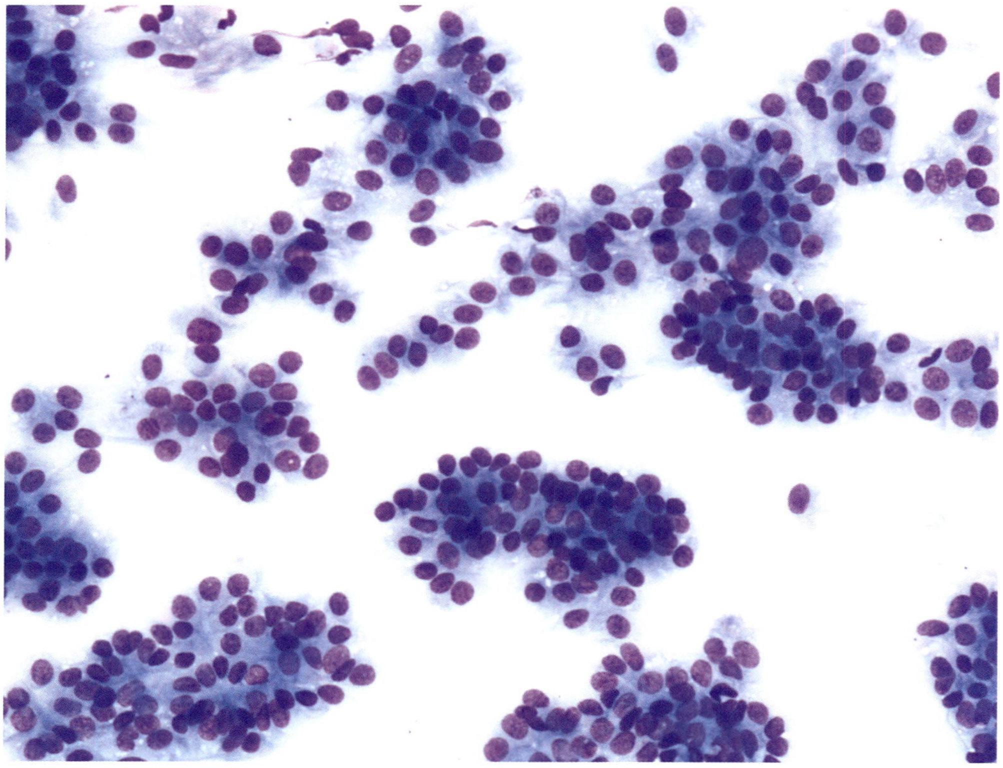

Figure 4.

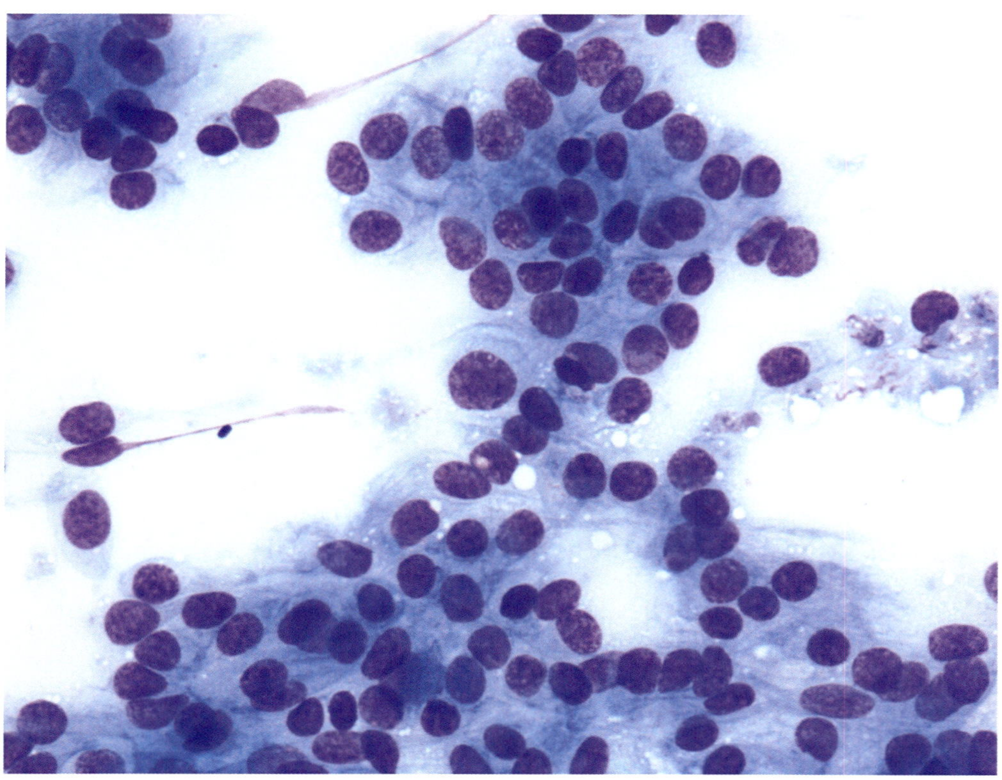

Figure 5.

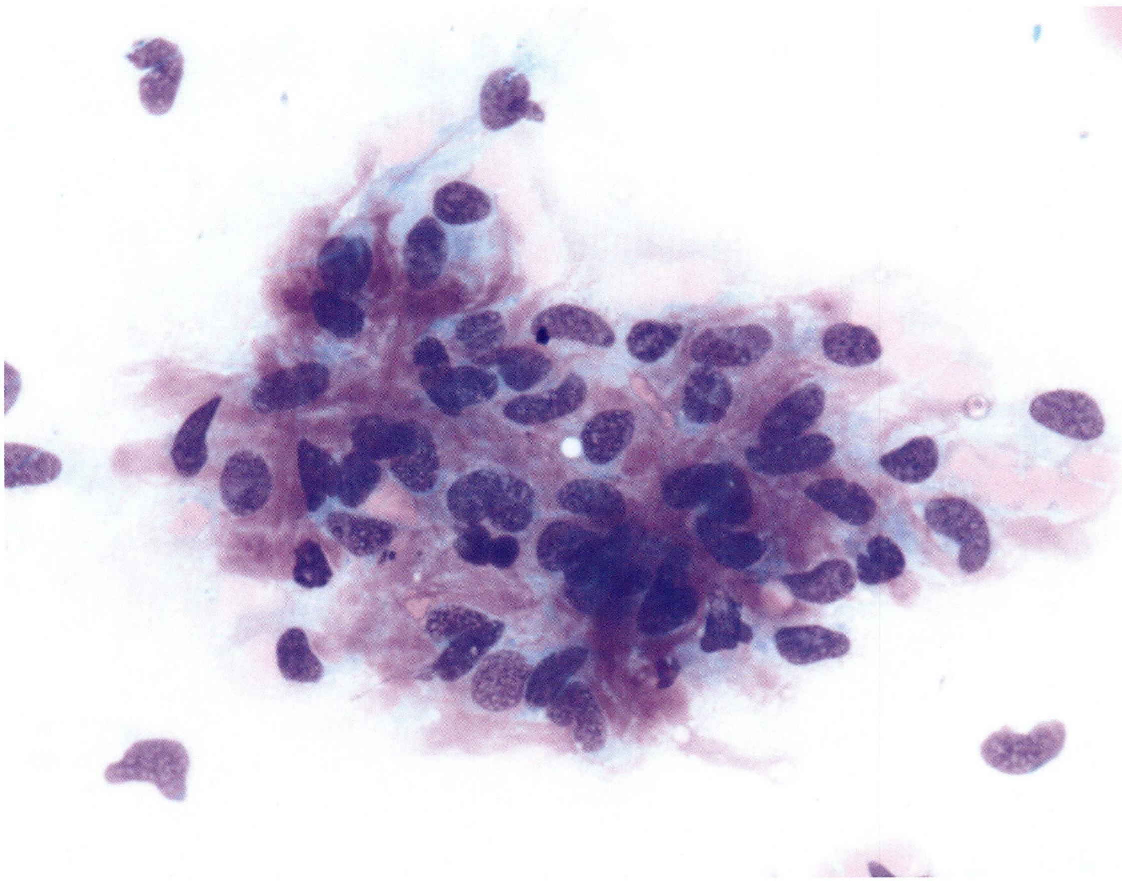

Figure 6. Low-grade sarcoma cells within a collagen matrix.

Figures 7–12. Images of low-grade sarcomas in which little or no relevant nuclear atypia is observed.

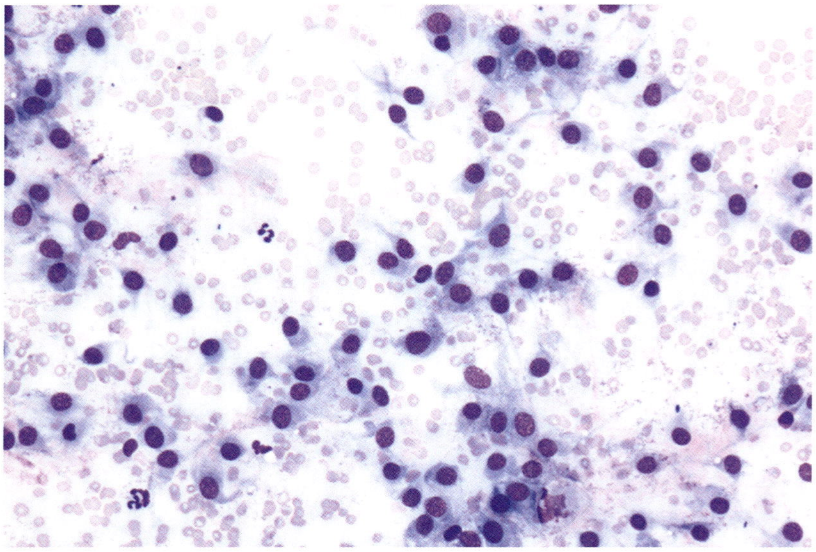

Figure 7.

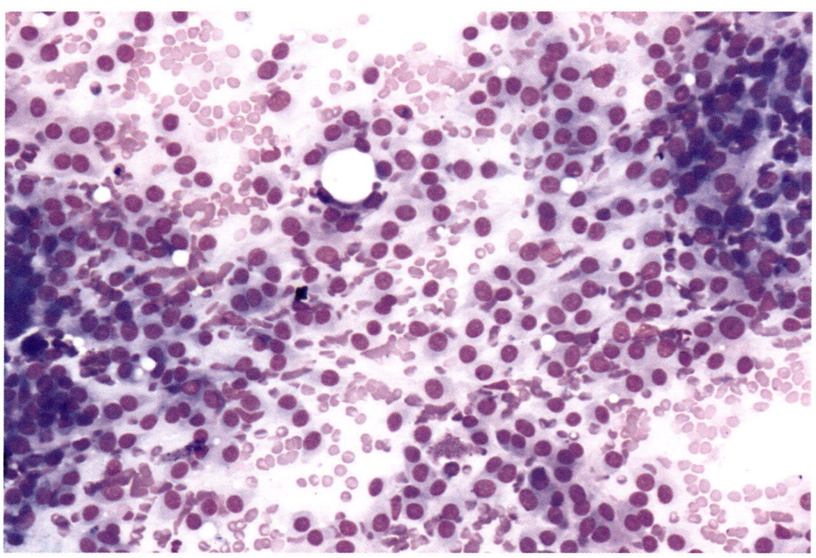

Figure 8.

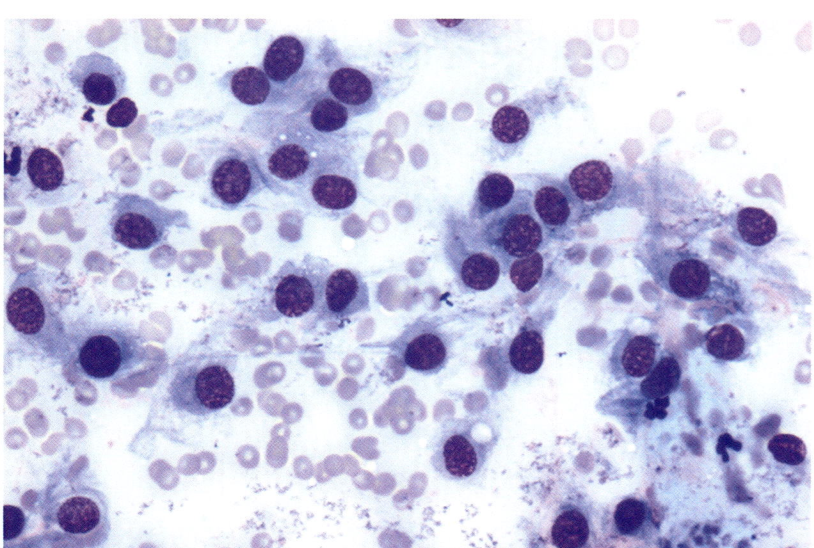

Figure 9.

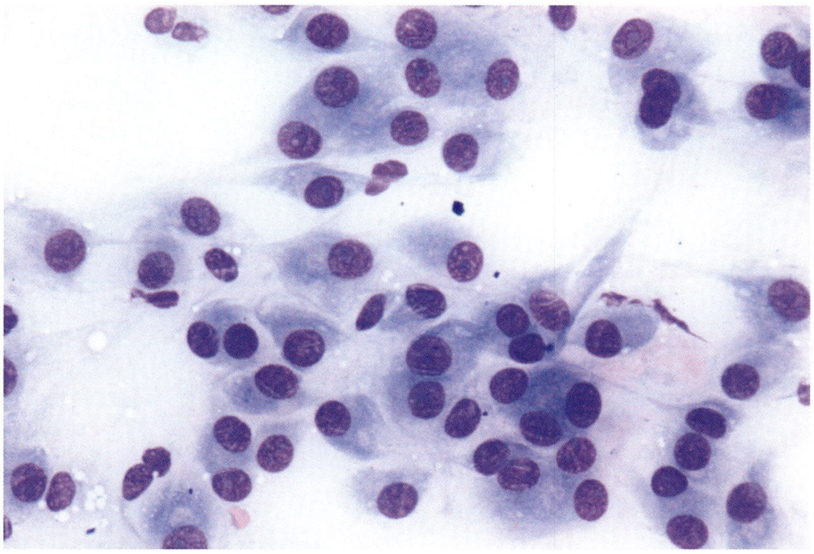

Figure 10.

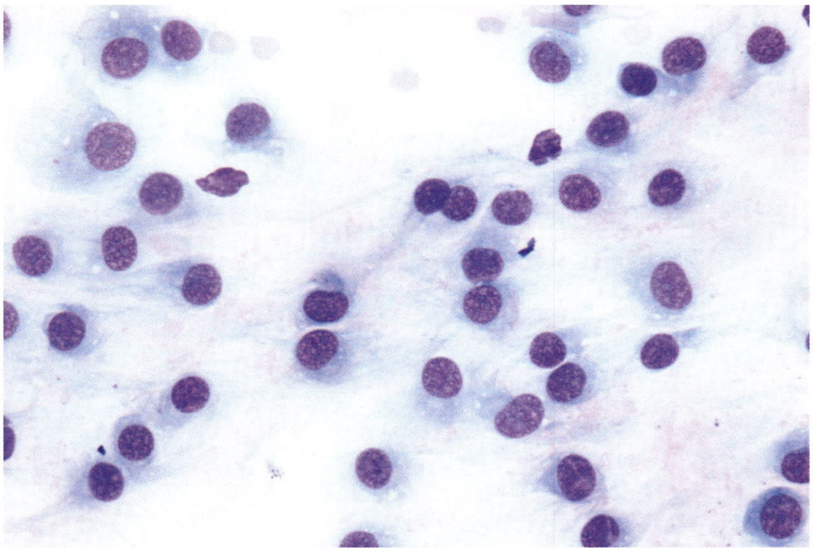

Figure 11.

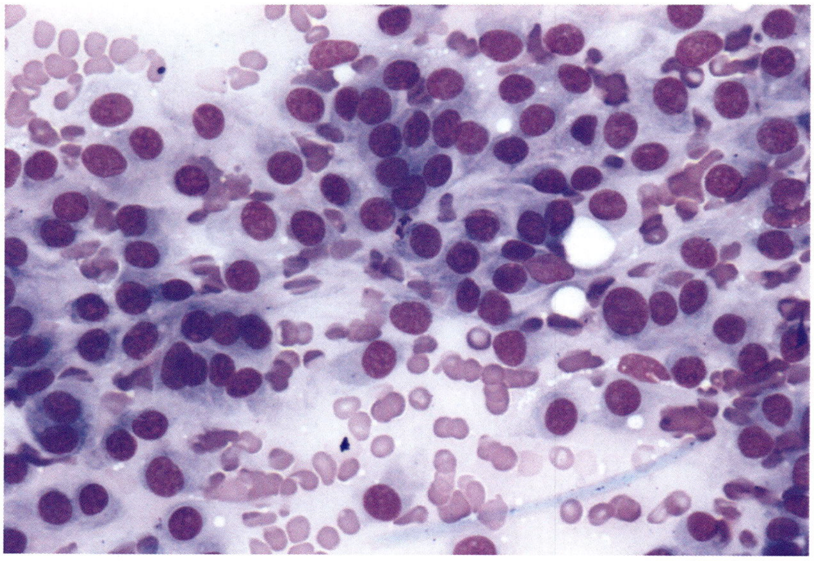

Figure 12.

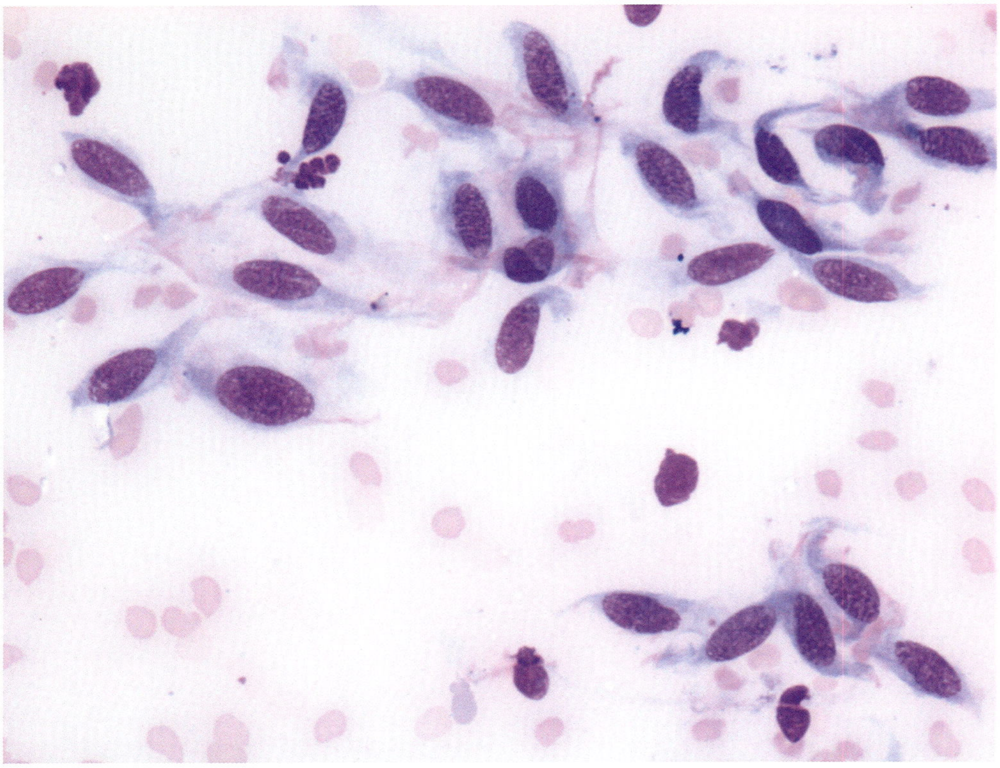

Figure 13. Mesenchymal proliferation. The cytological picture is very similar to that of low-grade sarcoma, although the cellularity of the entire preparation is lower.

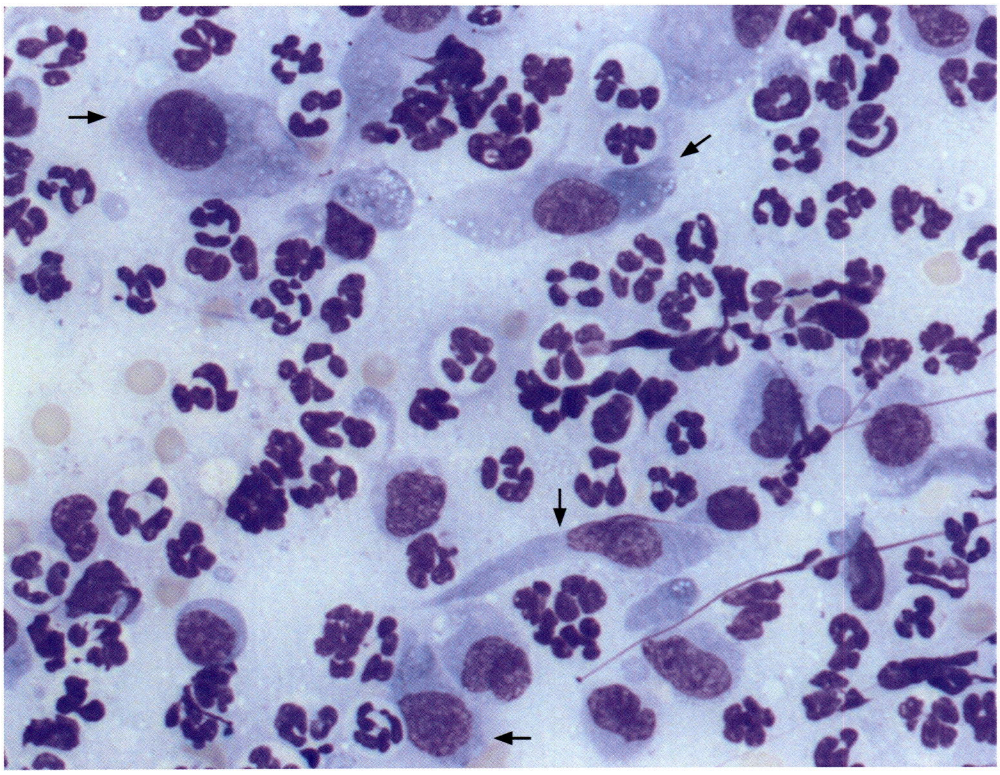

Figure 14. Pyogranulomatous inflammation in which activated conjunctive cells (arrows) are evident.

## HIGH-GRADE SARCOMA

Cytological preparations of high-grade sarcomas usually reveal a high degree of cellularity; large cells predominate, there is a significant increase in the nucleus:cytoplasm ratio, and the cytoplasm can be intensely basophilic. Although determination of a conjunctive origin is usually straightforward (except in cases of highly anaplastic tumours), marked cellular pleomorphism is observed. Numerous cells exhibit very evident nuclear atypia: marked anisokaryosis, with the presence of giant nuclei; prominent, multiple or large nucleoli; condensed chromatin with variable patterns throughout the population; and numerous binucleated or multinucleated cells (with intracellular anisokaryosis).

Mitoses are numerous and/or very atypical.

The cytological picture suggests malignity, since the population consists of very different cells with marked atypia (Figs. 15–20).

Although the presence of inflammatory cells is more frequent than in low-grade sarcoma, the high number of atypical tissue cells, which far exceeds the proportion of inflammatory cells, is usually sufficient to ensure diagnostic accuracy (Fig. 21).

Although unlikely, cases interpreted as compatible with high-grade sarcoma may constitute a false positive, even in the absence of inflammatory cells, if the lesion has an intense proliferative component (e.g. wound-healing processes) (Figs. 22–24).

## SARCOMA OF INDETERMINATE GRADE

Occasionally, cytological preparations of sarcomas can exhibit both high- and low-grade characteristics. These tend to be low-grade sarcoma samples in which some cells show more significant atypia than others (Fig. 25). In these cases, it is advisable to limit the diagnosis to “sarcoma”.

Figures 15–20. Images of high-grade sarcomas in which very marked cellular and nuclear atypia is observed (compare with Figs. 7–12). In Figure 17 numerous atypical mitoses are indicated.

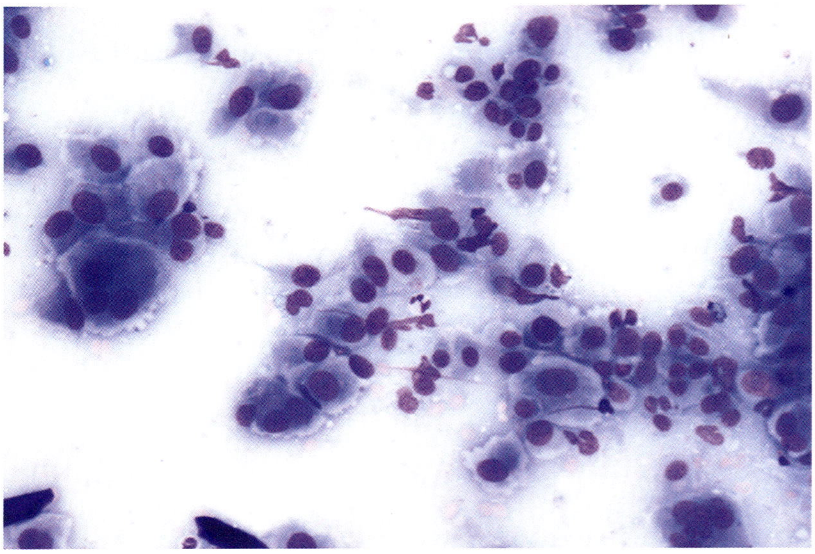

Figure 15.

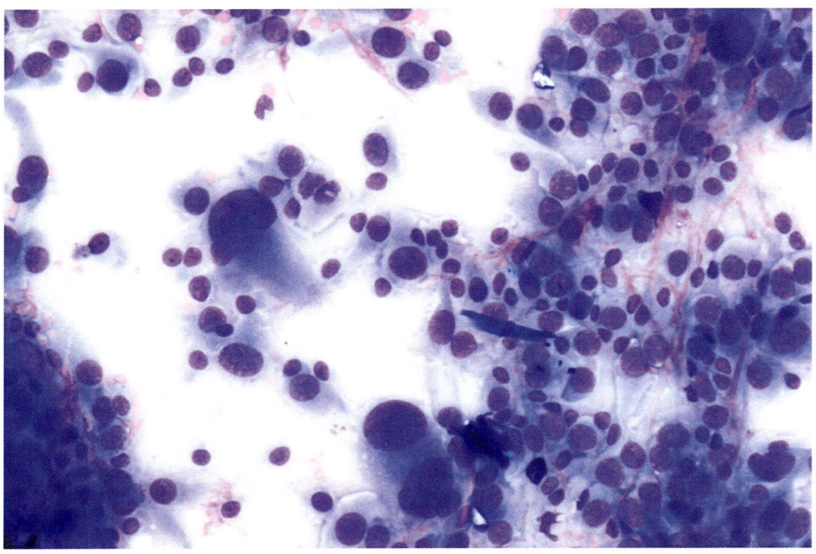

Figure 16.

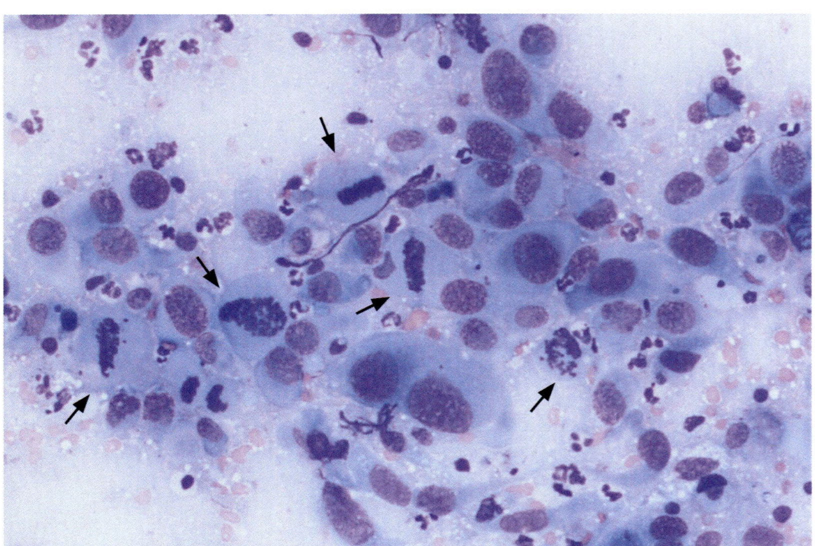

Figure 17.

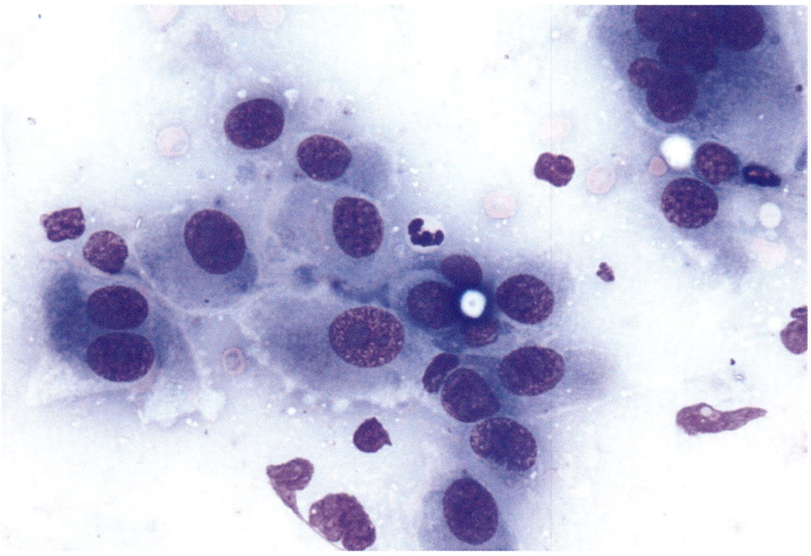

Figure 18.

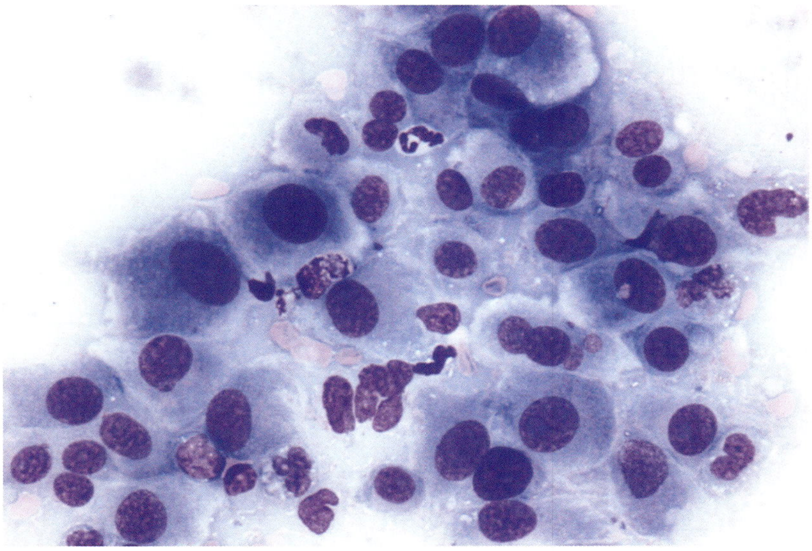

Figure 19.

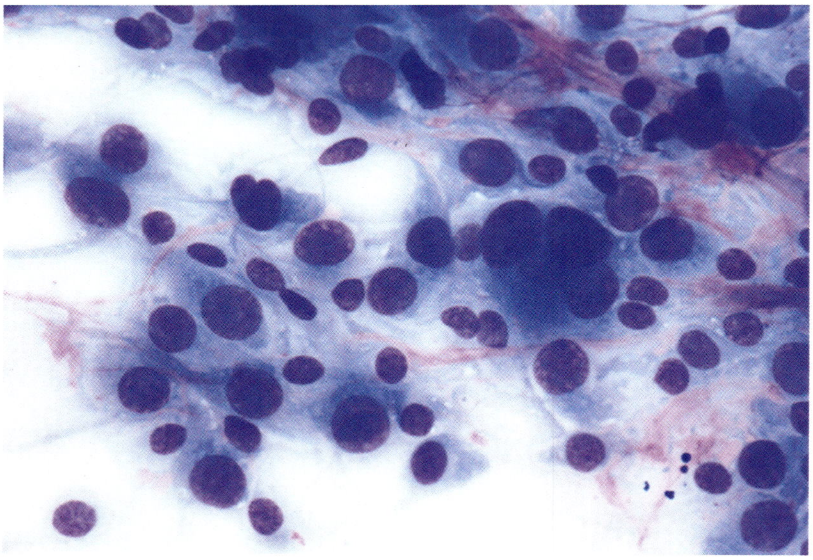

Figure 20.

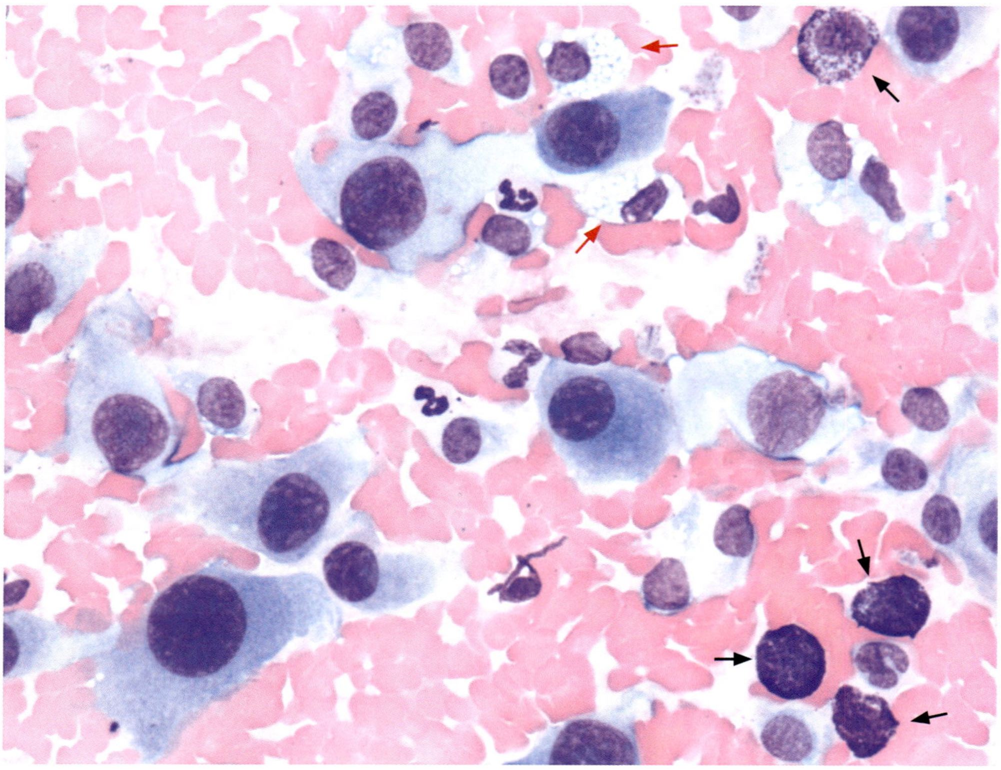

Figure 21. High-grade sarcoma with the presence of inflammatory cells. Black and red arrows indicate mast cells and macrophages, respectively.

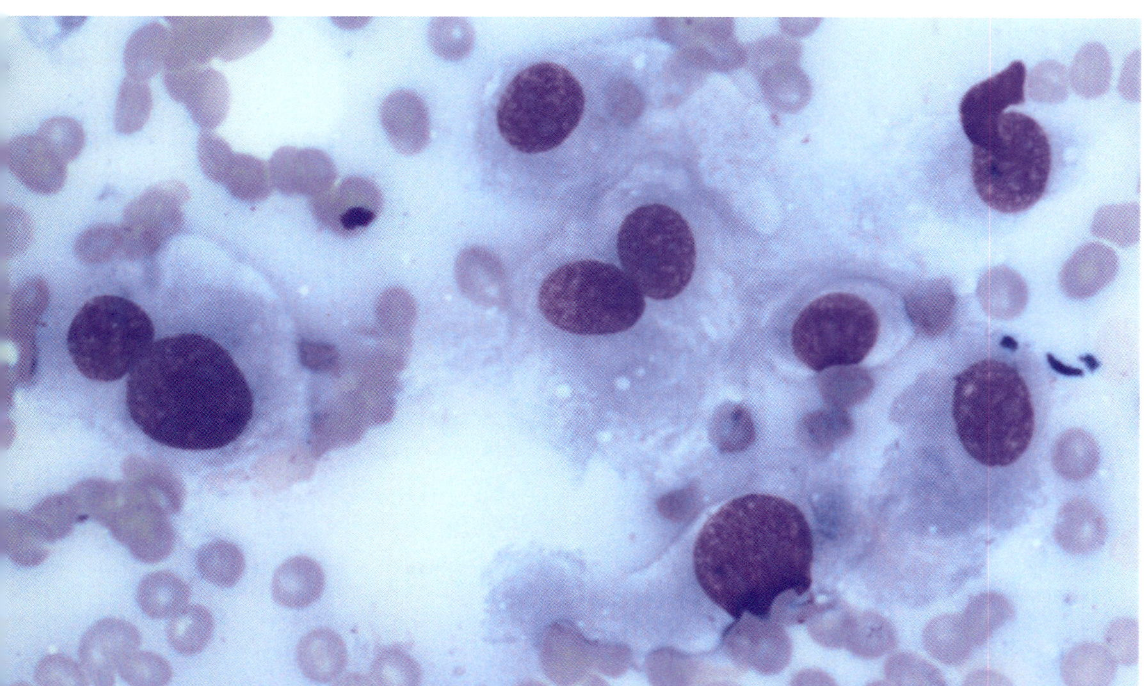

Figures 22–24. Different fields of the same skin cytology sample. Although characteristics compatible with high grade sarcoma are observed, this was identified as an intense mesenchymal proliferation (the lesion resolved without treatment).

Figure 22.

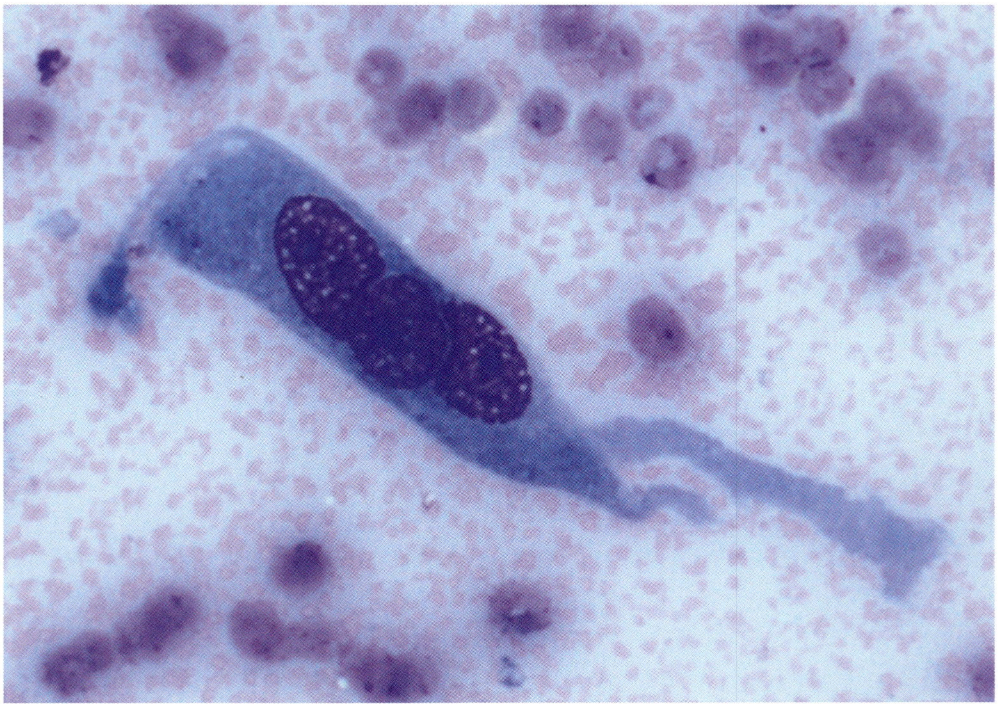

Figure 23.

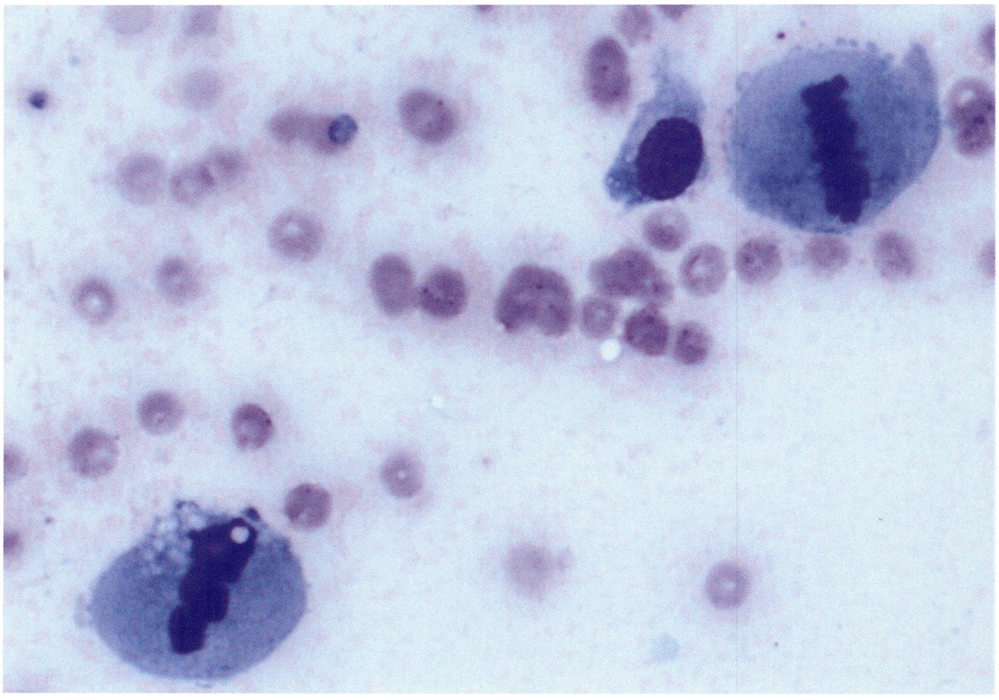

Figure 24.

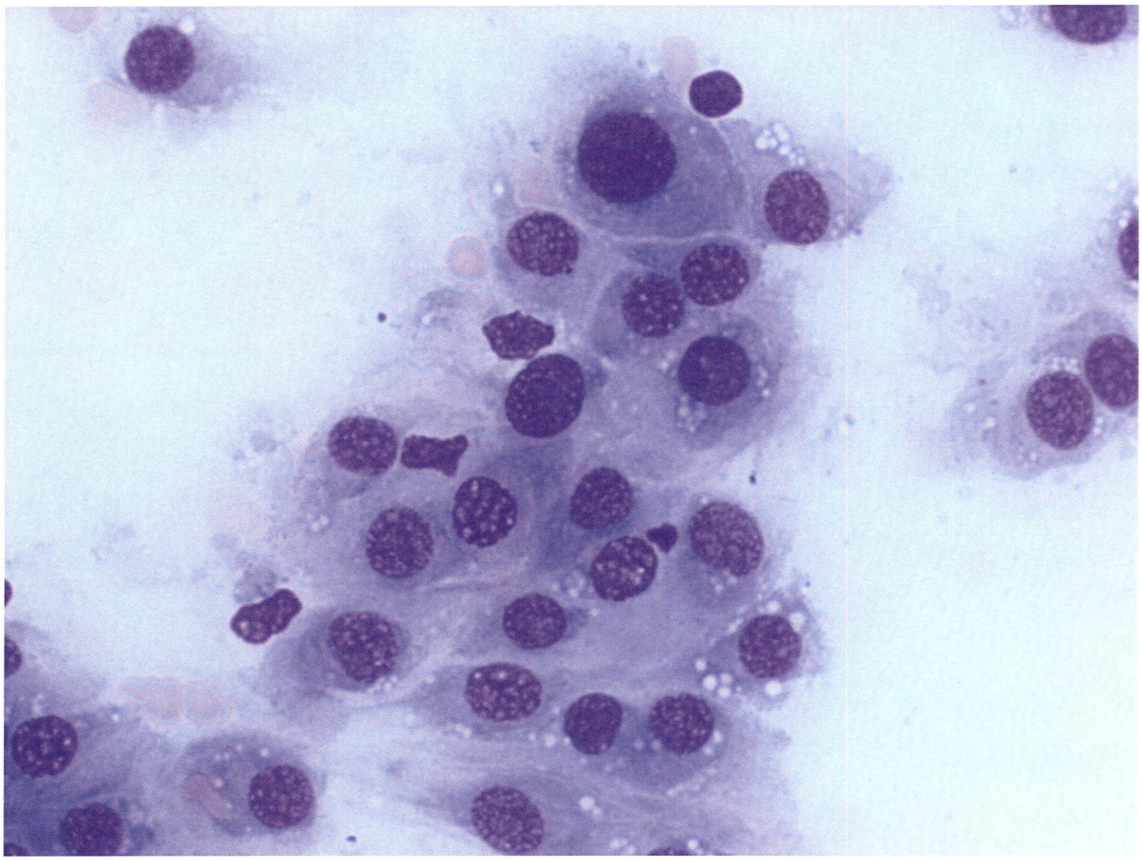

Figure 25. Sarcoma of indeterminate degree of differentiation. Some cells exhibit more marked nuclear atypia.

## DETERMINATION OF SARCOMA TYPE

Only in cases of tumours with highly differential features is a diagnosis more specific than sarcoma justified.

### VASCULAR TUMOURS AND NERVE SHEATH TUMOURS (HAEMANGIOPERICYTOMA AND SCHWANNOMA)

Both are classified as low-grade sarcomas and are often indistinguishable. The presence of cytoplasmic vacuoles is common. Multinucleated cells in which the nuclei are arranged in a circle in the cell periphery (crown cells) are characteristic of vascular tumours, in which the cells can also adhere to capillary structures. Their presence can increase diagnostic accuracy to up to 96 % (Figs. 26 and 27).[2,3]

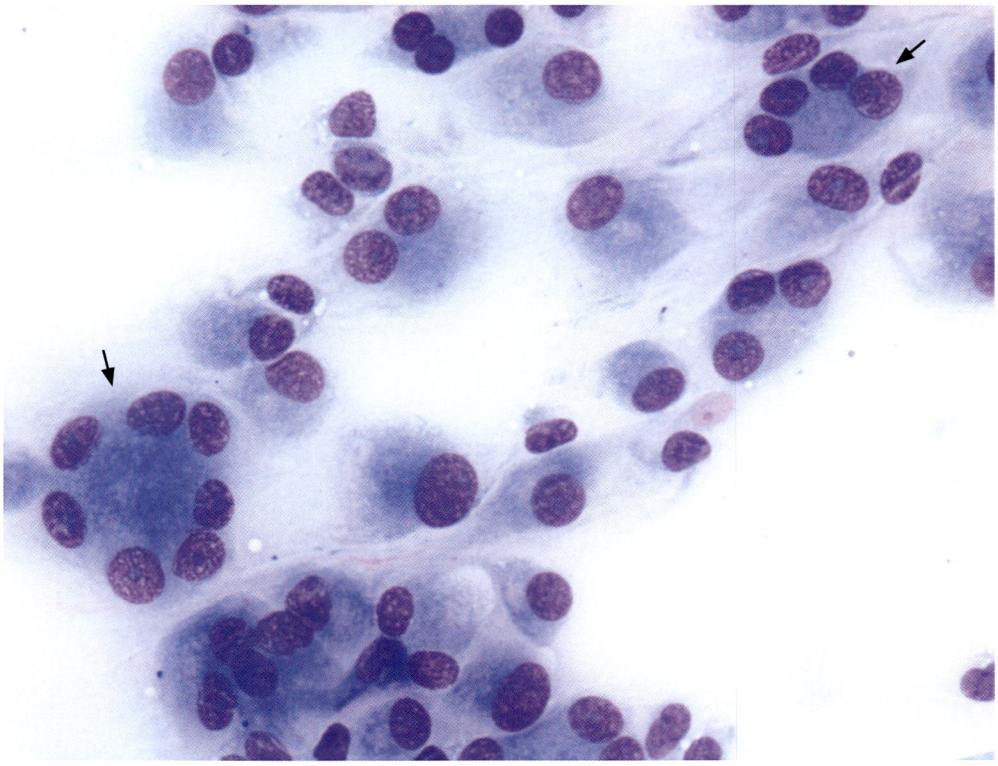

Figure 26. Crown cells (arrows) in a haemangiopericytoma.

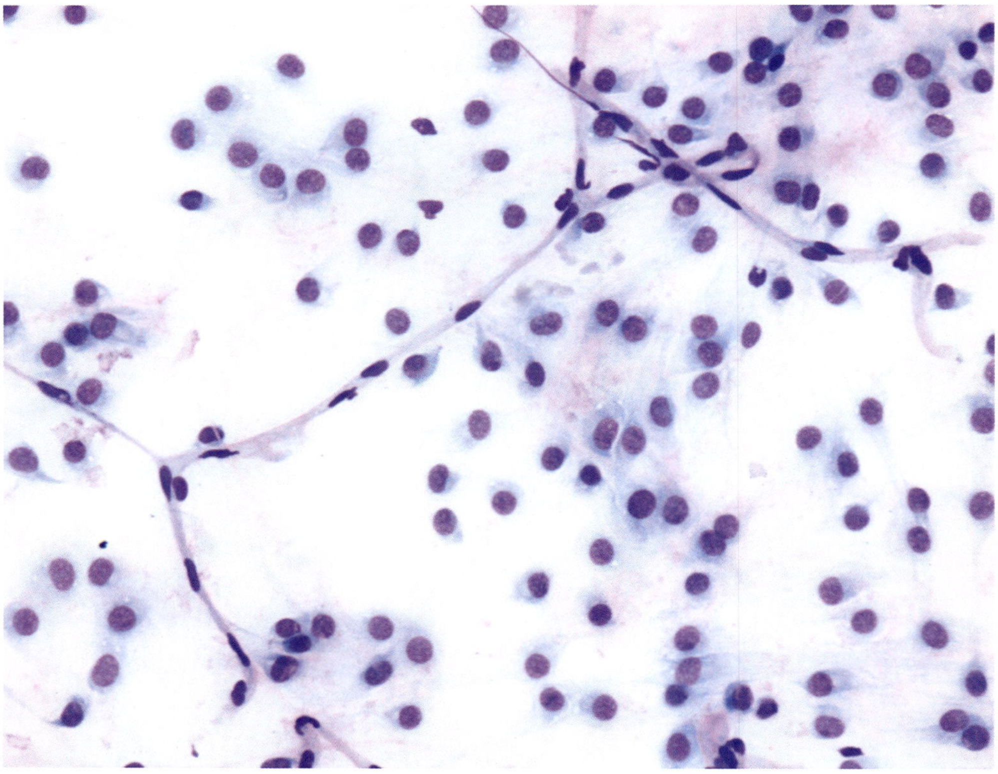

Figure 27. Presence of capillary cells (the most elongated cells) in a haemangiopericytoma.

## MYXOSARCOMA/SYNOVIAL SARCOMA

The stroma exhibits signs of viscosity, as evidenced by the presence of a granular and eosinophilic matrix (Fig. 28) and the alignment of erythrocytes and tissue cells.

## FELINE INJECTION-SITE SARCOMA

Cytology is of limited use for the diagnosis of this group of tumours, and is considered a reliable test in only 50 % of cases.

In many cases feline infection-site sarcomas (FISSs) do not exfoliate a sufficient number of cells. Furthermore, because these sarcomas are formed as a consequence of the neoplastic evolution of conjunctive cells in response to an intense inflammatory reaction, in samples in which the inflammatory component predominates (e.g. chronic panniculitis) it is impossible to determine whether the conjunctive cells are dysplastic or whether they have already acquired the neoplastic phenotype (Fig. 29).

In the 50 % of cases in which a cytological diagnosis can be established, most tumours tend to be high-grade (Figs. 30–34). However, cytology should not be used to estimate prognosis in cases of FISS.

Because these tumours often contain viscous fluid, extracellular matrix and cell alignment can be observed (Fig. 35). Another common finding is the presence of numerous multinucleated giant cells (Fig. 36).

In some cases, in addition to spindle and giant cells, a population of round histiocyte-like cells is observed. This cellular mixture is also observed in giant cell sarcoma (previously known as malignant fibrous histiocytoma) in dogs (Fig. 37).

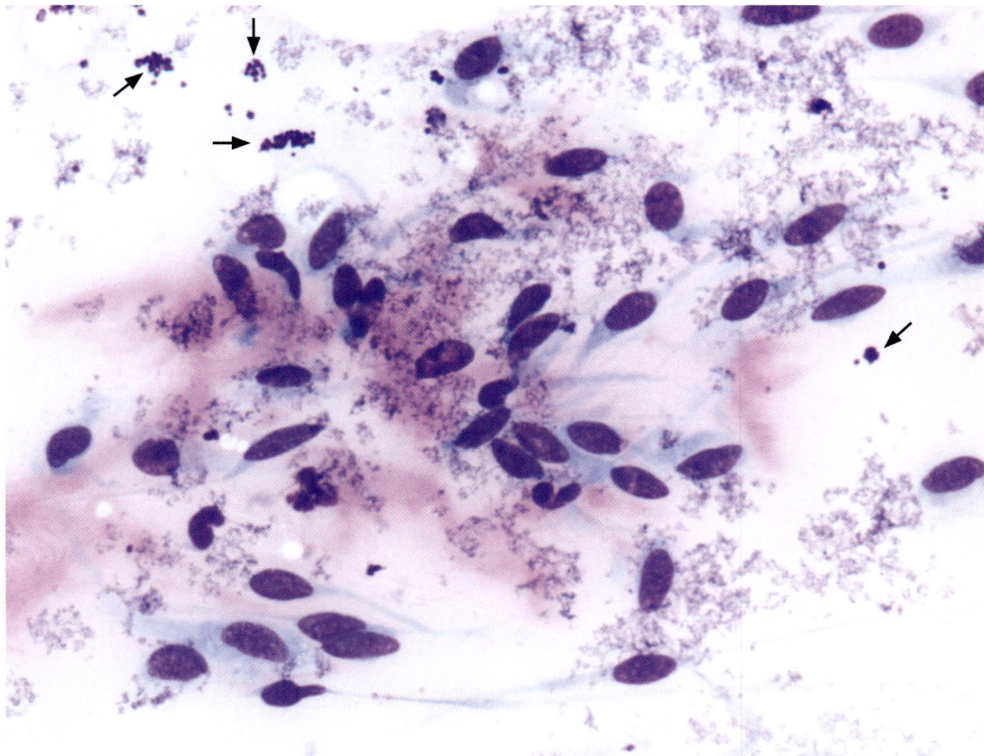

Figure 28. Synovial sarcoma An abundant protein matrix is evident (not to be confused with ultrasound gel precipitate, which is indicated with arrows).

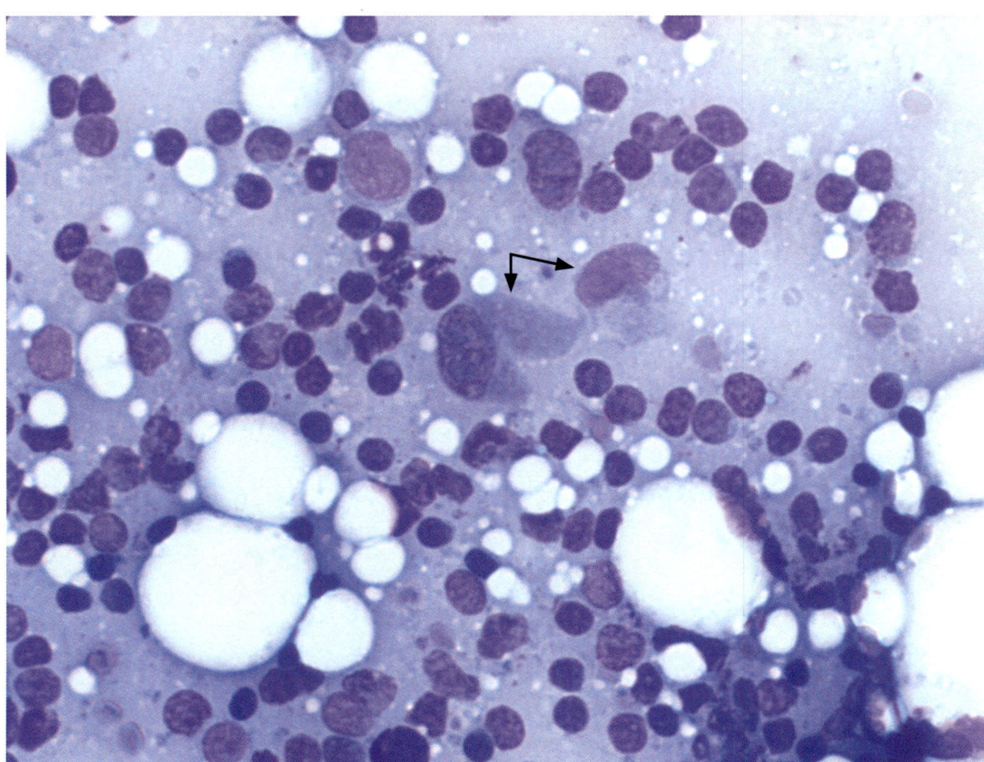

Figure 29. Feline panniculitis caused by an injection reaction. Arrows indicate activated conjunctive cells. Whether they are already neoplastic cannot be determined.

Figures 30–34. Images of feline injection-site sarcomas, including lymph node metastasis (34).

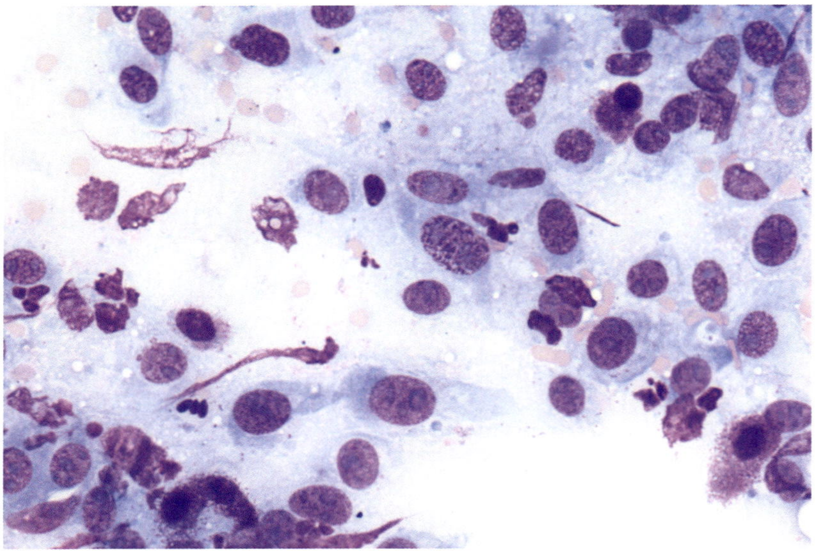

Figure 30.

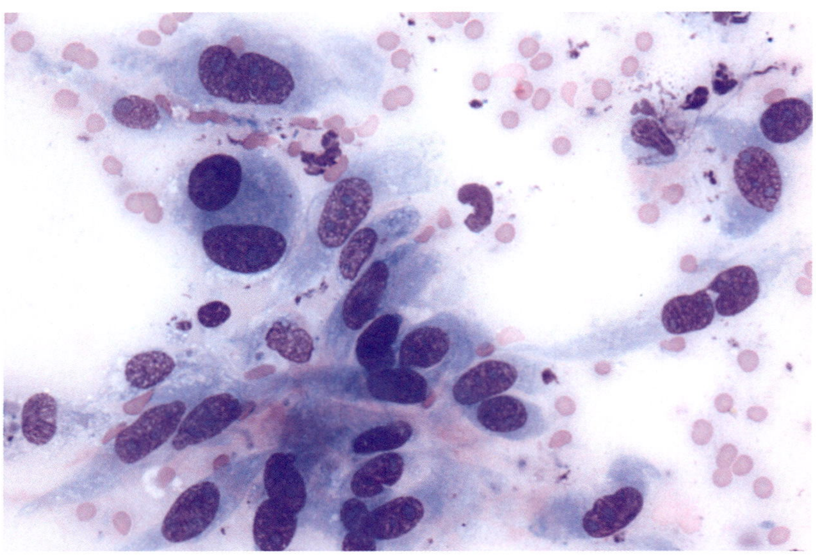

Figure 31.

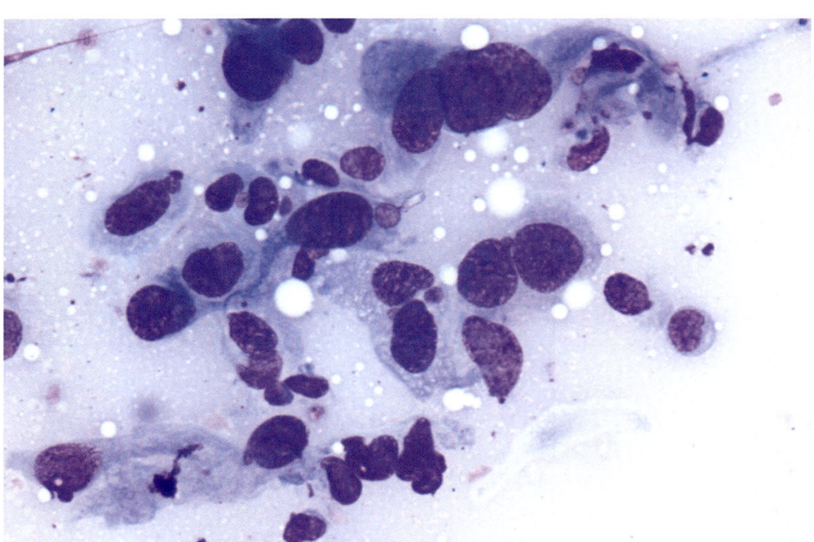

Figure 32.

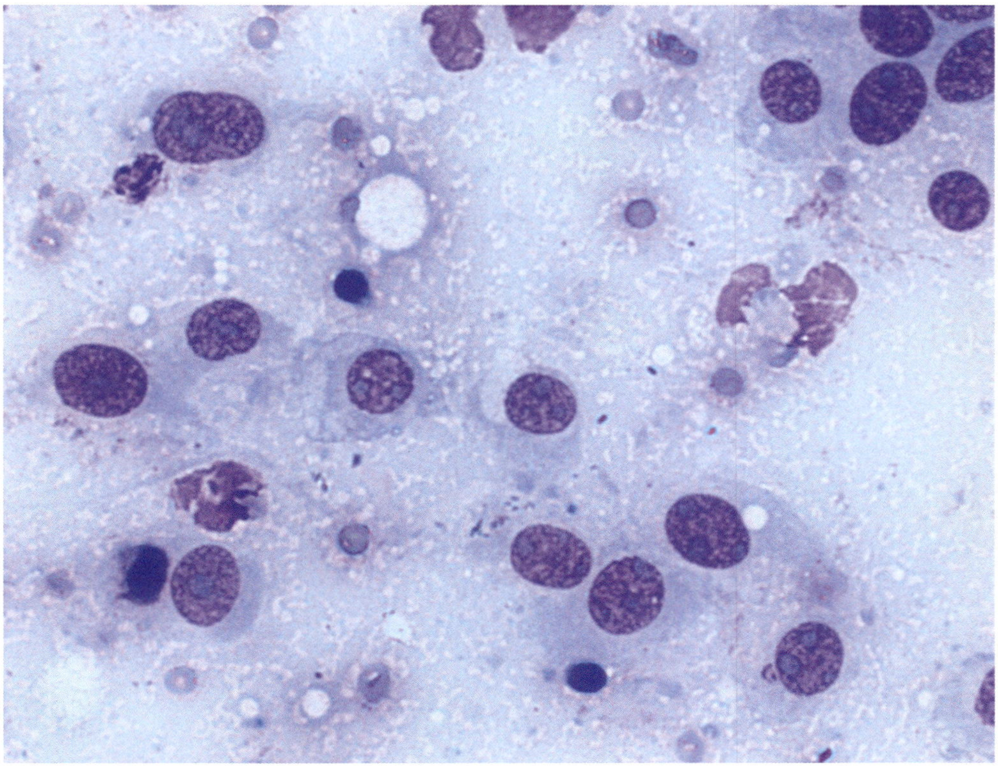

Figure 33.

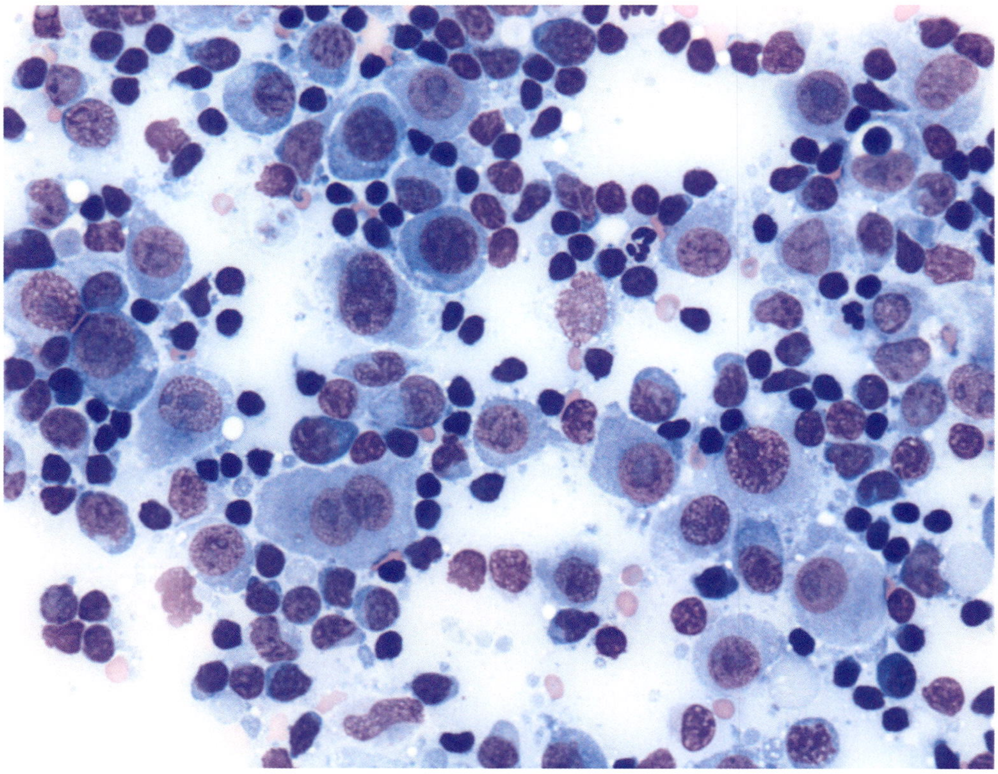

Figure 34.

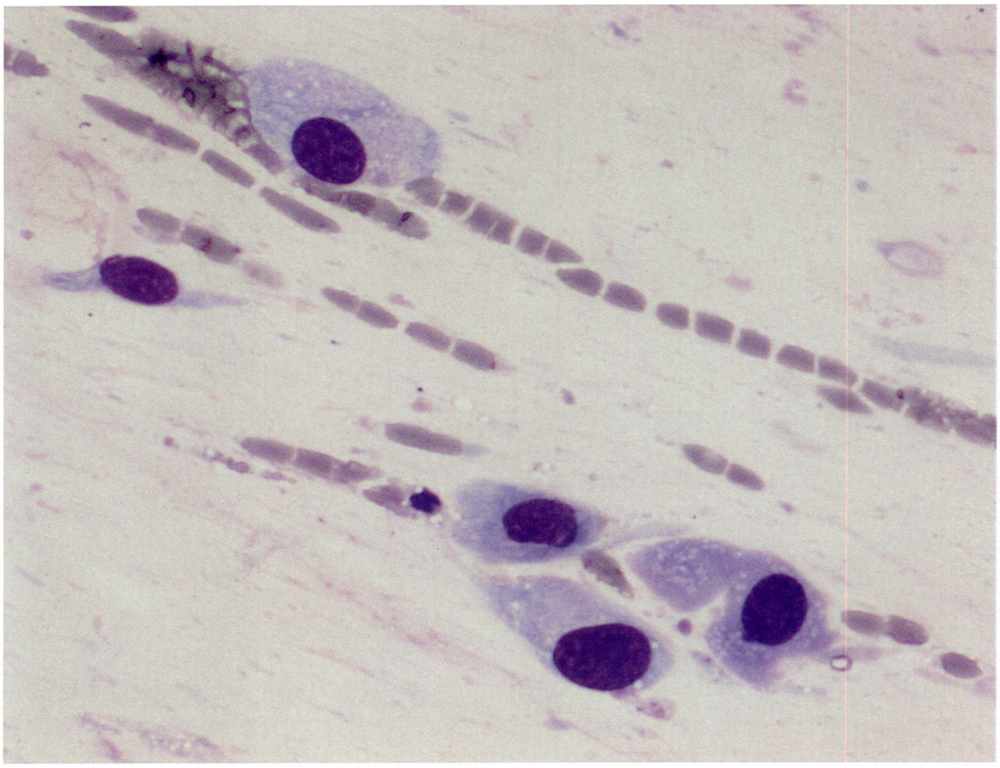

Figure 35. Cellular alignment, caused by the viscous fluid present in a feline injection-site sarcoma.

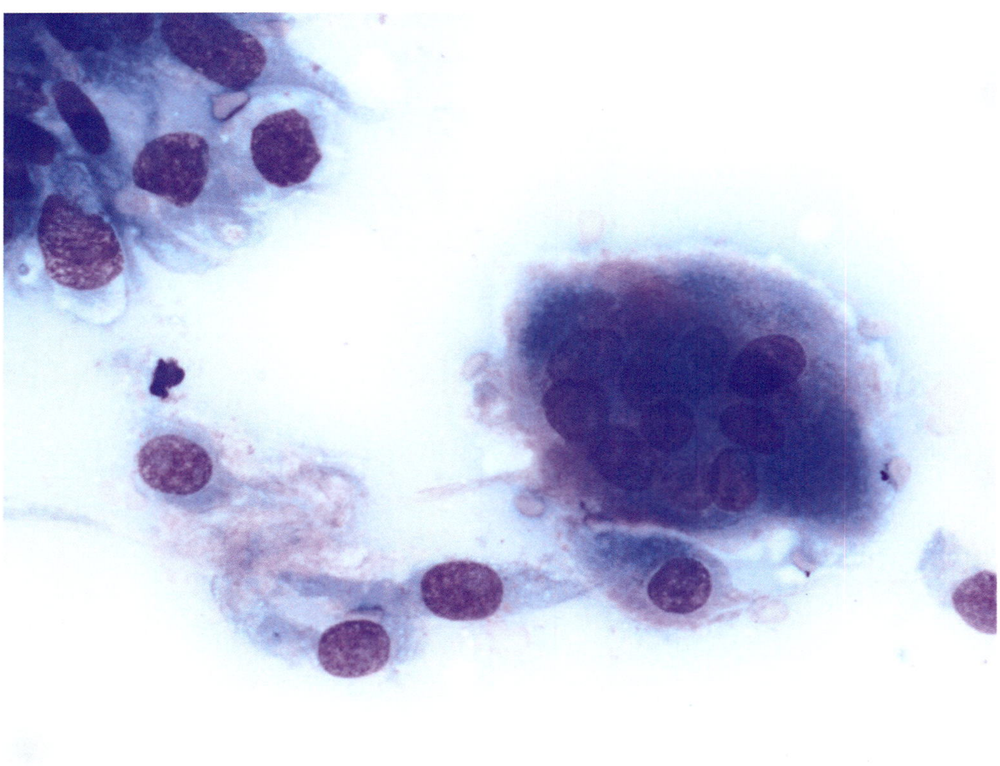

Figure 36. Cytology of a feline injection-site sarcoma in which a giant multinucleated cell is clearly evident.

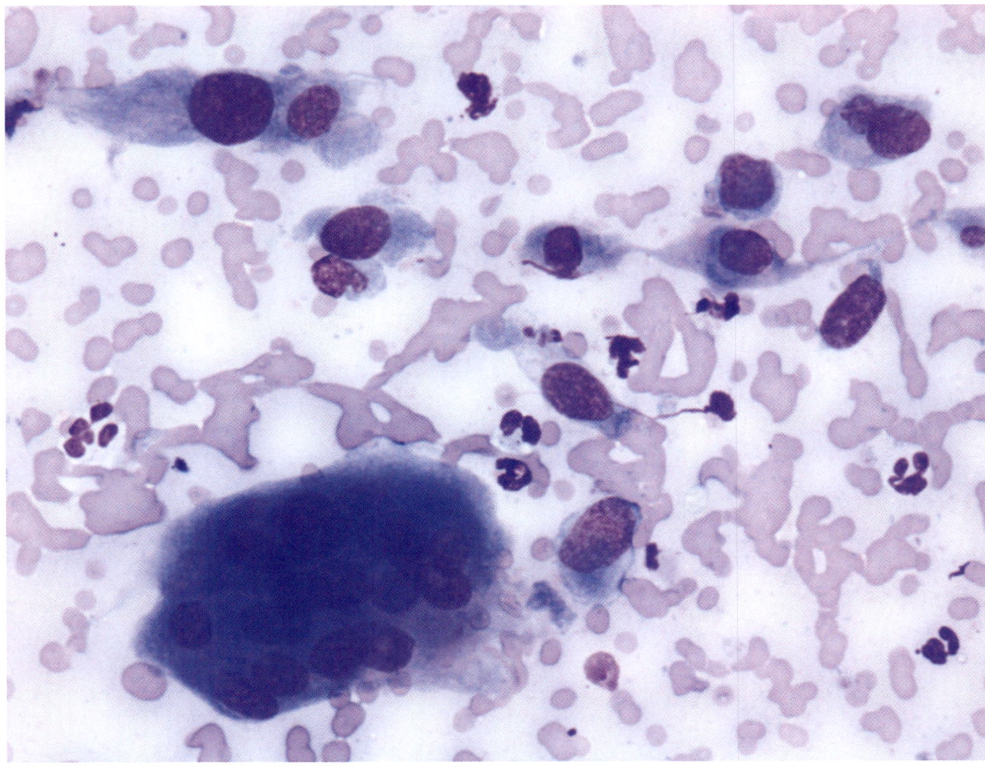

Figure 37. Giant cell sarcoma in a dog. The cytological picture is very similar to that commonly observed in feline injection-site sarcomas.

## LIPOSARCOMA

The cytological picture of this type of sarcoma is highly characteristic, consisting of numerous rounded, hyperchromatic and apparently naked nuclei (with a variable degree of atypia depending on the degree of differentiation) within a matrix in which adipose vacuoles predominate, enabling differentiation from a neuroendocrine tumour (Figs. 38–40). In some cases, well-defined cells with abundant vacuoles can be distinguished.

The main differential diagnosis is chronic panniculitis, since the presence of conjunctive cells and fat vacuoles can cause confusion. The main differential criterion is cellularity, which is scarce in panniculitis (Fig. 41).

It is not possible to mistake a liposarcoma for a lipoma or for normal adipose tissue. Lipoma and normal adipose tissue (which are indistinguishable from one other) contain large clusters of cells with a thin membrane surrounding a large volume of clear cytoplasm, with a small, eccentric nucleus, which may be deformed by the fat vacuoles. Owing to the size of the cells, the cytological picture is highly characteristic at low magnification (Fig. 42).

Figures 38–40. Images showing cutaneous (38 and 39) and splenic (40) liposarcomas.

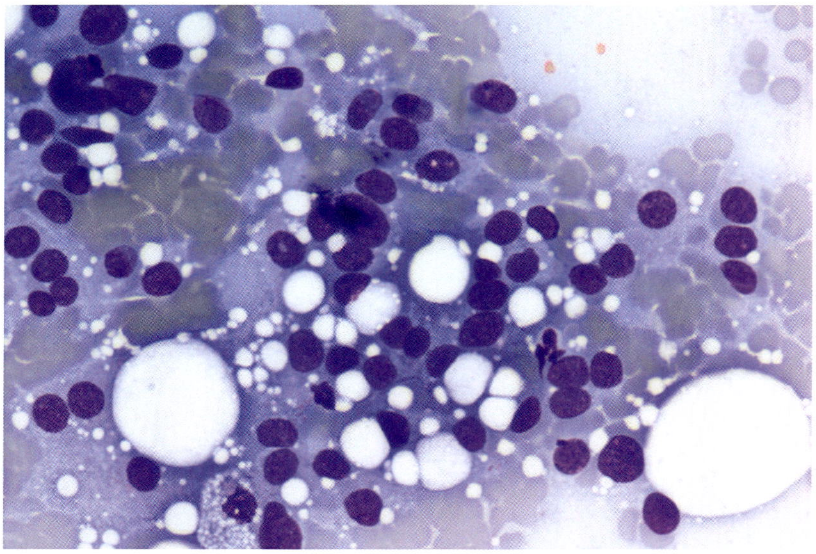

Figure 38.

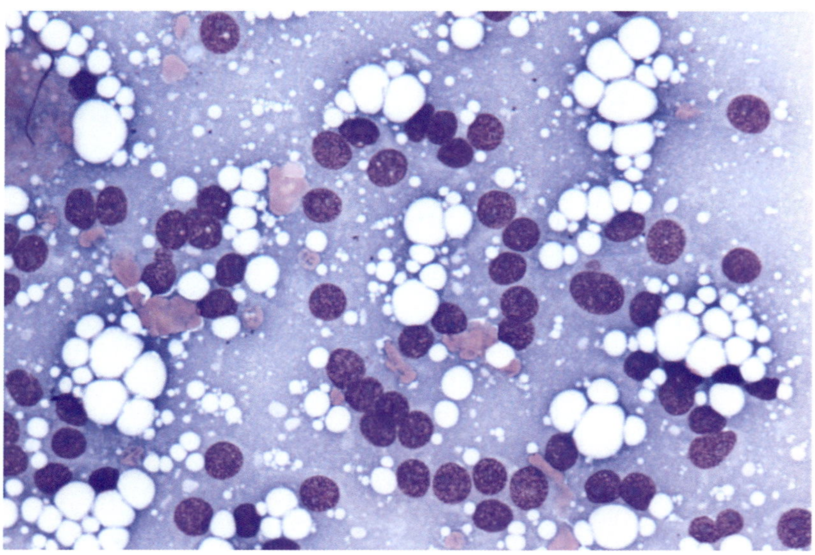

Figure 39.

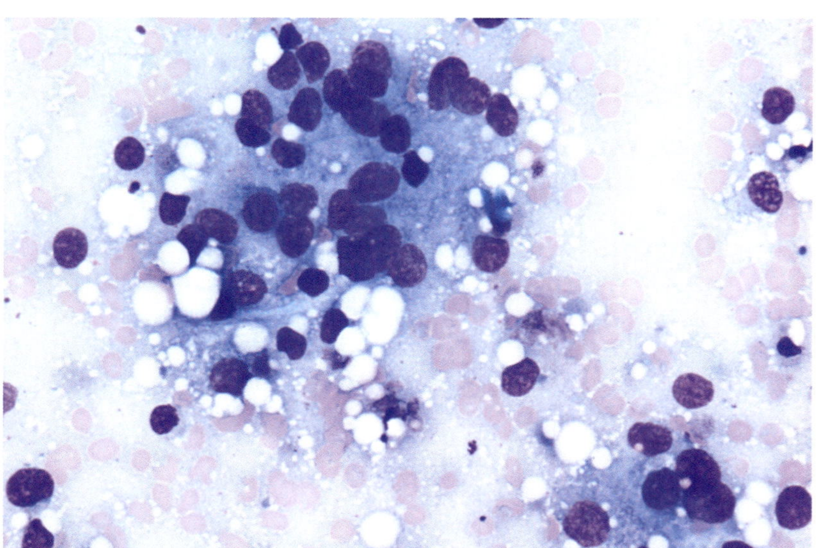

Figure 40.

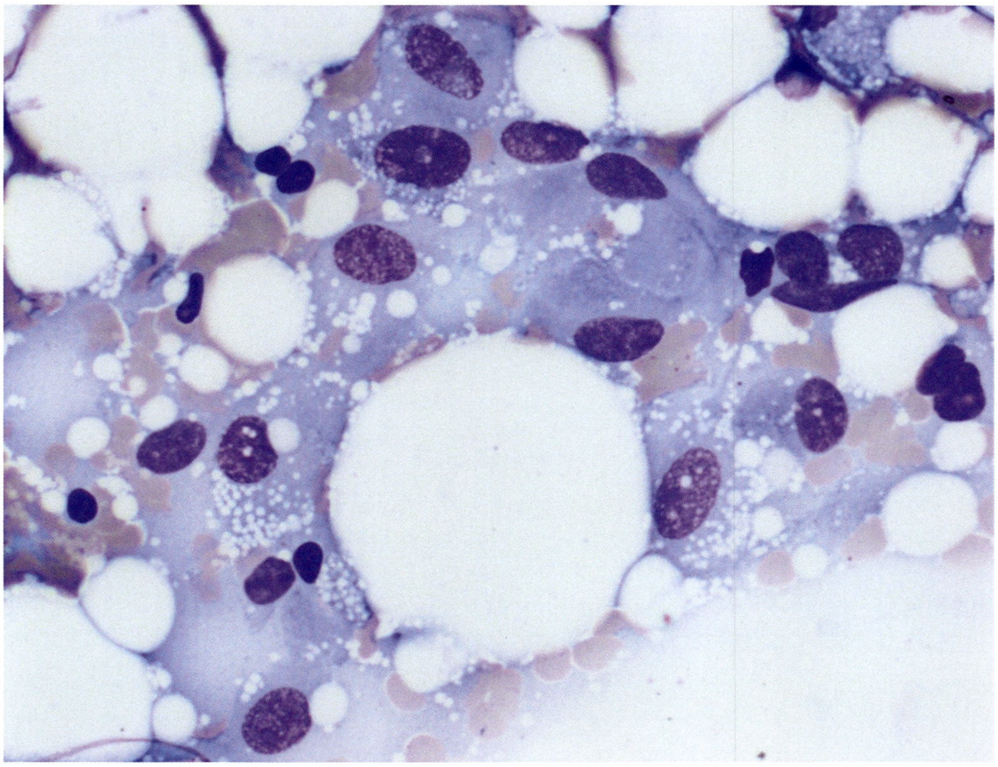

Figure 41. Chronic panniculitis. Differentiation from liposarcoma is necessary, although there is a lower degree of cellularity in chronic panniculitis.

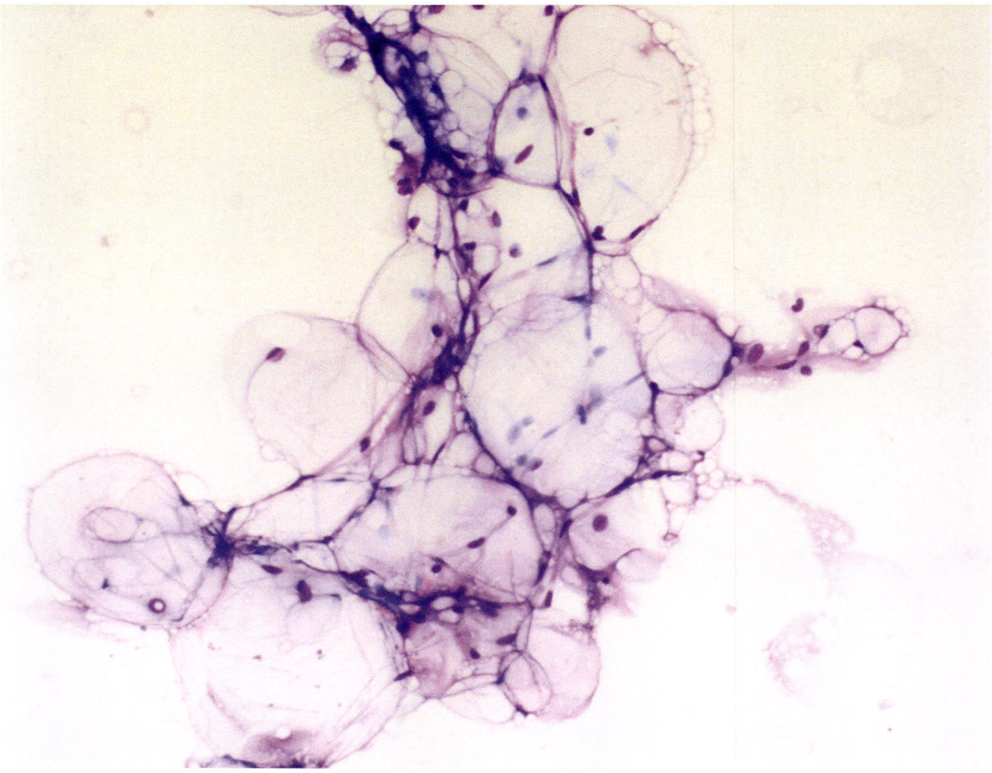

Figure 42. Low-magnification image of adipose tissue (lipoma). This tumour cannot be mistaken for a liposarcoma.

## MUSCLE TUMOURS

Well-differentiated leiomyosarcomas usually exfoliate extremely elongated cells with very oblong nuclei (Fig. 43). High-grade muscle tumours cannot be distinguished from other sarcomas.

There is no specific cytological pattern characteristic of rhabdomyosarcoma (Fig. 44), in which cells of varying morphologies (polygonal, fusiform, elongated, round) can be observed.

## OSTEOSARCOMA

Cytology offers very high diagnostic accuracy for the diagnosis of osteosarcoma (70–90 %, even reaching 100 % if alkaline phosphatase stains are used).[10] At a minimum, cytology can be used to rule out other differential diagnoses (e.g. osteomyelitis, other bone tumours).

> Cytological evaluation is recommended as the first step in the diagnostic protocol for all bone lesions compatible with osteosarcoma.

Osteoblasts, which resemble plasma cells (Fig. 45), are small- to medium-sized round or oval cells with an eccentric oval nucleus and basophilic cytoplasm (Fig. 46). They may contain eosinophilic vacuoles or cytoplasmic granules with an osteoid matrix. They are rarely fusiform. Thus, if this cell type predominates in bone cytology it is unlikely that it corresponds to an osteosarcoma (Fig. 47).

In addition to neoplastic osteoblasts (Figs. 48–50), osteosarcomas feature a bright pink extracellular osteoid matrix (Fig. 51), around which neoplastic cells are arranged (unlike chondrosarcomas, in which the cells are observed within the matrix), as well as osteoclasts and multinucleated giant cells (Fig. 52).

Owing to the morphological similarity between osteoblasts and plasma cells, plasmacytoma should be included in the differential diagnosis of osteosarcoma (Fig. 53).

## HAEMANGIOSARCOMA

Cytology of lesions in affected organs or of effusions resulting from tumour rupture is not particularly useful for the diagnosis of haemangiosarcoma. Only in 25 % of cases are there sufficient cells exhibiting the characteristics of high-grade sarcoma (Figs. 54–56). In the remainder, haemodilution is so severe that the neoplastic cells cannot be visualised, although erythrophagocytosis, indicating chronic haemorrhage, may be observed.

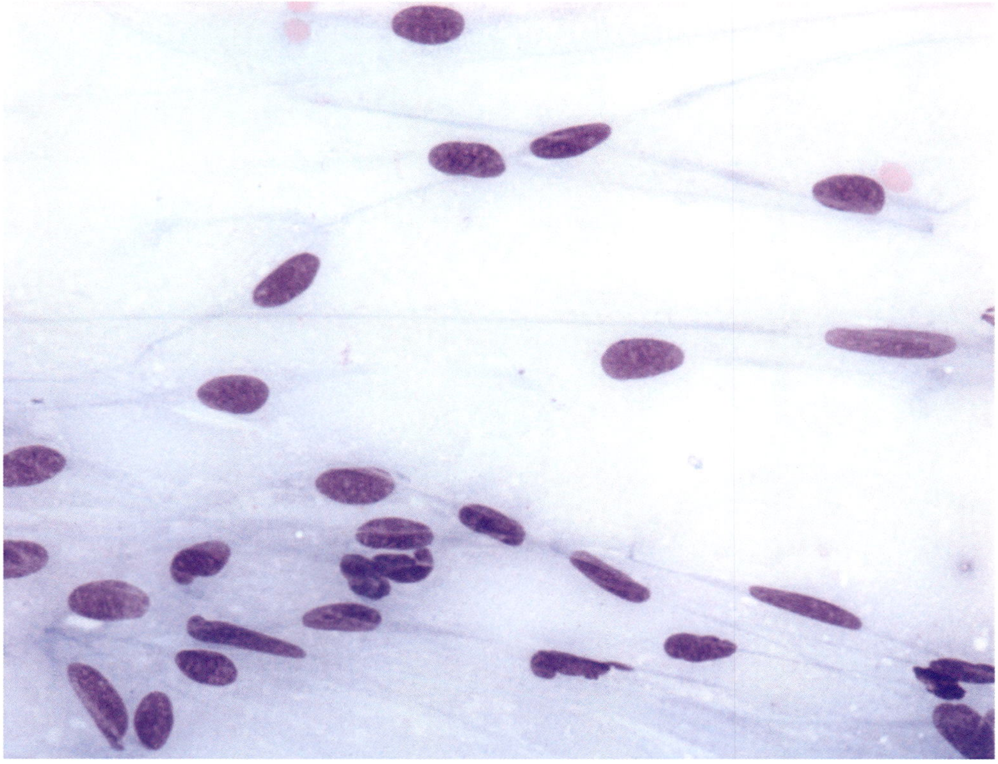

Figure 43. Hepatic metastasis of a (well differentiated) leiomyosarcoma.

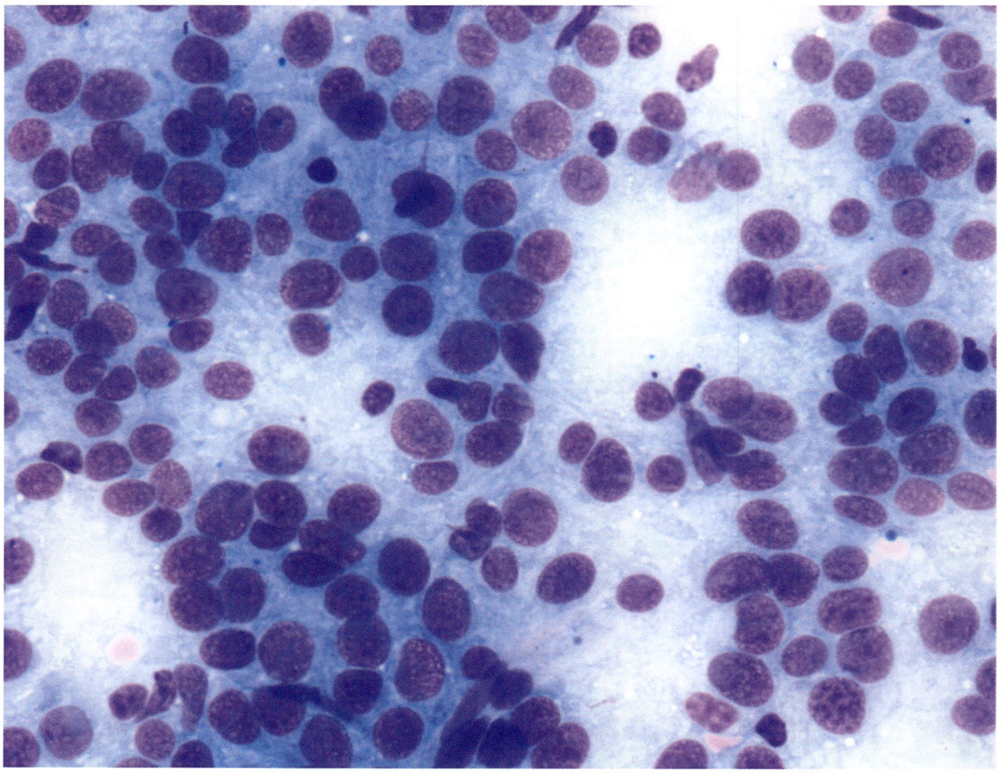

Figure 44. Rhabdomyosarcoma (histologically confirmed). There is no cytological pattern that enables diagnosis of this tumour type.

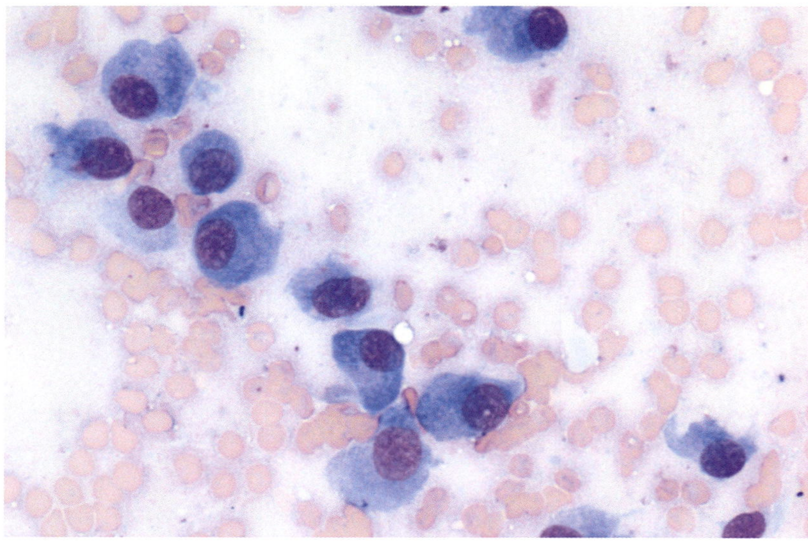

Figure 45. Neoplastic osteoblasts that resemble plasma cells.

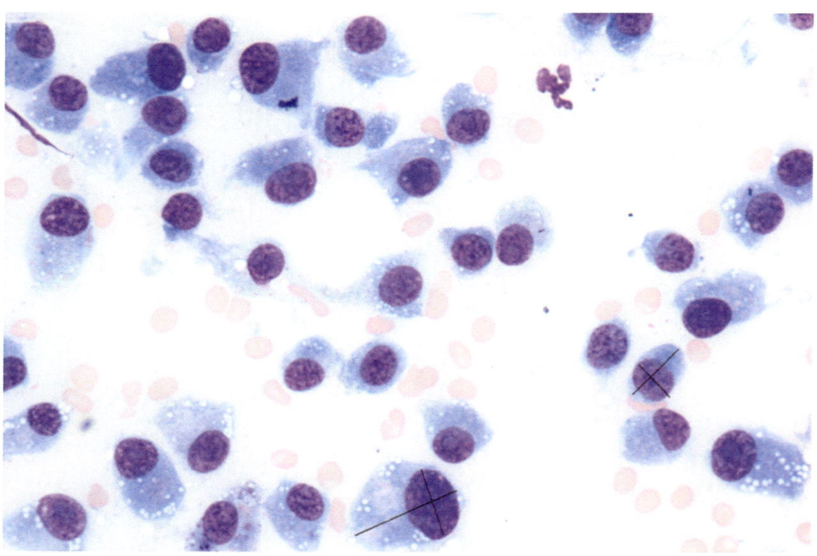

Figure 46. Neoplastic osteoblasts. The major axis of the oval nucleus is perpendicular to the major axis of the cell.

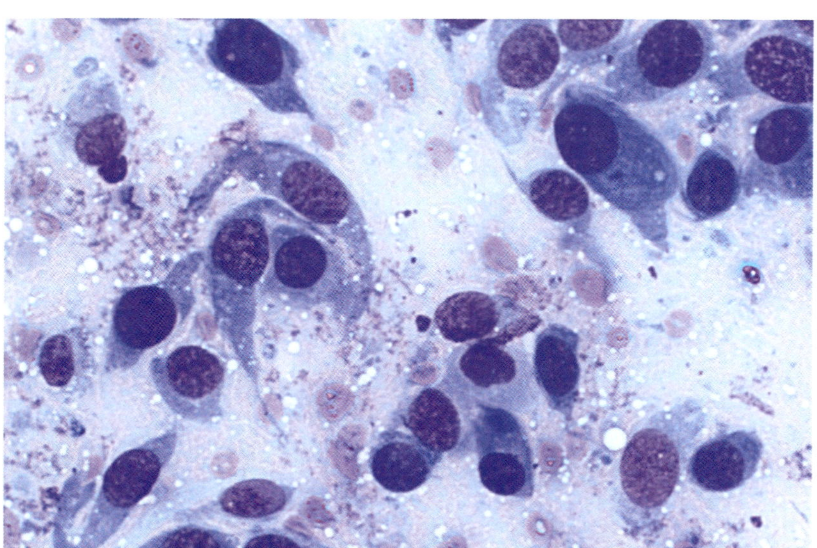

Figure 47. Cytology of an osteolytic lesion. The predominantly fusiform cell morphology is uncommon in osteosarcoma. A histological diagnosis of fibroblastic osteosarcoma was established.

Figures 48–50. Images of osteosarcoma: osseous (48), mammary (49), and cutaneous (50). In these cases differential diagnosis with round cell tumour is necessary.

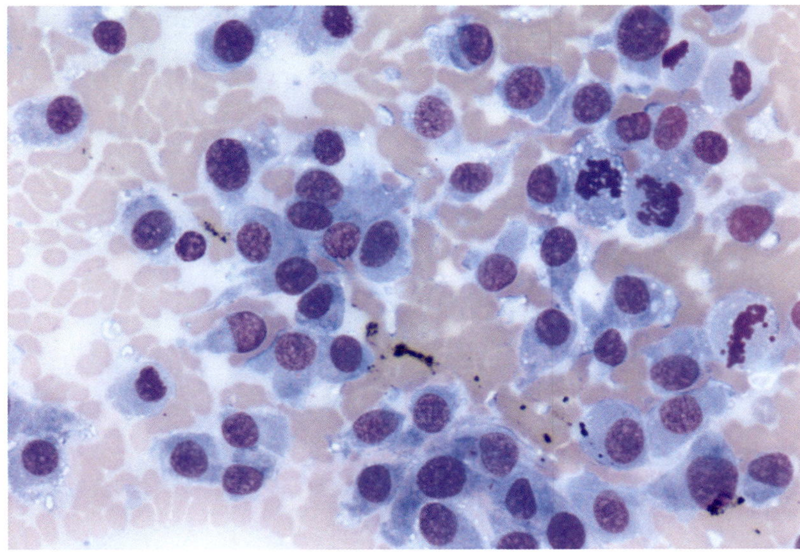

Figure 48.

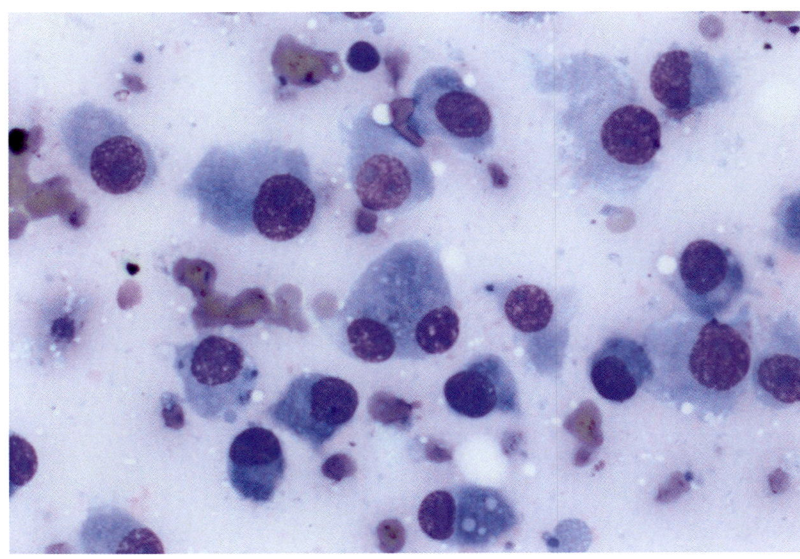

Figure 49.

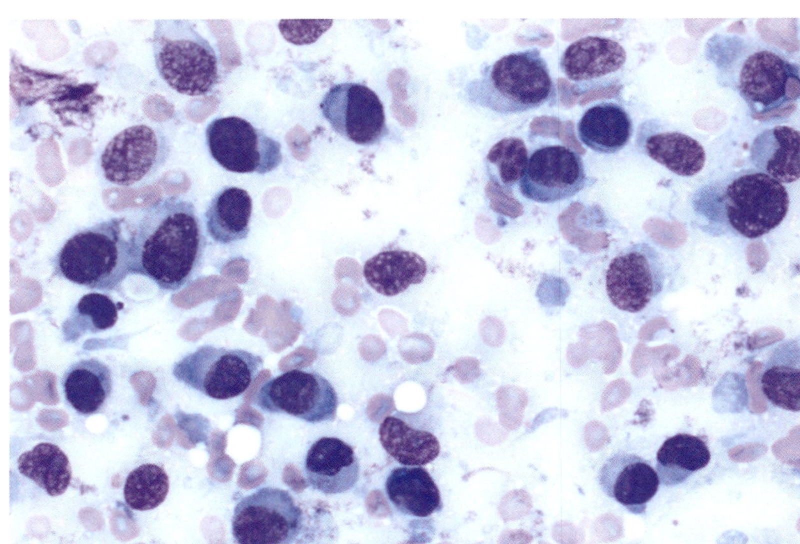

Figure 50.

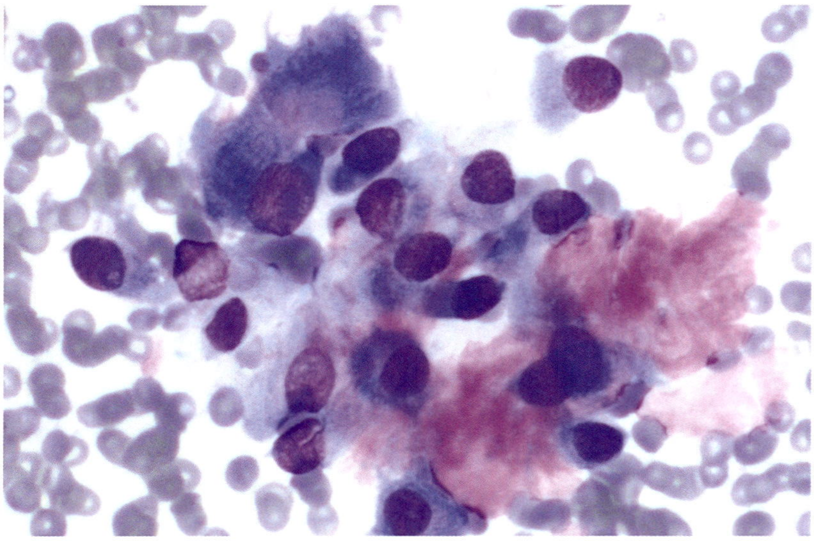

Figure 51. Osteoblasts around the osteoid matrix.

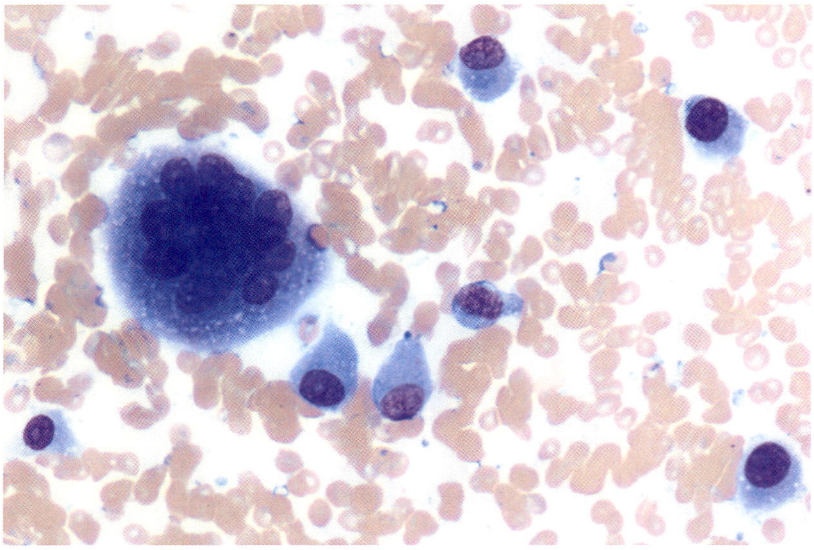

Figure 52. Neoplastic osteoblasts and an osteoclast.

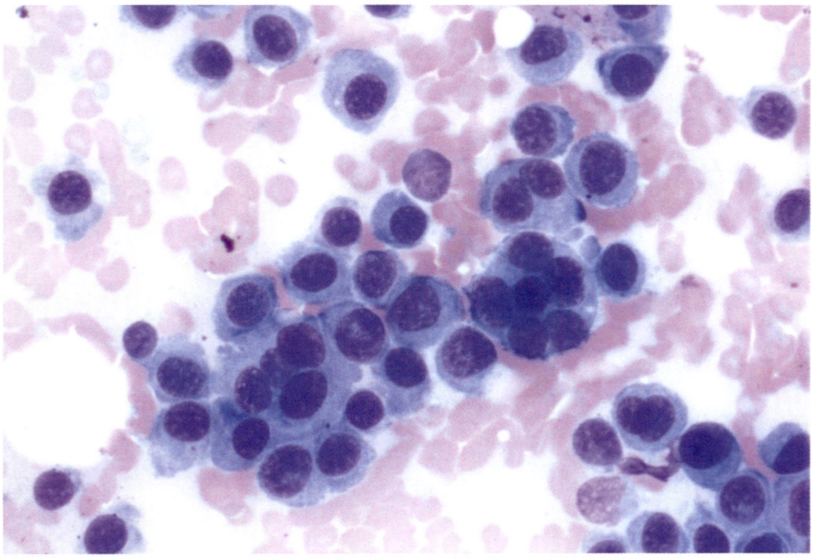

Figure 53. Extramedullary bone plasmacytoma. The cytological picture can be confused with that of an osteosarcoma.

Figures 54–56. Haemangiosarcoma in the spleen (54) and kidney (55), and lymph node metastasis (56).

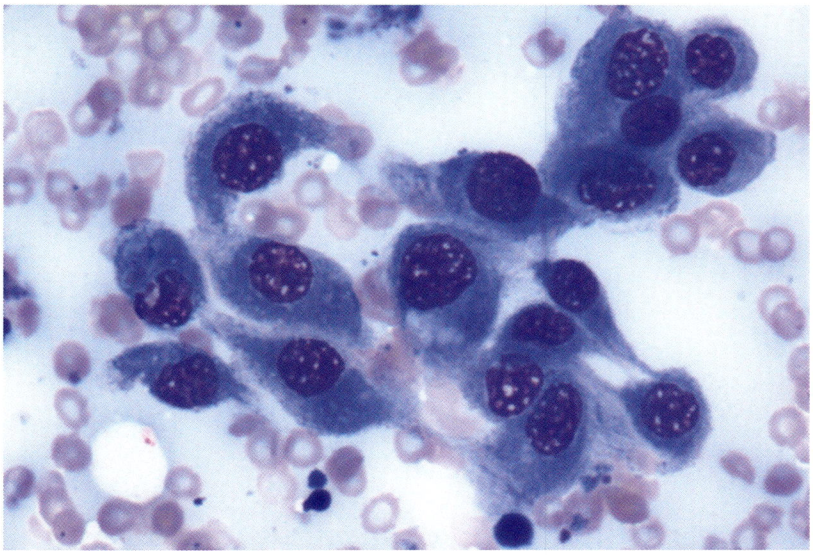

Figure 54.

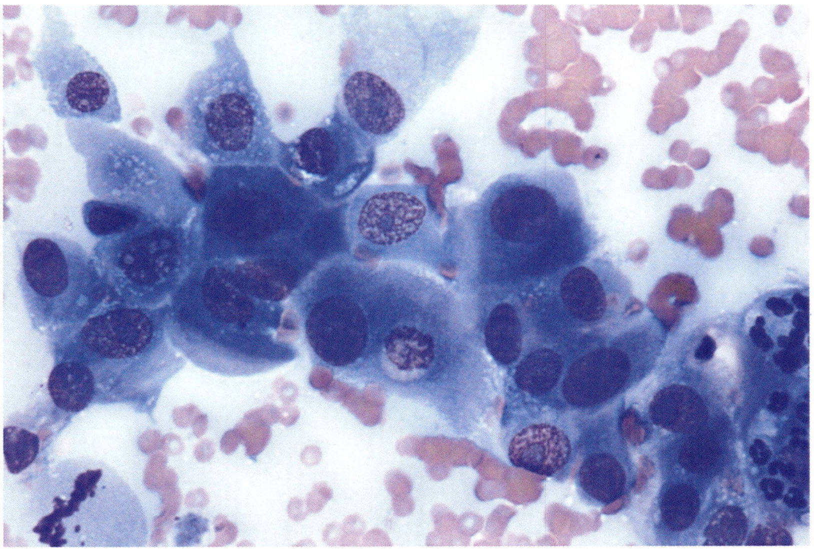

Figure 55.

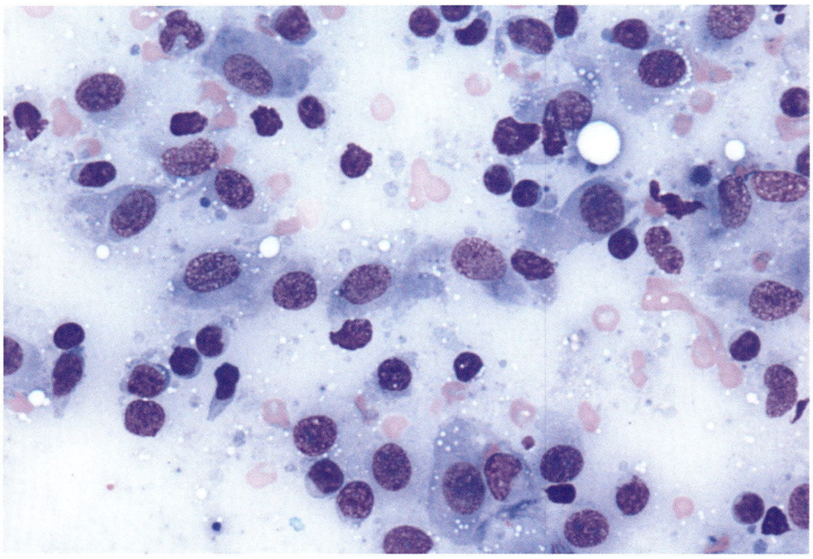

Figure 56.

# 07

# Cytology of epithelial tumours

# Cytology of epithelial tumours

Epithelial tumours, affecting the skin or other organs, are very common in both cats and dogs. Cytological recognition of epithelial lesions is simple, except in cases of highly undifferentiated tumours.

The following characteristics should be evaluated in samples, which typically exhibit a high degree of cellularity:

1. Cell disposition.
2. Cell morphology.
3. Cytoplasmic vacuoles.
4. Malignancy criteria.

## CELL DISPOSITION

The most characteristic feature of the epithelial tissue is the distribution of cells in groups, visible even at low magnification, consisting of variable numbers of cells. Cells may also be arranged in cords, palisades, or acini (Figs. 1–4).

If these groups are very large, the cellular characteristics should be evaluated in the most peripheral cells, since the central areas consist of multiple overlapping layers (Fig. 5).

In some epithelia (e.g. prostate or stomach), the organised groups form honeycomb-like structures in which the cell borders are clearly delimited (Figs. 6 and 7).

There are exceptions to this typical arrangement of cells in groups:

- In normal conditions, the squamous cells have already disintegrated. Therefore, in squamous cell carcinomas (SCCs), individual cells or poorly cohesive clusters predominate (Figs. 8 and 9).
- A similar cytological picture is observed for neuroendocrine tumours, regardless of their location (e.g. thyroid, adrenal medulla, chemoreceptors, pancreatic beta cells, gastrointestinal tract, liver, or anal sac): abundant free, round or oval nuclei within a poorly basophilic matrix derived from cytoplasm of the lysed cells, with no clearly identifiable individual cellular elements ("naked nuclei"). Acinar structures or groups, in which the cytoplasmic borders are poorly defined, may also be observed (Figs. 10–15).
- In anaplastic carcinomas these grouped structures disintegrate, and therefore this trait, which enables differentiation from other tumour types, is lost (Fig. 16).
- Resting mesothelial cells of the pleura, peritoneum, and pericardium exfoliate to form small clusters of strongly cohesive, epithelial-like cells (Fig. 17), which in dogs are arranged around an acidophilic hyaline matrix (Fig. 18).

Figures 1–4. Epithelial cells arranged in groups, palisades (ciliated cells in a tracheal wash), or acinar structures.

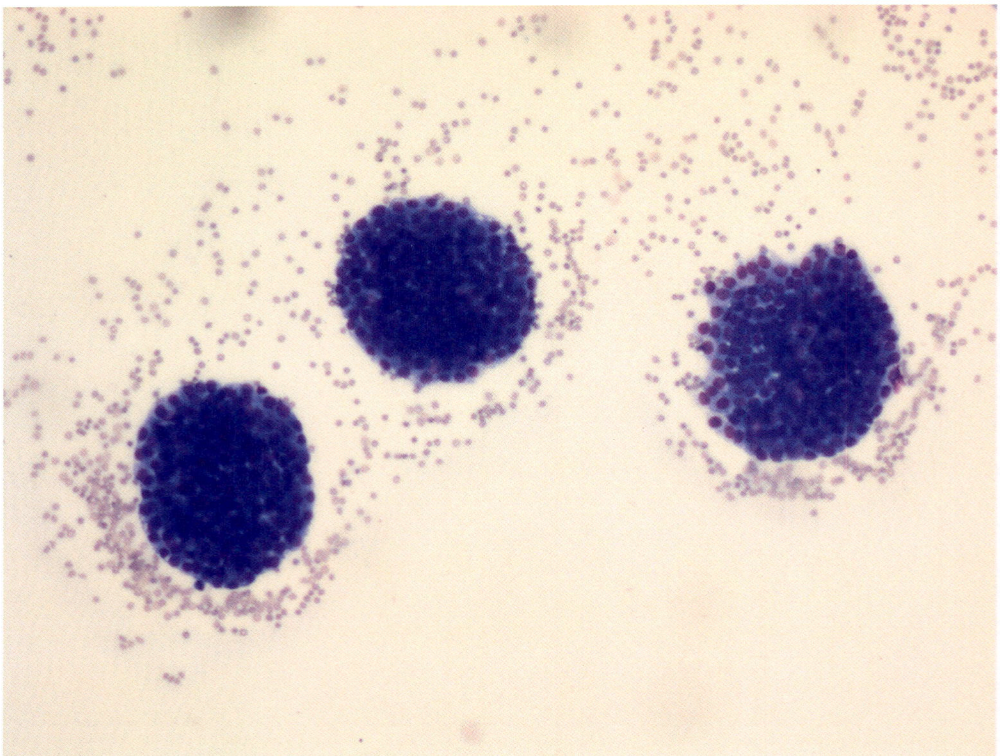

Figure 1.

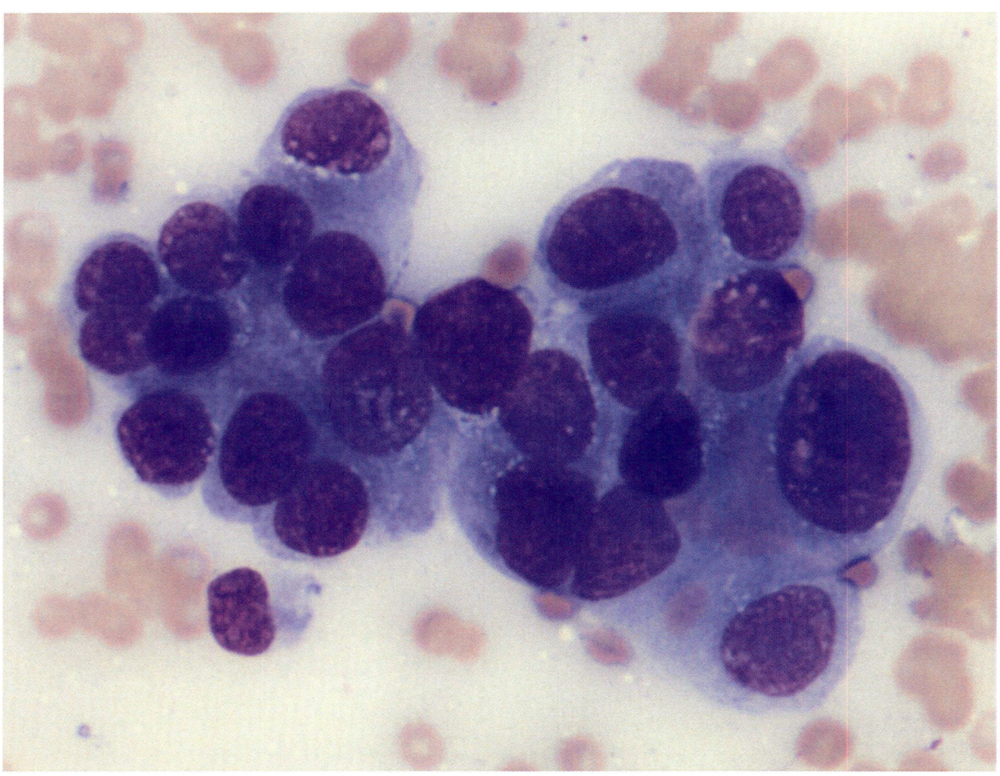

Figure 2.

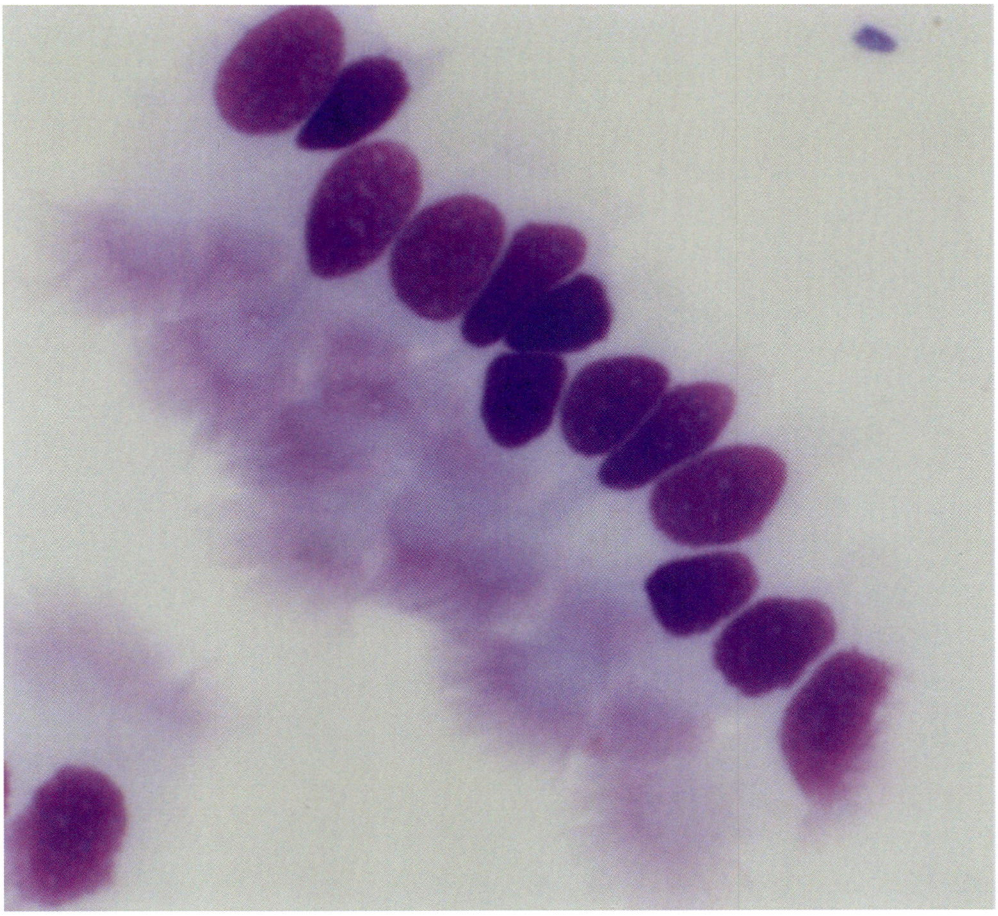

Figure 3.

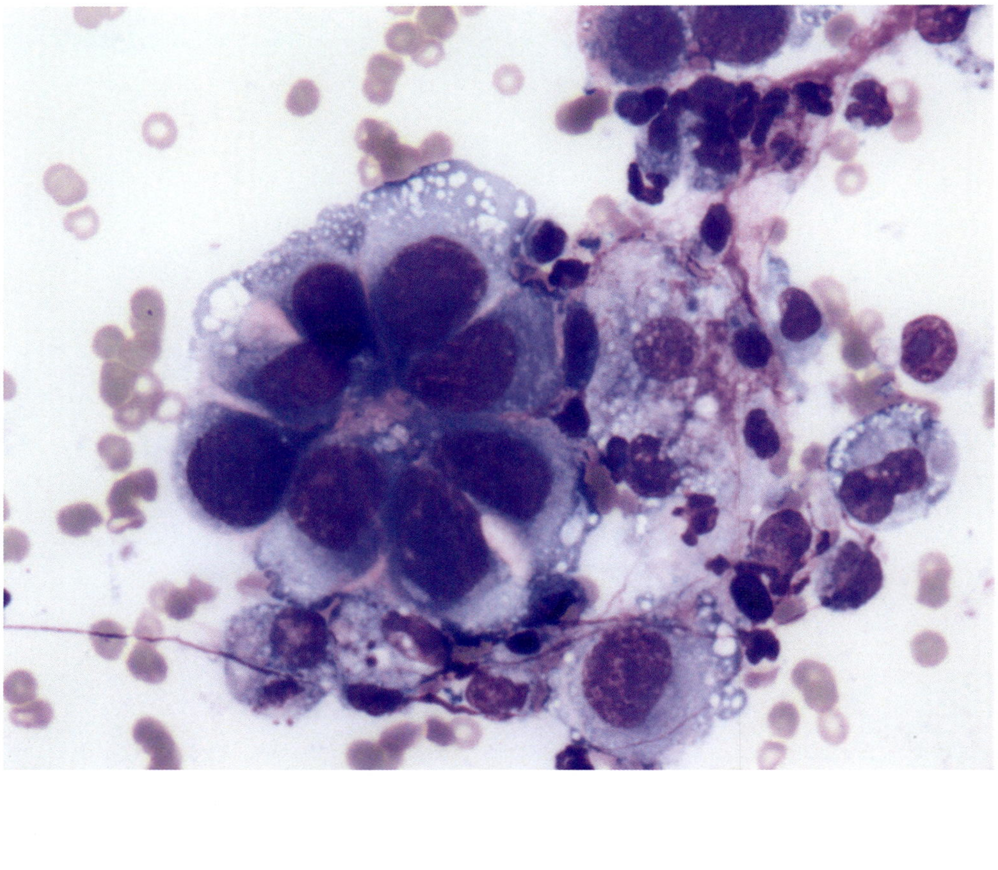

Figure 4.

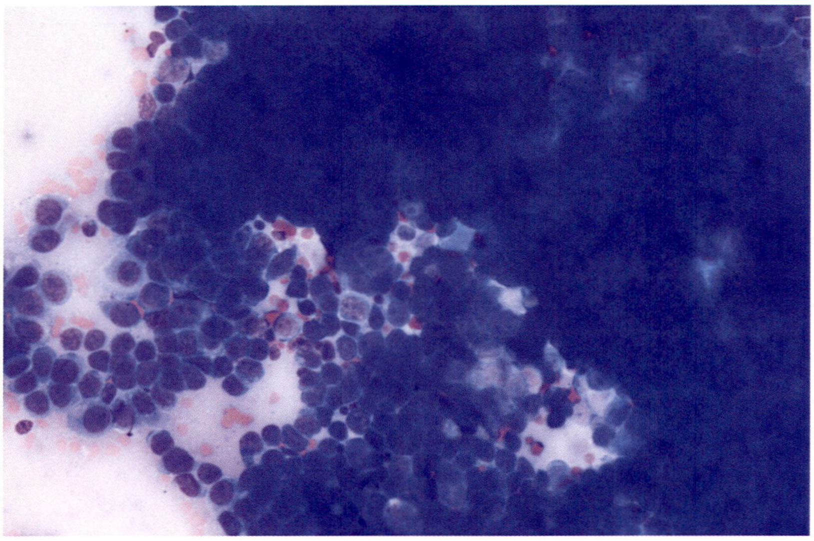

Figure 5. Transitional cell carcinoma. Cytological interpretation should be based on analysis of a monolayer. The central areas consisting of bulky groups of cells are not appropriate for evaluation.

Figures 6 and 7. Normal prostatic (6) and gastric (7) epithelium, in which a honeycomb pattern can be observed.

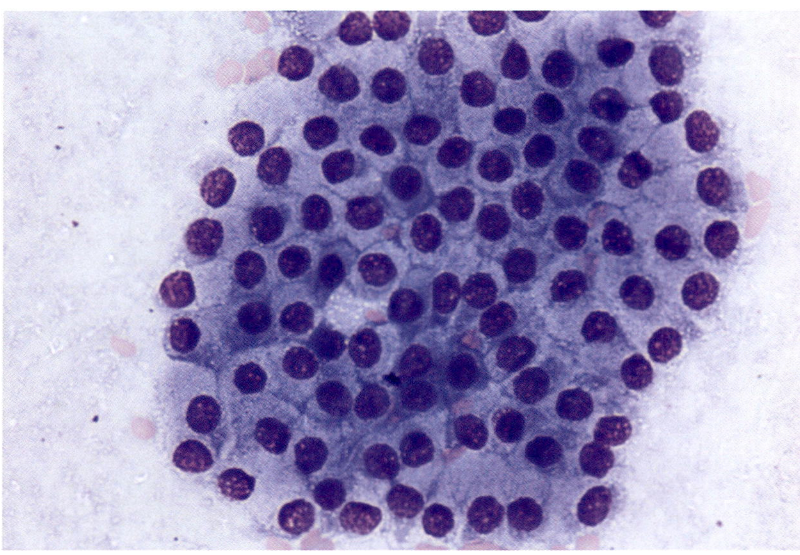

Figure 6.

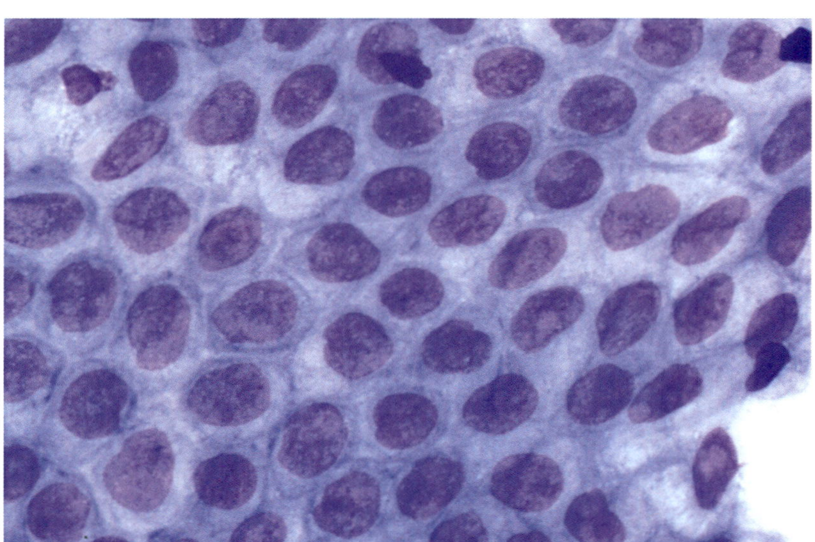

Figure 7.

Figures 8 and 9. Squamous cell carcinomas. Cells exfoliate individually or in groups without intercellular bridges.

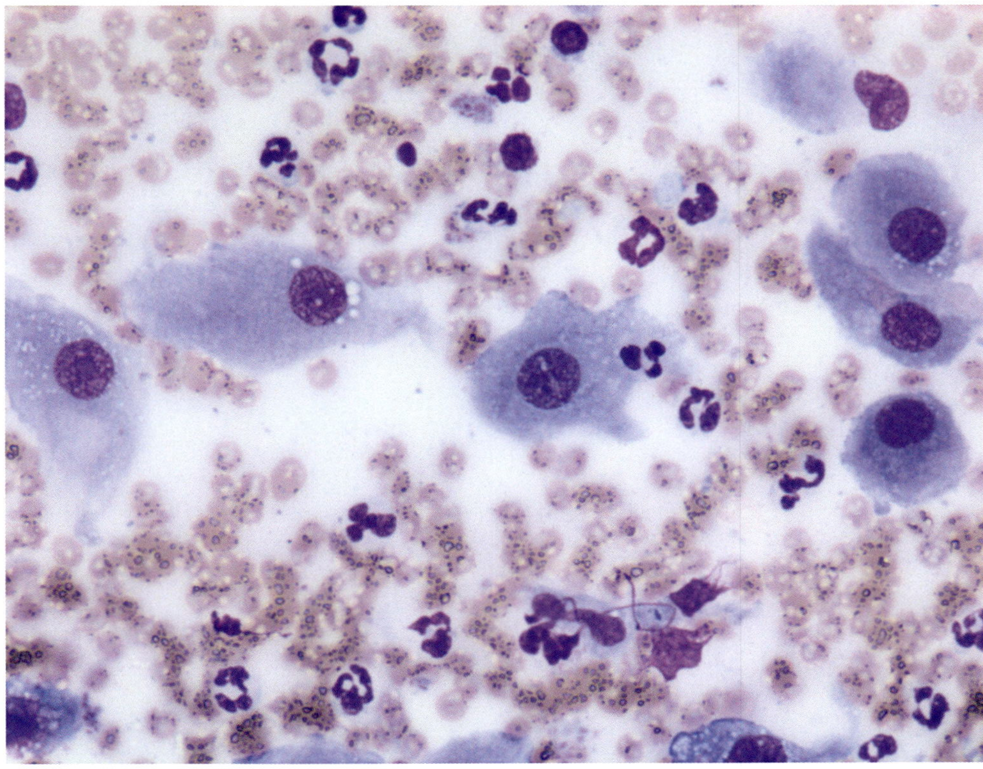

Figure 8.

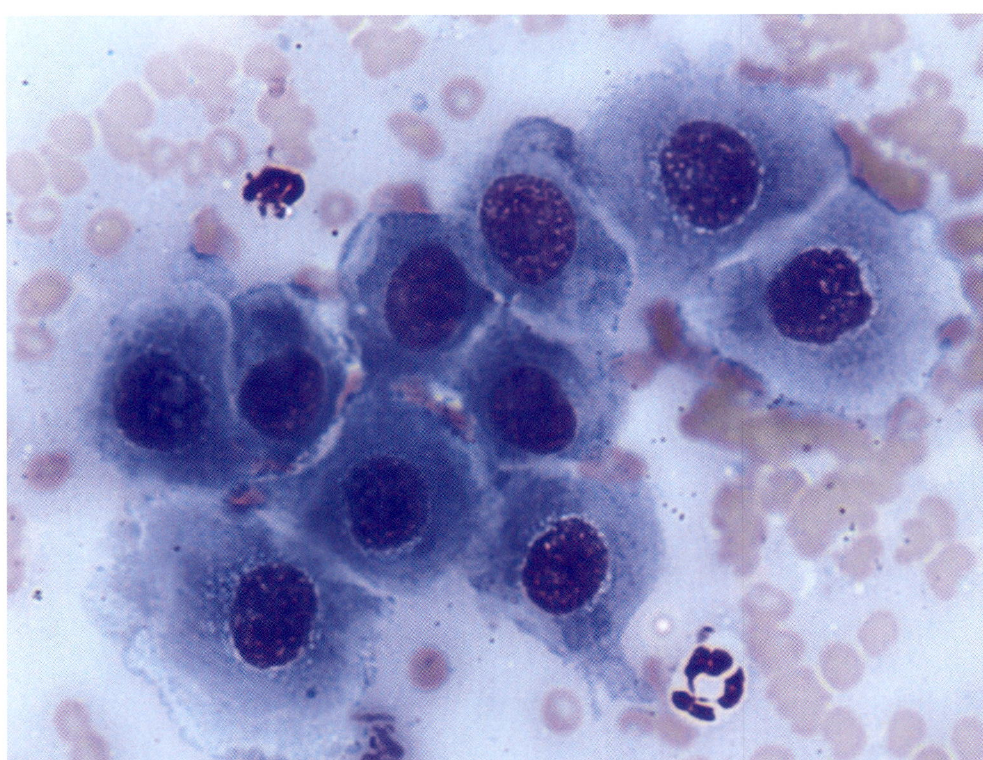

Figure 9.

Figures 10–15. Different neuroendocrine tumours with a similar cytological picture: thyroid carcinoma (10, 14), pheochromocytoma (11), hepatic carcinoid tumour (12), anal sac carcinoma (13), and insulinoma (15).

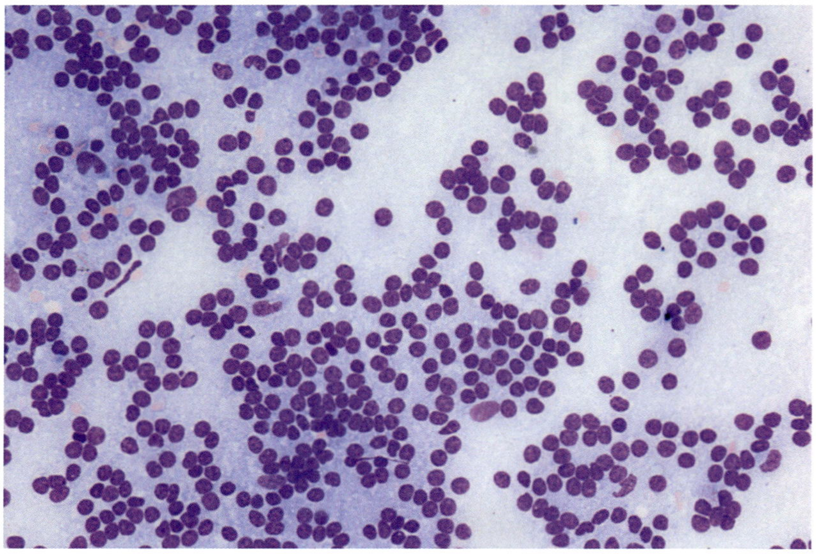

Figure 10.

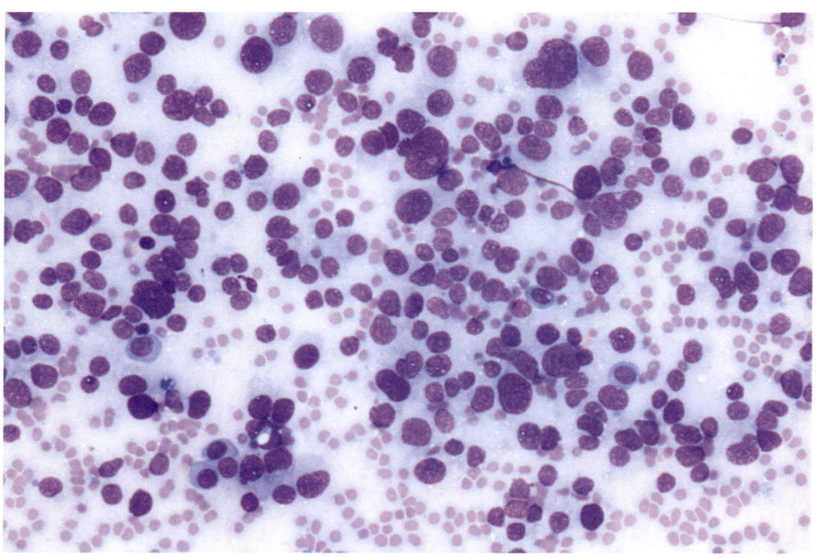

Figure 11.

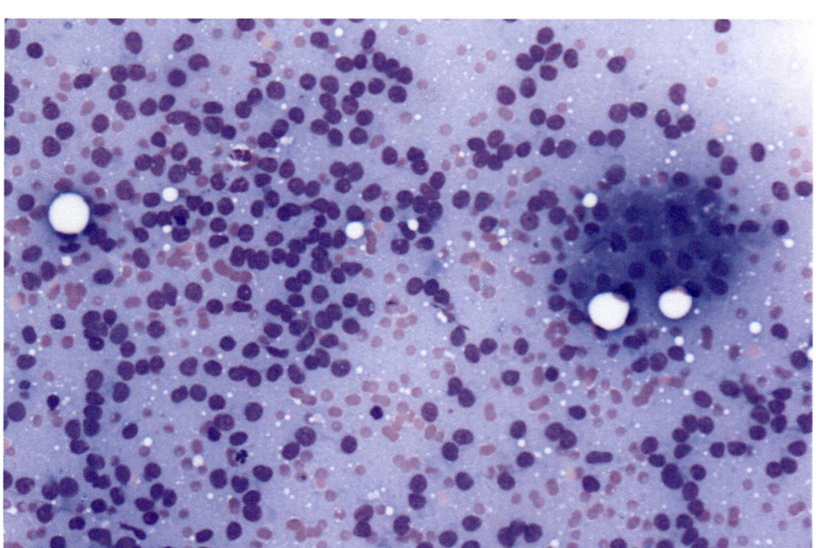

Figure 12.

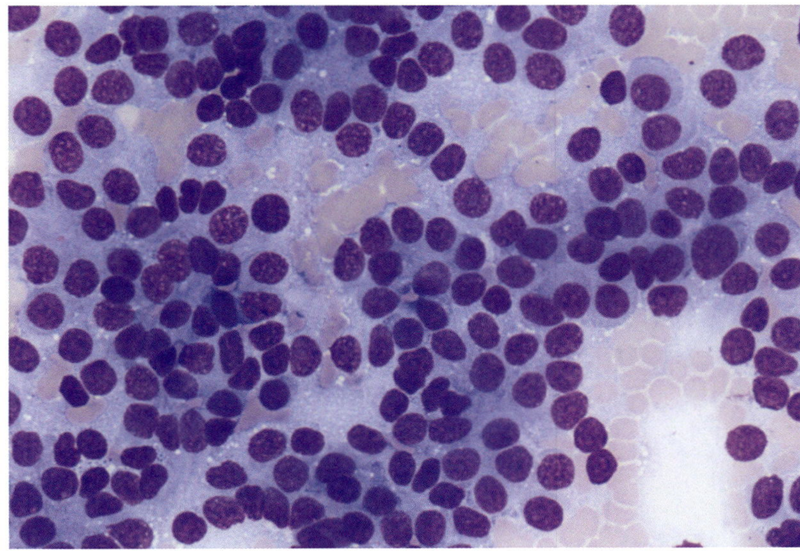

Figure 13.

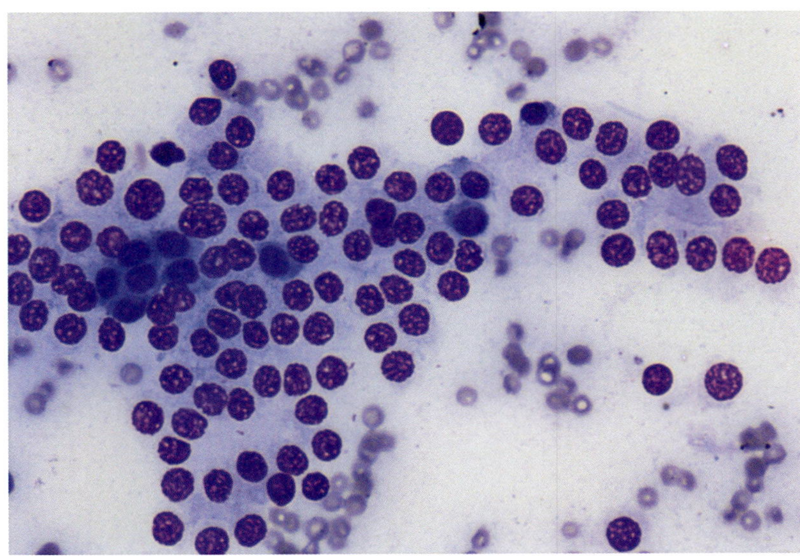

Figure 14.

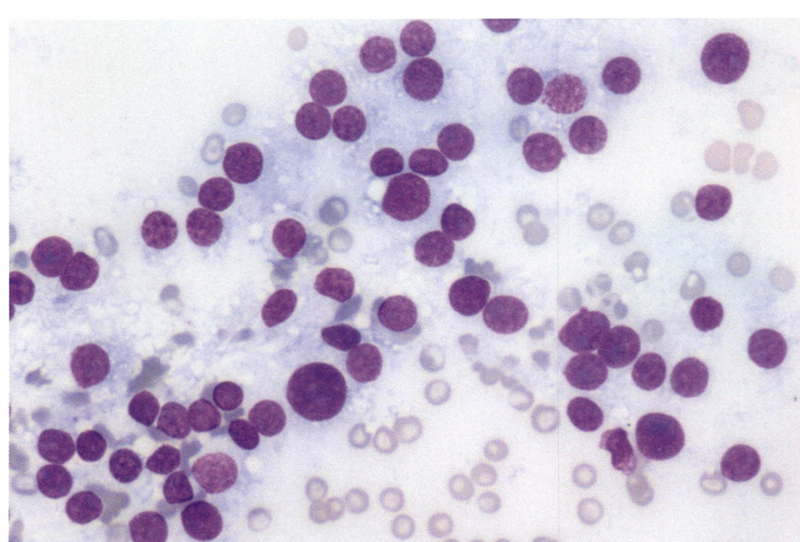

Figure 15.

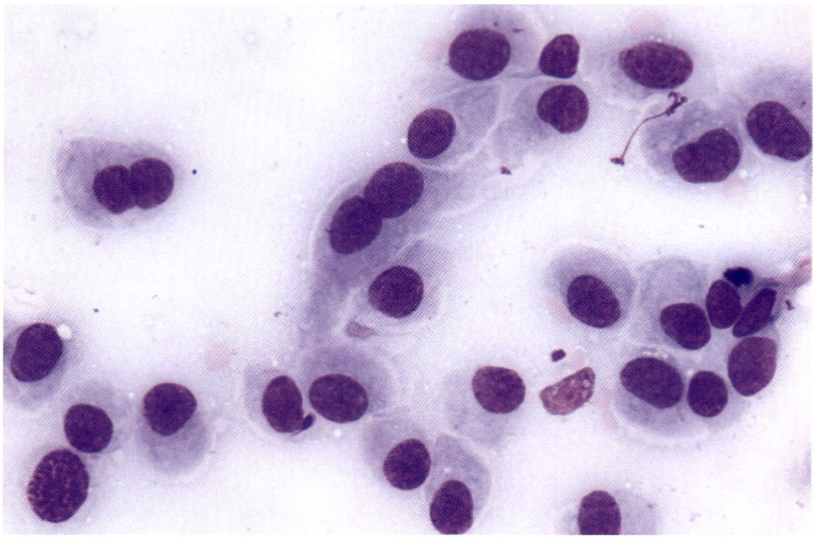

Figure 16. Anaplastic carcinoma (histopathological diagnosis). Cytologically, epithelial cells cannot be identified.

Figures 17 and 18. Groups of resting mesothelial cells, with and without a hyaline matrix, in abdominal and pleural fluid cytology samples, respectively.

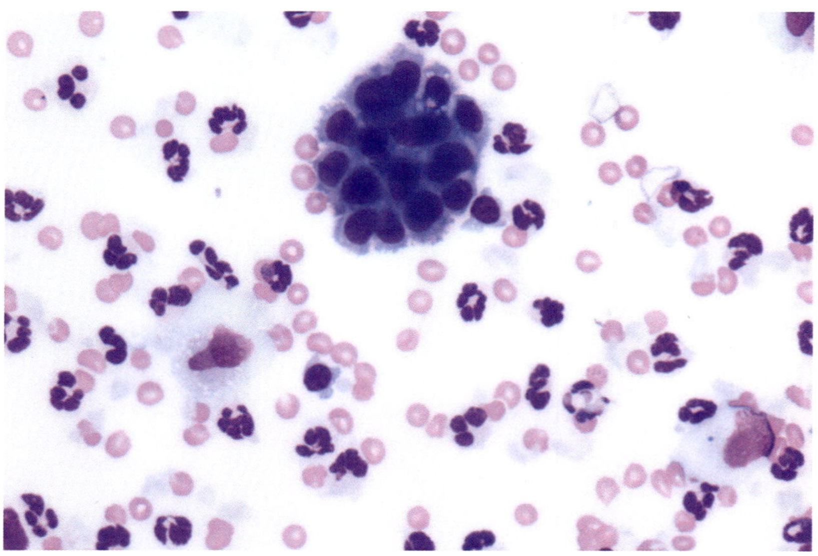

Figure 17.

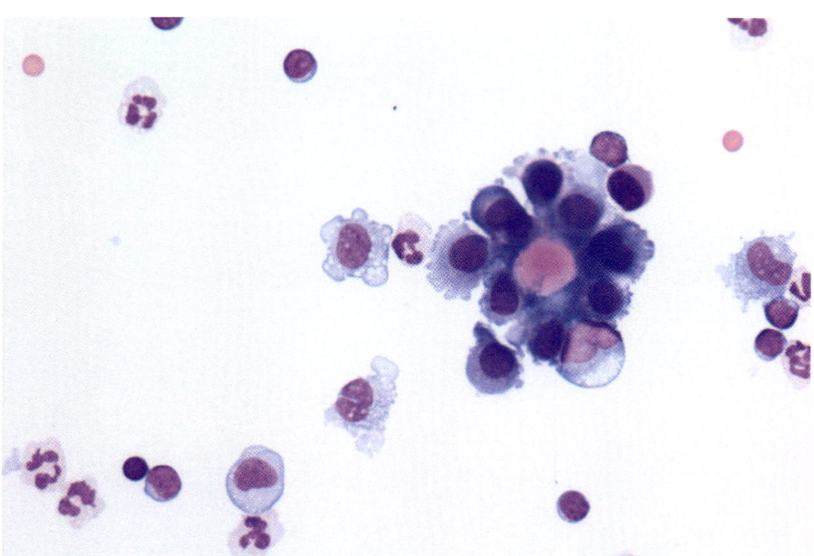

Figure 18.

## CELL MORPHOLOGY

Although epithelial cells are described as large, polygonal cells, their morphology (size, shape, and quantity and type of cytoplasm) varies depending on the dermal layer or organ to which they belong:

- Rounded, small- to medium-sized cells with a very high nucleus:cytoplasm ratio. This morphology is typical of the basal cells of the dermis (Fig. 19) or the biliary epithelium (Fig. 20). If observed individually, these cells can be mistaken for round, lymphoid-like cells (Fig. 21). Resting mesothelial cells are very similar.
- Polygonal, medium- to large-sized cells, with variable amounts of cytoplasm. This is the most common morphology in glandular cells, the intermediate strata of the dermis, and the cuboidal cells of the respiratory and gastrointestinal epithelia (Figs. 22–24).
- Normal squamous cells are characterised by their large size, large amount of basophilic cytoplasm, and small, pyknotic nucleus (in normal conditions). The most differentiated cells are polygonal and may be folded (Fig. 25), but in SCC can be rounded, globose, or elongated (Figs. 26–27).

In the transitional epithelia of the urinary system several different morphologies can be observed simultaneously (Fig. 28). These cells can contain large eosinophilic granular inclusions or magenta glycosaminoglycan inclusions (Fig. 29).

The epithelia of the respiratory and intestinal tract contain elongated columnar cells, which should not be confused with conjunctive cells: the former are more polygonal, with the nucleus located at one of the poles, and tend to form groups or palisades. Cilia may be attached to the opposite pole to the nucleus, but often detach due to handling of the sample (Fig. 30).

Figures 19 and 20. Epithelial cells with high nucleus:cytoplasm ratio: basal cells (19) and biliary epithelium (arrow) together with atypical hepatocytes (20).

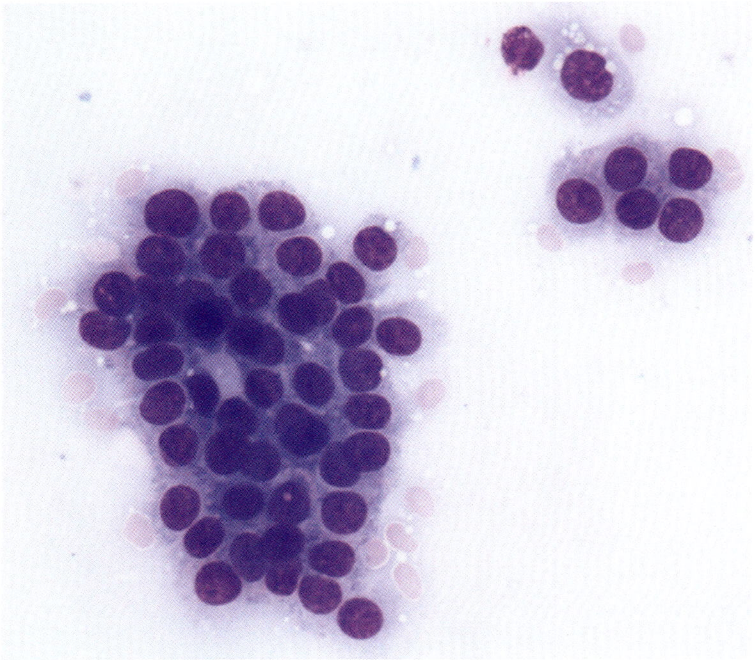

Figure 19.

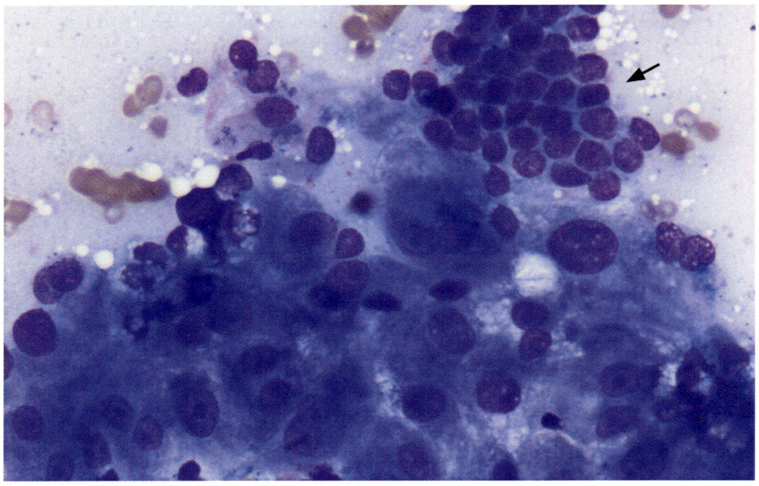

Figure 20.

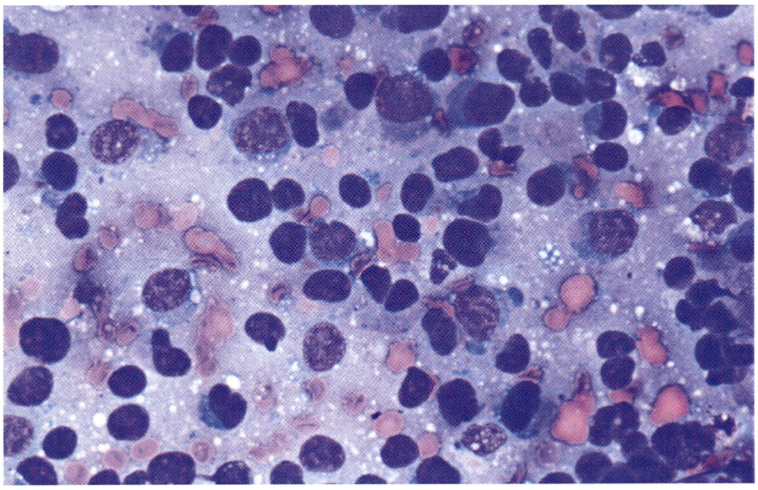

Figure 21. Cholangiocarcinoma. Bile cells have been exfoliated individually and resemble lymphoid cells.

Figures 22–24. Epithelial cells with moderate/abundant cytoplasm: lung carcinoma (22), adrenal cortex carcinoma (23), and cuboidal cells from a nasal carcinoma (24).

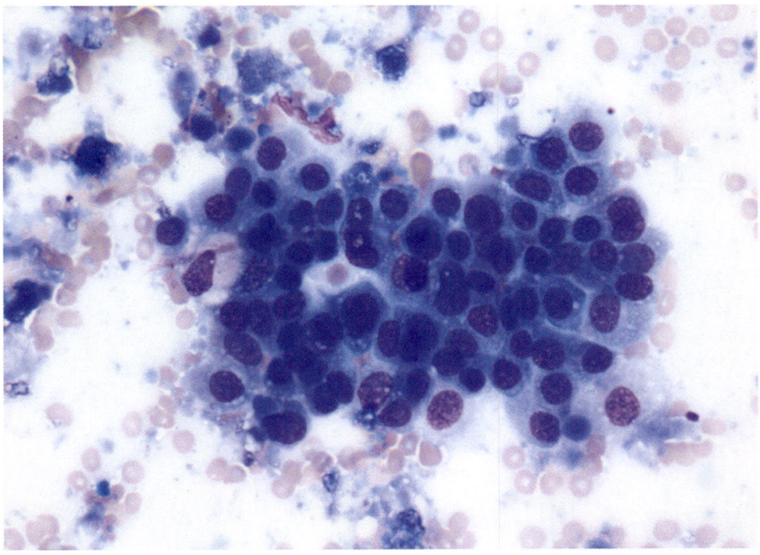

Figure 22.

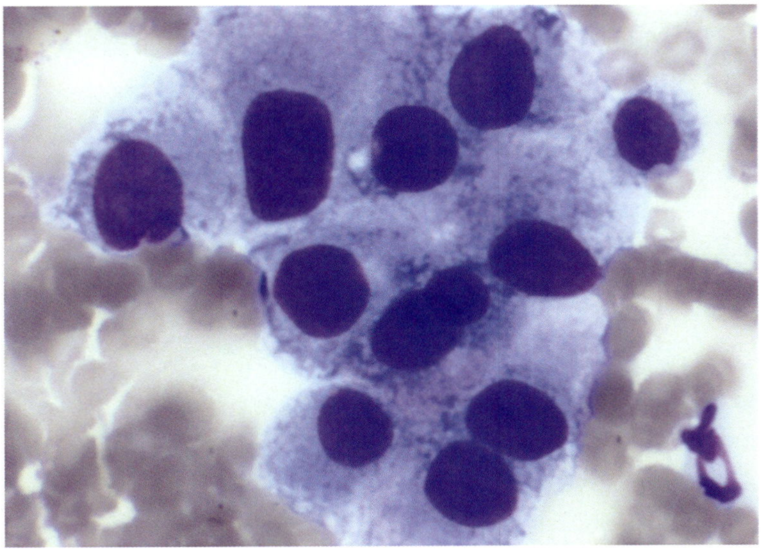

Figure 23.

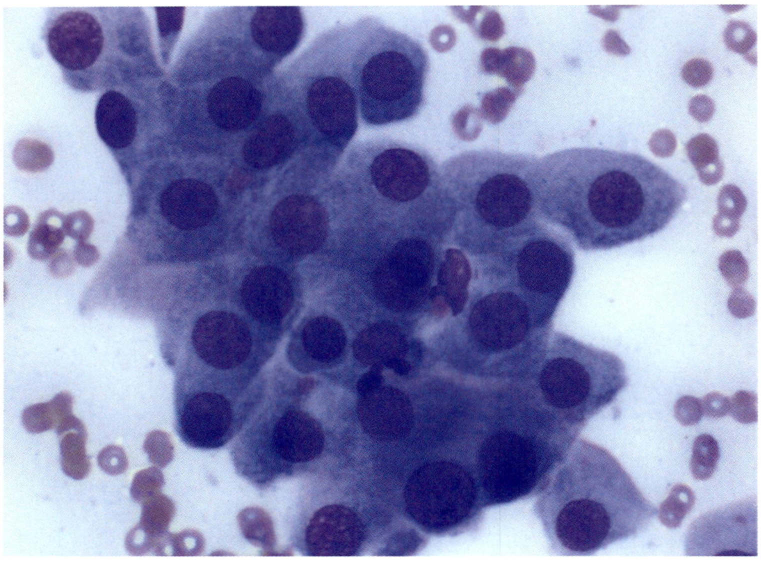

Figure 24.

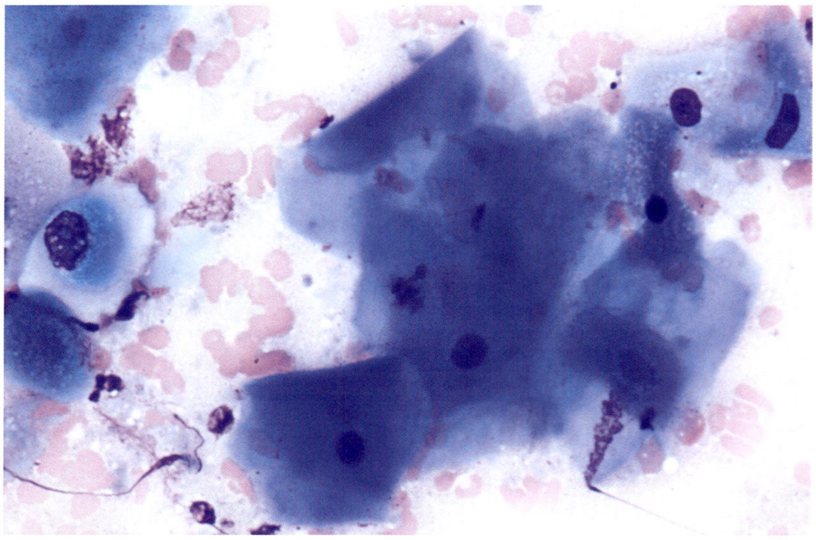

Figure 25. Normal, polygonal, and folded squamous cells, with a pyknotic nucleus.

Figures 26 and 27. Squamous cell carcinoma. Cells exhibit a globose (26) and polygonal/elongated (27) morphology.

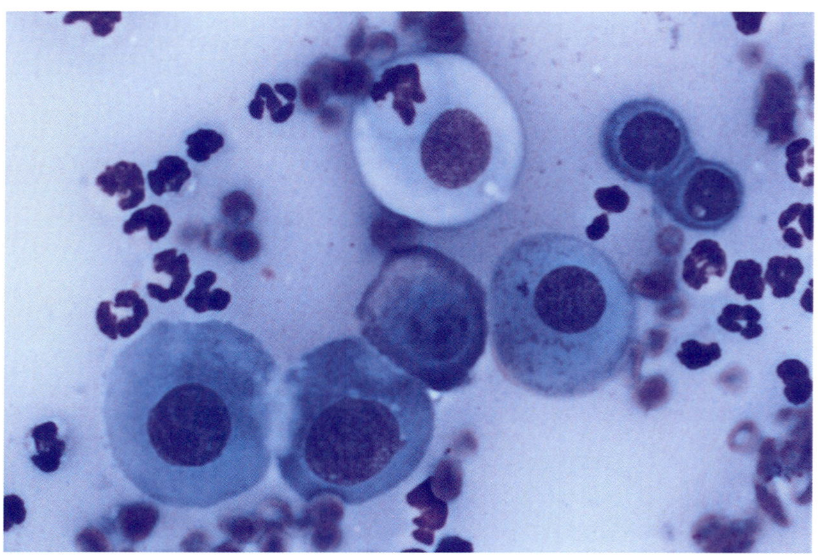

Figure 26.

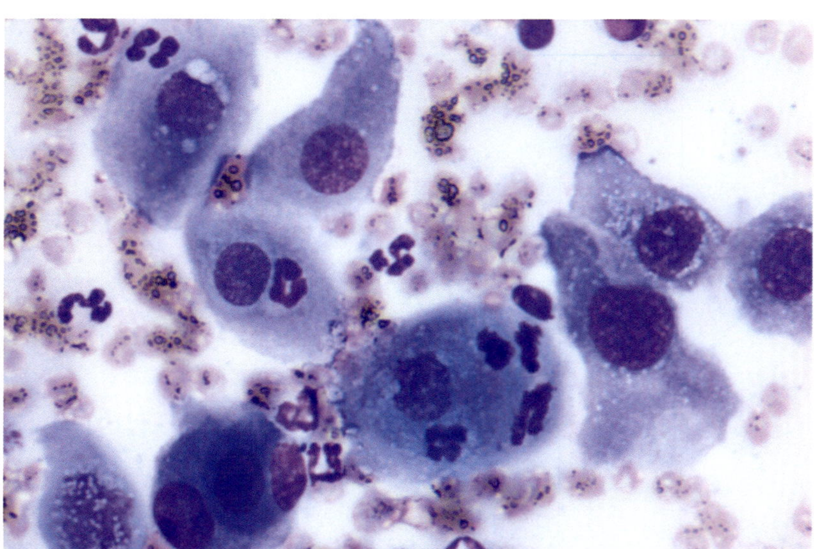

Figure 27.

Figure 28. Transitional cell carcinoma sample in which cells from different strata are observed.

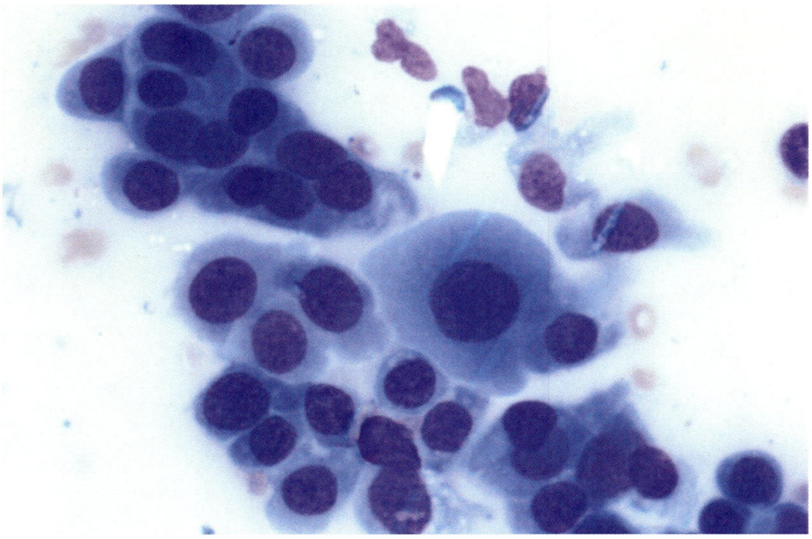

Figure 29. Glycosaminoglycan inclusions (arrows) in cells from a transitional cell carcinoma.

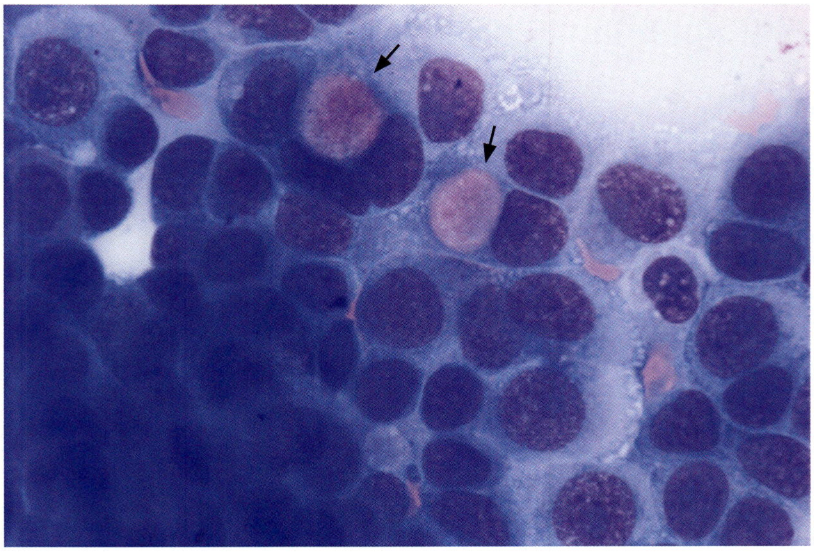

Figure 30. Ciliated columnar cells from the respiratory epithelium (nasal wash sample).

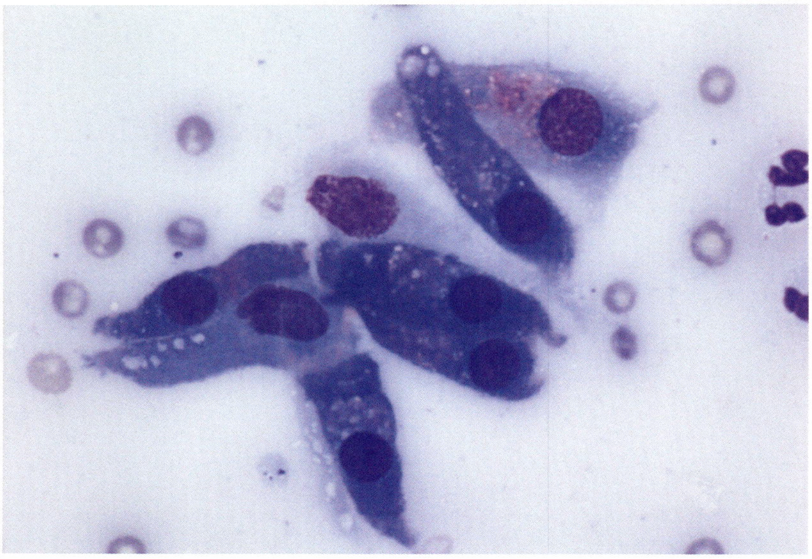

## CYTOPLASMIC VACUOLES

Glandular epithelia are defined by the presence of cytoplasmic vacuoles. Occasionally, a mixed population of glandular cells and reserve basal cells may be observed (Fig. 31).

The cells of most glands contain macrovacuoles, the number and size of which can vary depending on the structure in question and the degree of cellular differentiation (Figs. 32 and 33). Vacuole size and number will vary amongst cells in a given cytological preparation (Fig. 34).

Occasionally, glandular cells acquire a signet-ring morphology, characterised by the presence of a single large vacuole that compresses and displaces the nucleus to the periphery (Fig. 35). This morphology may also be observed in macrophages (Fig. 36).

The presence of microvacuoles, which lend the cytoplasm a characteristic moth-eaten or granular appearance, is typical of the perianal gland (Fig. 37) and hepatocytes (Fig. 38), and is also observed in the prostate. Although hepatocytes acquire macrovacuoles during degenerative processes, the moth-eaten appearance of the rest of the cytoplasm is maintained (Fig. 39).

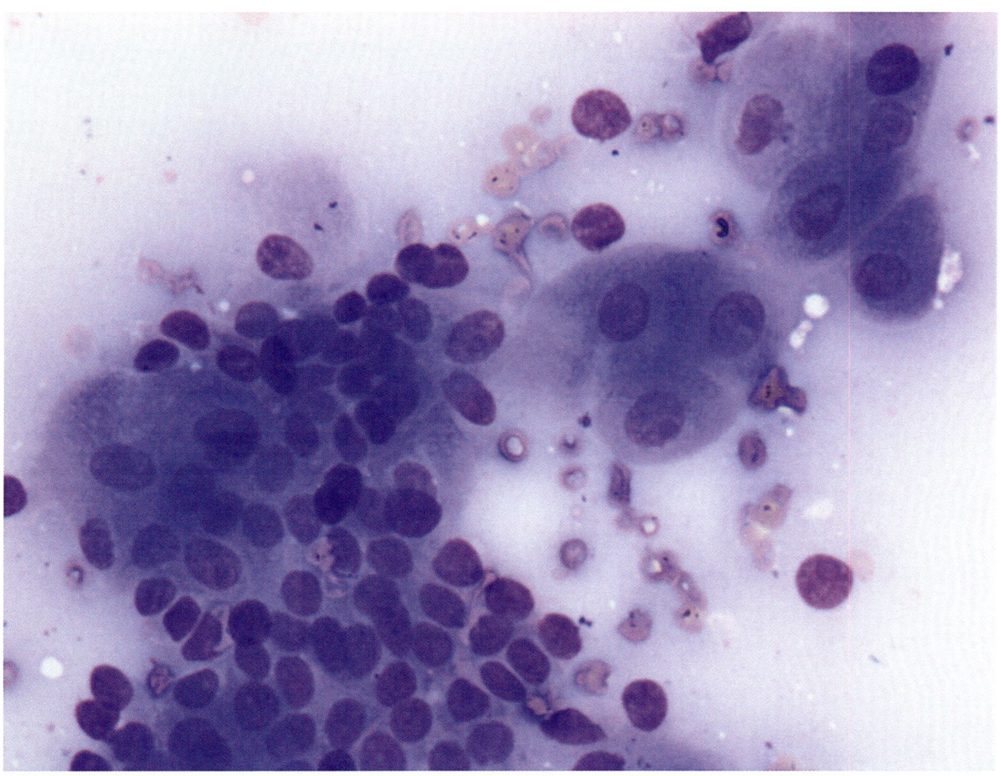

Figure 31. Glandular and reserve basal cells in a perianal tumour cytology sample.

Figures 32 and 33. Sebaceous cell adenoma (32) and adenocarcinoma (33). The number of vacuoles in the cells depends on the degree of differentiation.

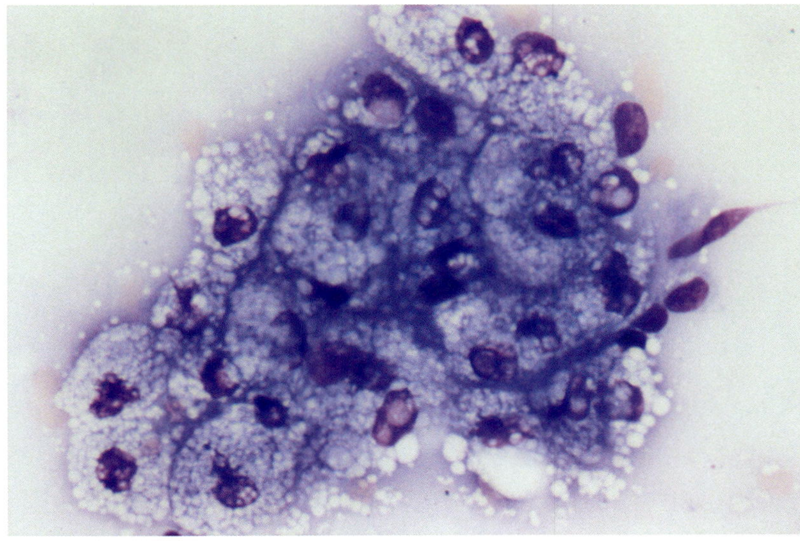

Figure 32.

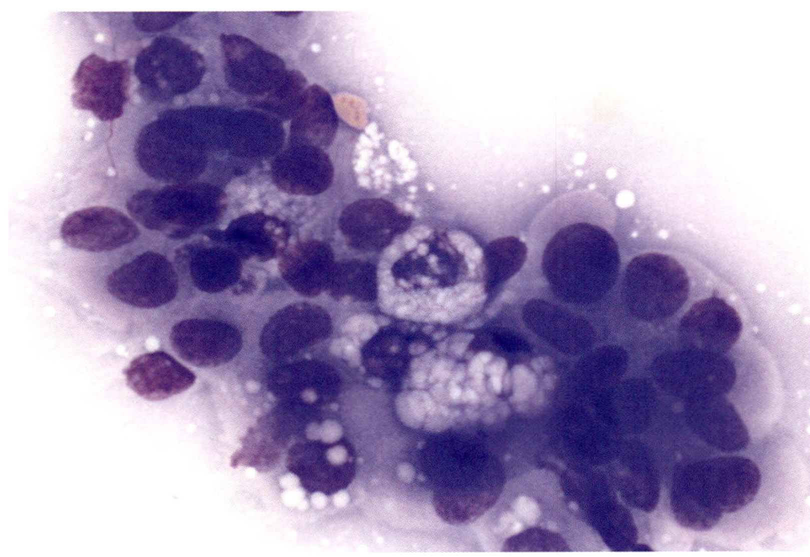

Figure 33.

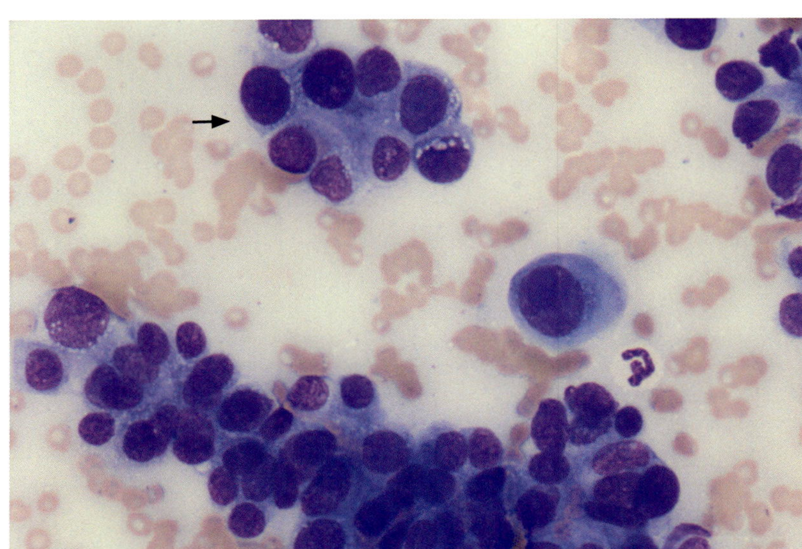

Figure 34. Cutaneous adenocarcinoma. In addition to cytoplasmic vacuoles (not present in all cells), the acinar structure (arrow) enables identification of a glandular origin.

Figures 35 and 36. Signet-ring cells in a sebaceous adenocarcinoma sample (35) and a macrophage in a tracheal wash sample (36).

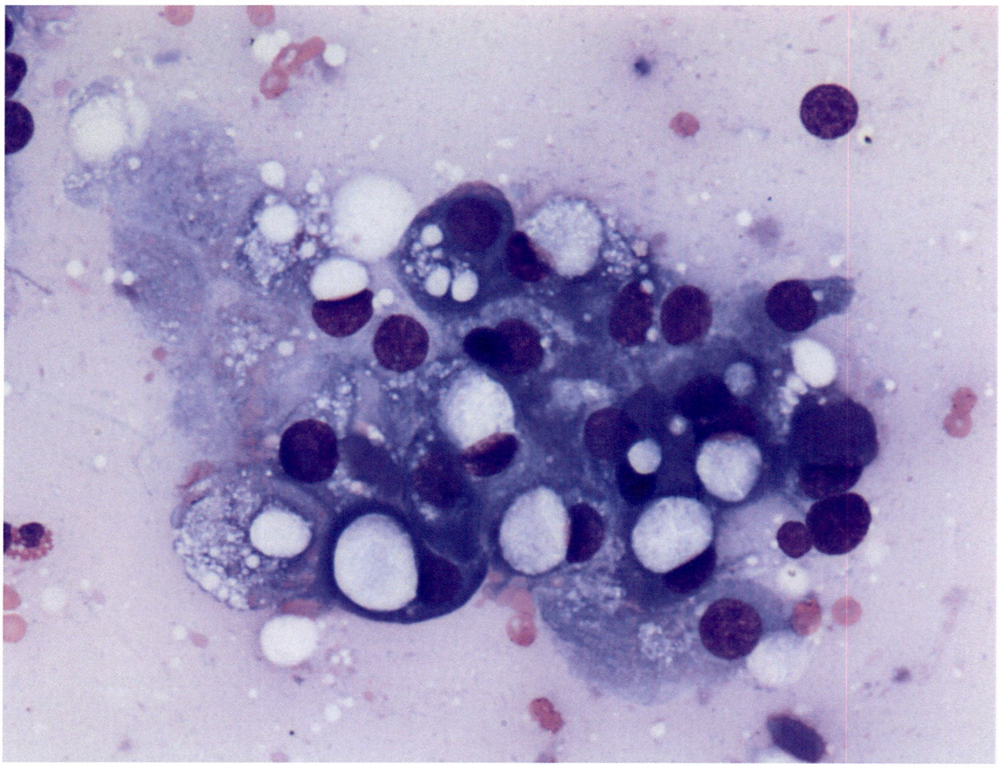

Figure 35.

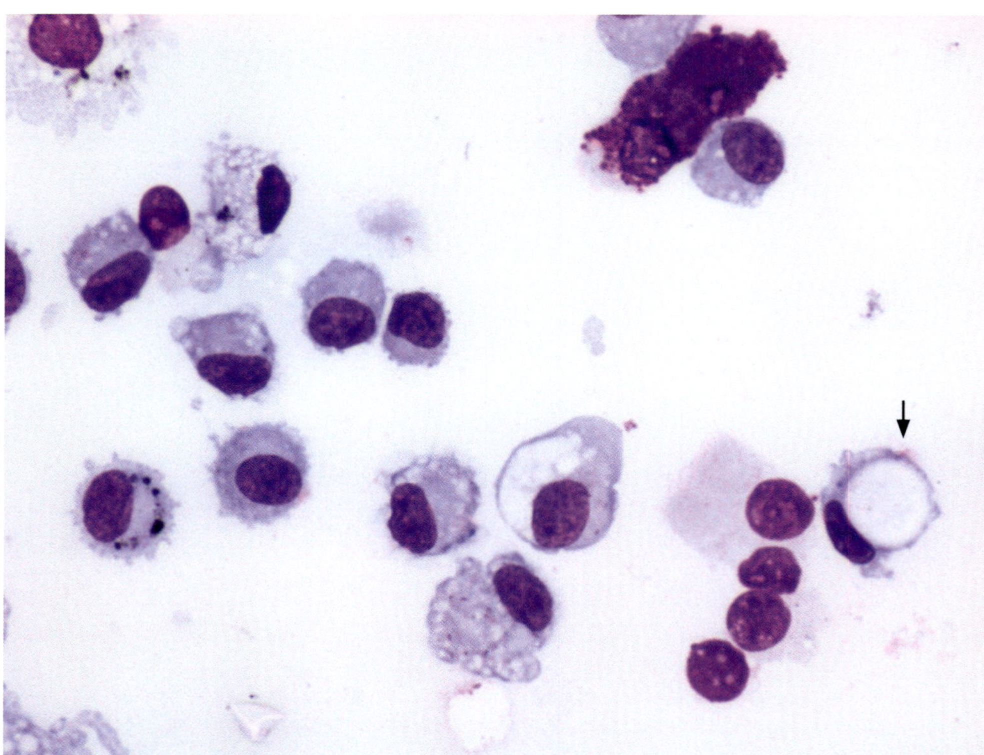

Figure 36.

Figures 37 and 38. Perianal gland cells (37) and hepatocytes (38) in which microvacuolated, moth-eaten cytoplasm is evident.

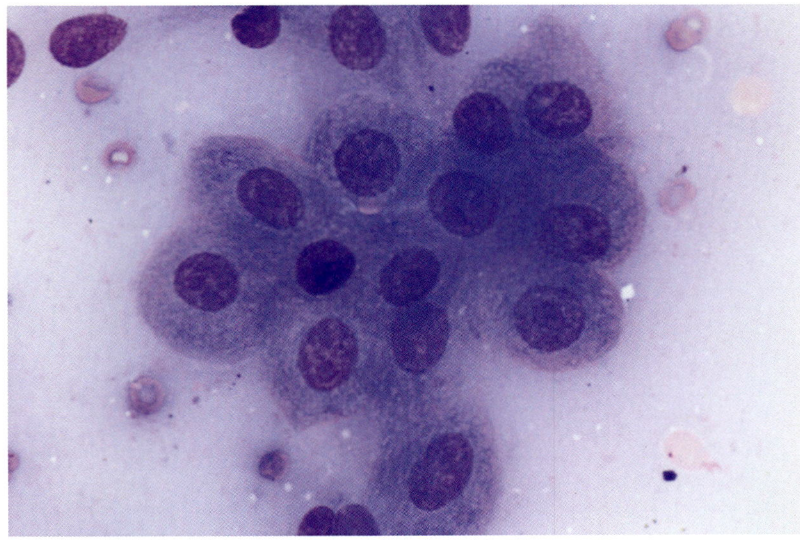

Figure 37.

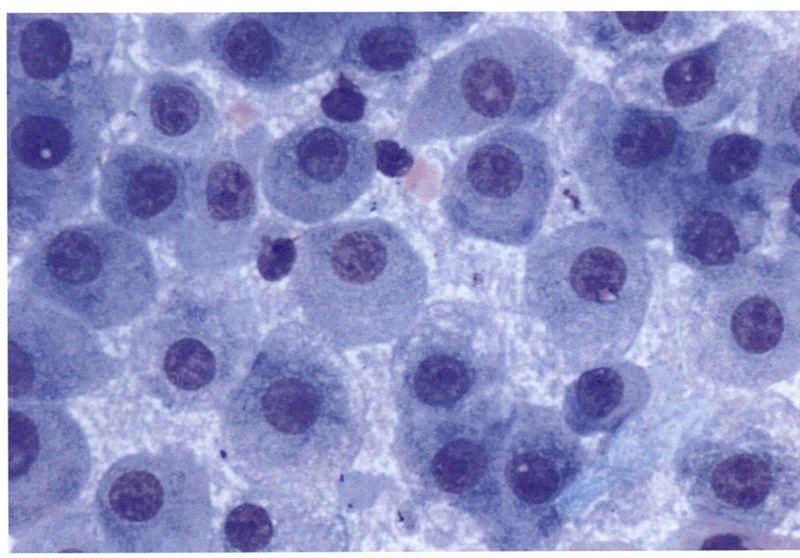

Figure 38.

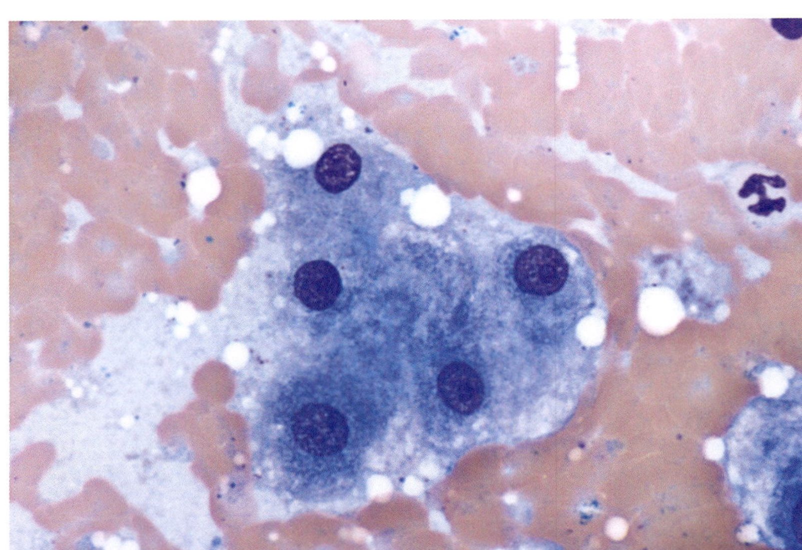

Figure 39. Hepatocytes exhibiting lipid vacuolar degeneration (macrovacuoles) and the remaining microvacuolated cytoplasm.

## CRITERIA FOR MALIGNANCY

In general, the criteria for malignancy for epithelial tumours are the same as those applied to other tumour types (Fig. 40). However, there are some specific criteria.

In some cases, the presence of abundant epithelial cells is sufficient to establish a diagnosis of malignancy. In normal conditions, renal cytology reveals few epithelial cells, which in cats may contain lipid vacuoles (Fig. 41). In pulmonary cytology, the predominant cell is the macrophage (Fig. 42). In hepatic cytology, groups of biliary cells are only observed occasionally (Fig. 20). Regardless of whether the criteria for malignancy are fulfilled, a high degree of cellularity indicates that the primary differential diagnosis should be renal, pulmonary, or biliary carcinoma (Figs. 43–45).

In normal conditions, the groups of cells should be well organised, such that a nucleus-cytoplasm-nucleus-cytoplasm sequence is observed (Fig. 46). Alterations in this sequence imply tissue disorganisation, and are indicative of malignancy (Fig. 47).

### The differences in certain structures between normal and neoplastic tissues are indicative of malignancy (Fig. 48).

Two particular malignancy criteria are applied to SCCs. The first is asynchronous maturation; large cells with abundant cytoplasm lack the pyknotic nucleus that should correspond to their degree of differentiation, and remain intact, large, and active. The second is perinuclear vacuolisation, which reflects atypical keratinisation (Figs. 49 and 50).

Many epithelial tumours, especially SCC, transitional cell carcinoma (TCC), and nasal carcinoma, are accompanied by intense inflammation. An apparently malignant, mixed inflammatory and tissue component should be interpreted with caution, since the observed changes may be dysplastic (Fig. 51). A carcinoma can only be identified if nuclear atypia are observed in the absence of inflammatory cells or if the atypia is so intense that it cannot be attributed to activation phenomena (Figs. 52 and 53).

In some epithelial tumours it is possible to observe inconsistencies between the cytological picture and the degree of malignancy:

- Neuroendocrine tumours do not usually exhibit marked nuclear atypia. In most cases, the nuclei are usually relatively homogeneous, although this does not imply that the tumour is benign (Fig. 54).
- In perianal gland tumours, cytology is the ideal technique to determine cellular origin (based on the presence of a characteristic microvacuolated cytoplasm). However, it does not allow differentiation of adenomas from carcinomas, both of which have a similar cytological picture, characterised by mild nuclear atypia, prominent nucleoli, and mild to moderate anisokaryosis (Fig. 55).
- Benign basal cell tumours may exhibit mild nuclear atypia, which, in this case, is not indicative of malignancy but is characteristic of active, immature cells (Fig. 56).

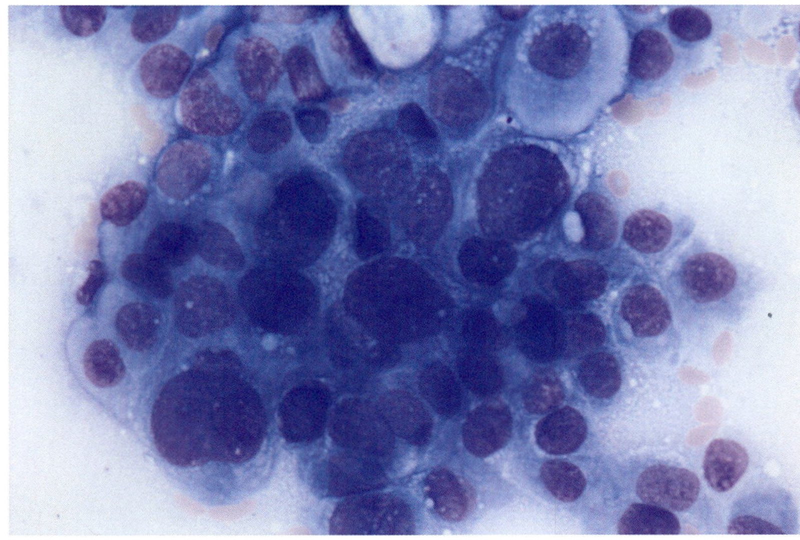

Figure 40. Transitional cell carcinoma in which nuclear atypia is observed.

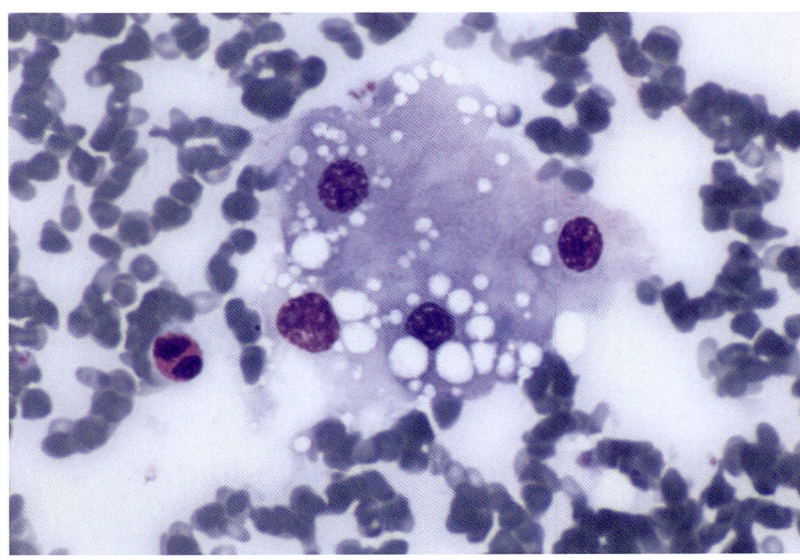

Figure 41. Renal epithelial cells with lipid vacuoles.

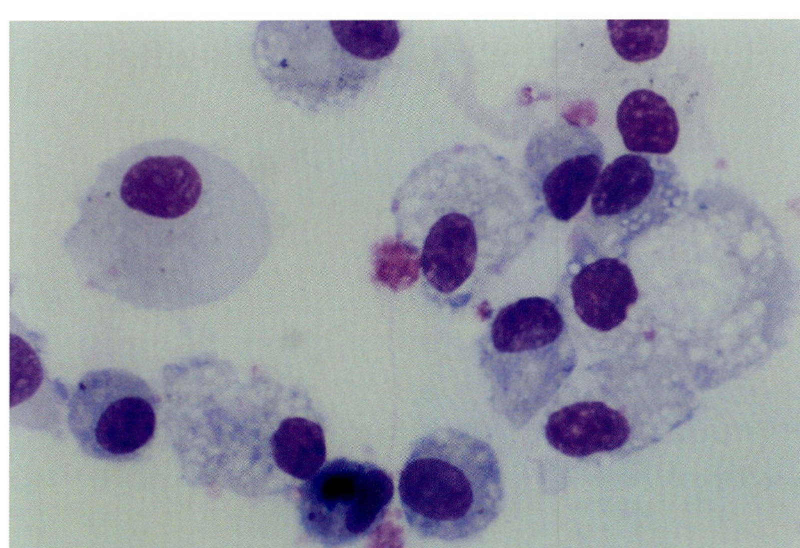

Figure 42. Tracheal wash sample containing multiple macrophages (normal cell population of the pulmonary alveolus).

Figures 43–45. Renal carcinoma (43), lung carcinoma (44), and cholangiocarcinoma (45). The high degree of cellularity is a criterion of malignancy.

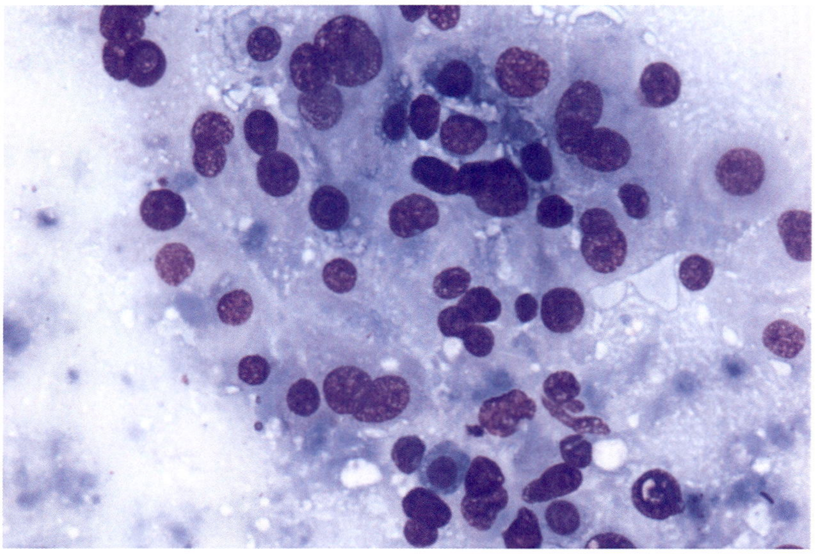

Figure 43.

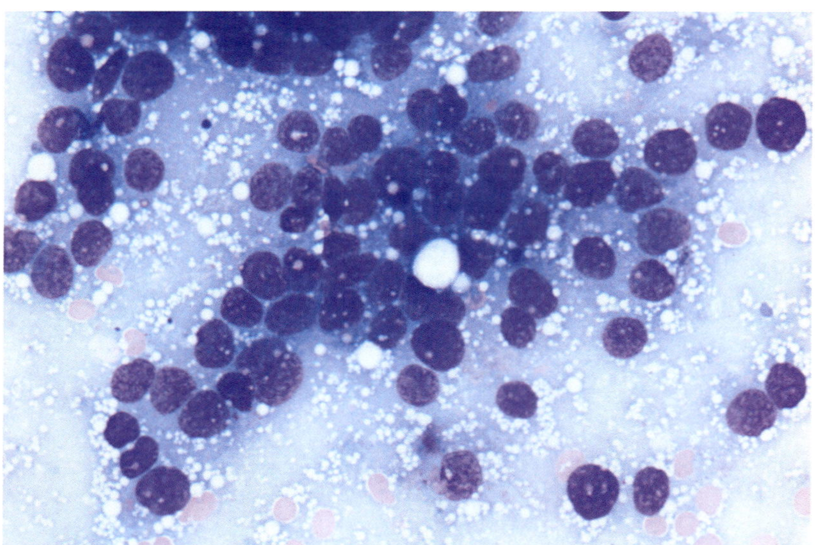

Figure 44.

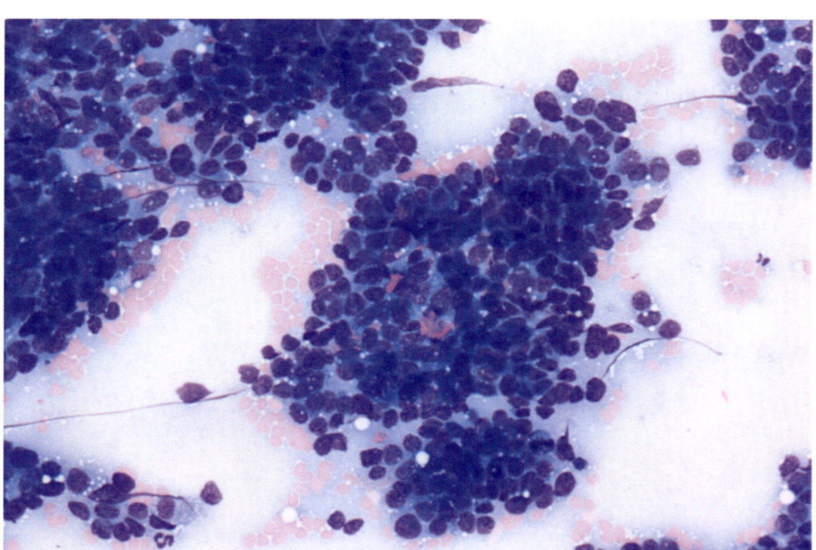

Figure 45.

Figures 46 and 47. Differences in cell group structure in a benign epithelial tumour (46) and a salivary adenocarcinoma (47).

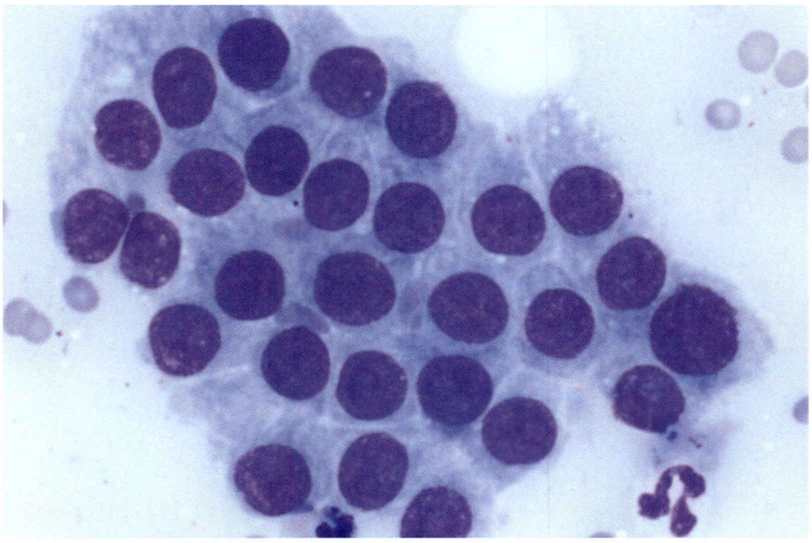

Figure 46.

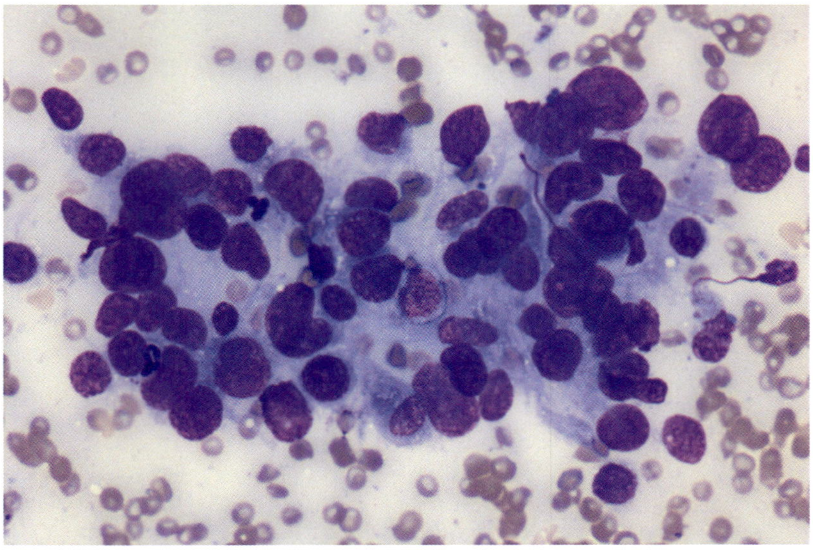

Figure 47.

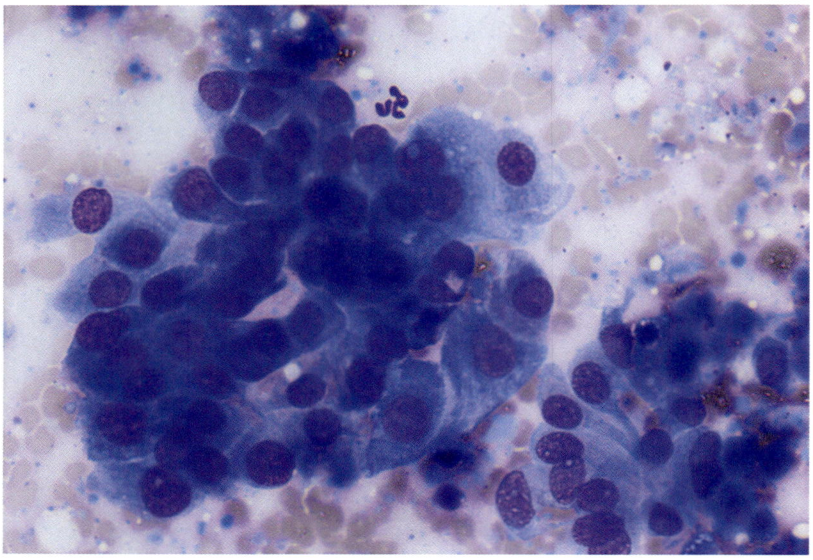

Figure 48. Prostatic carcinoma. The cells are very atypical, and exhibit a pattern that differs from the normal epithelial honeycomb pattern.

Figures 49 and 50. Squamous cell carcinomas in which asynchronous maturation and perinuclear vacuolisation are evident.

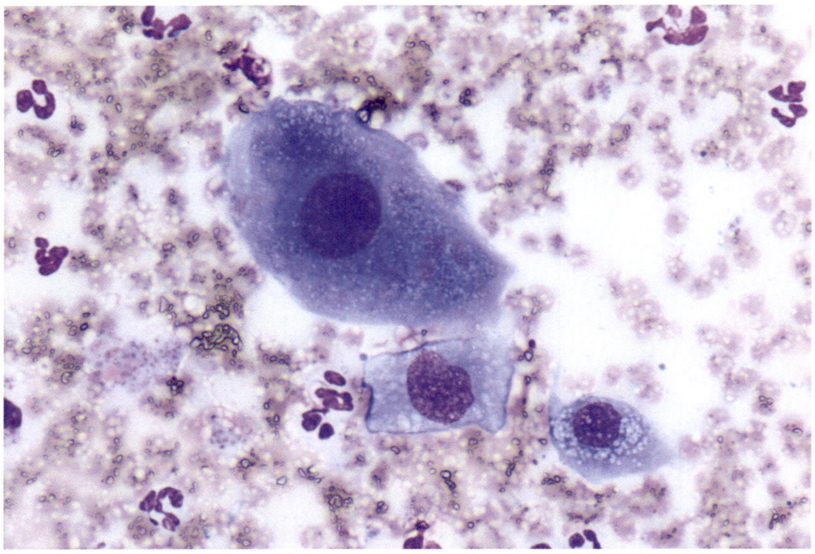

Figure 49.

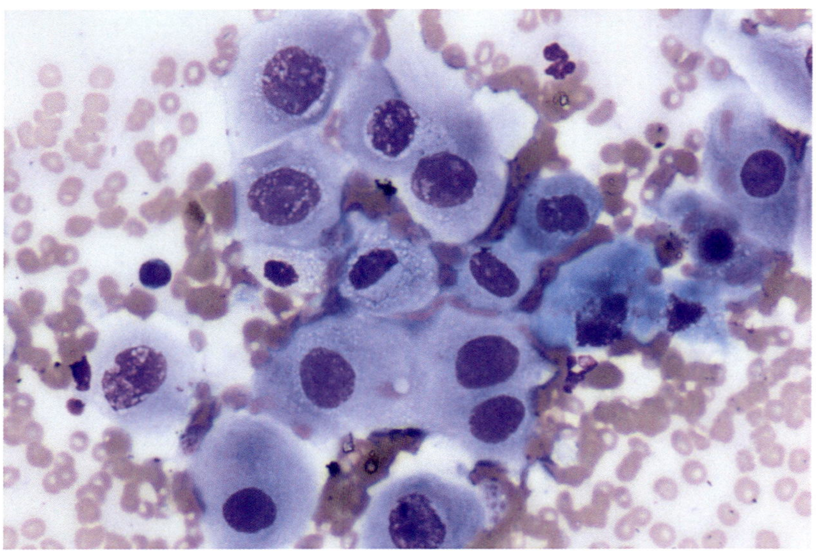

Figure 50.

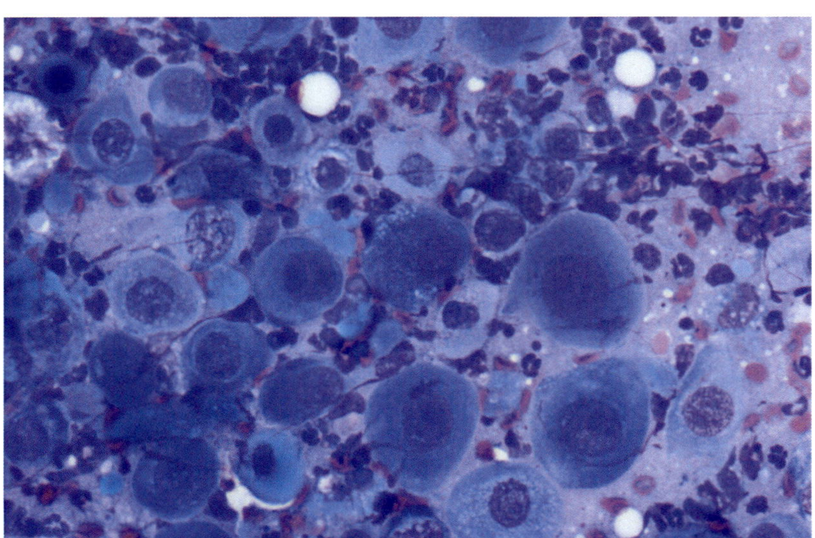

Figure 51. Squamous cell carcinoma accompanied by an intense inflammatory component. This cytological picture should be interpreted with caution.

Figures 52 and 53. Transitional cell carcinomas. Marked atypia in the absence of inflammation enables diagnosis.

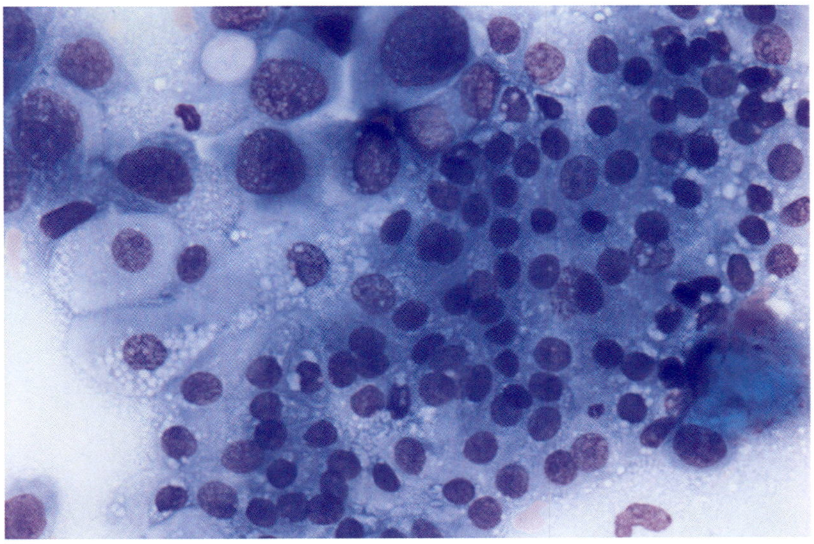

Figure 52.

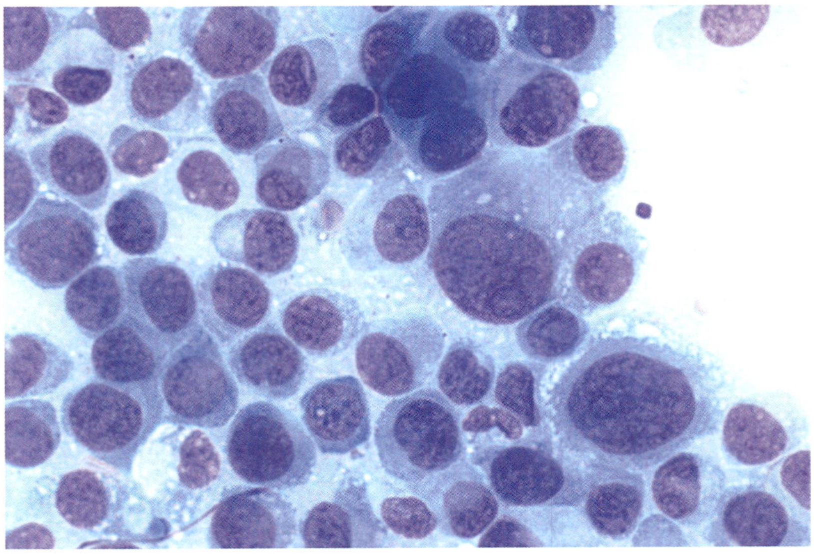

Figure 53.

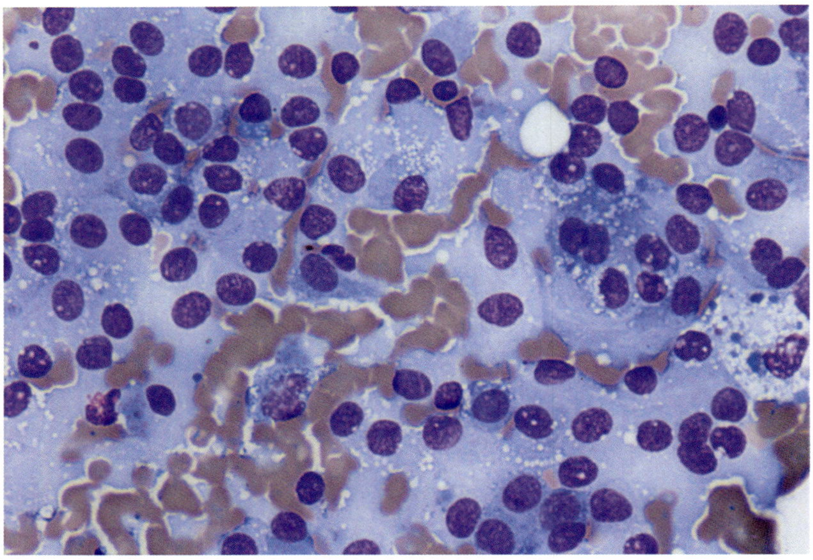

Figure 54. Lymph node metastasis of an anal sac carcinoma. Despite their malignancy, neuroendocrine tumours may exhibit little nuclear atypia.

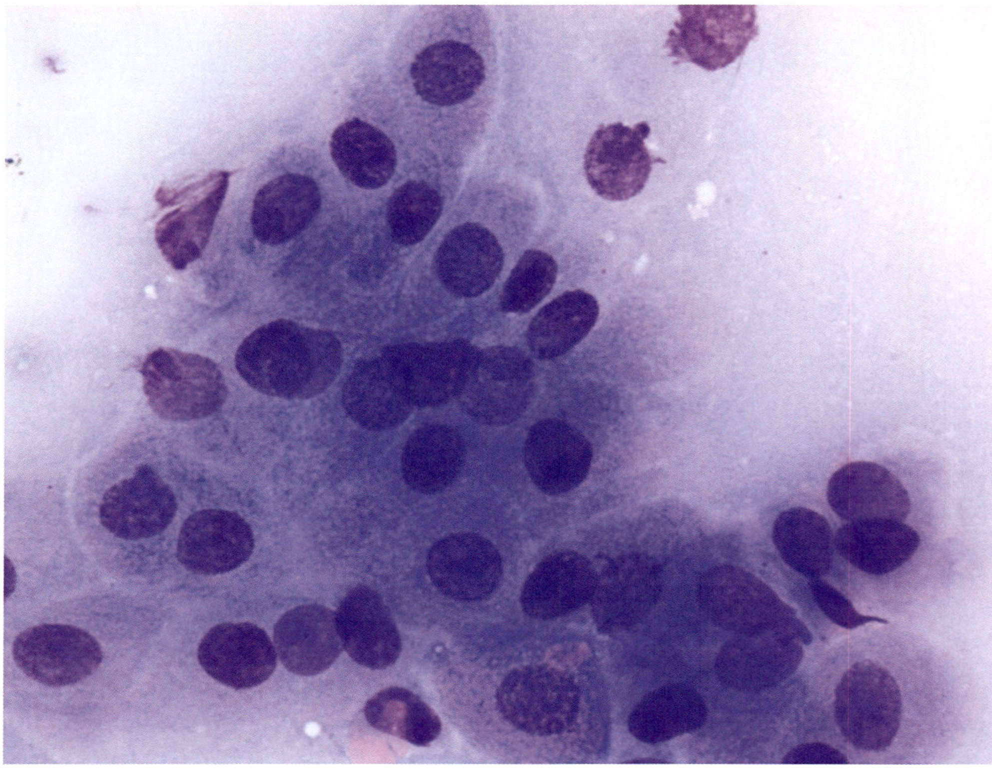

Figure 55. Perianal gland tumour. Adenoma and adenocarcinoma are cytologically indistinguishable.

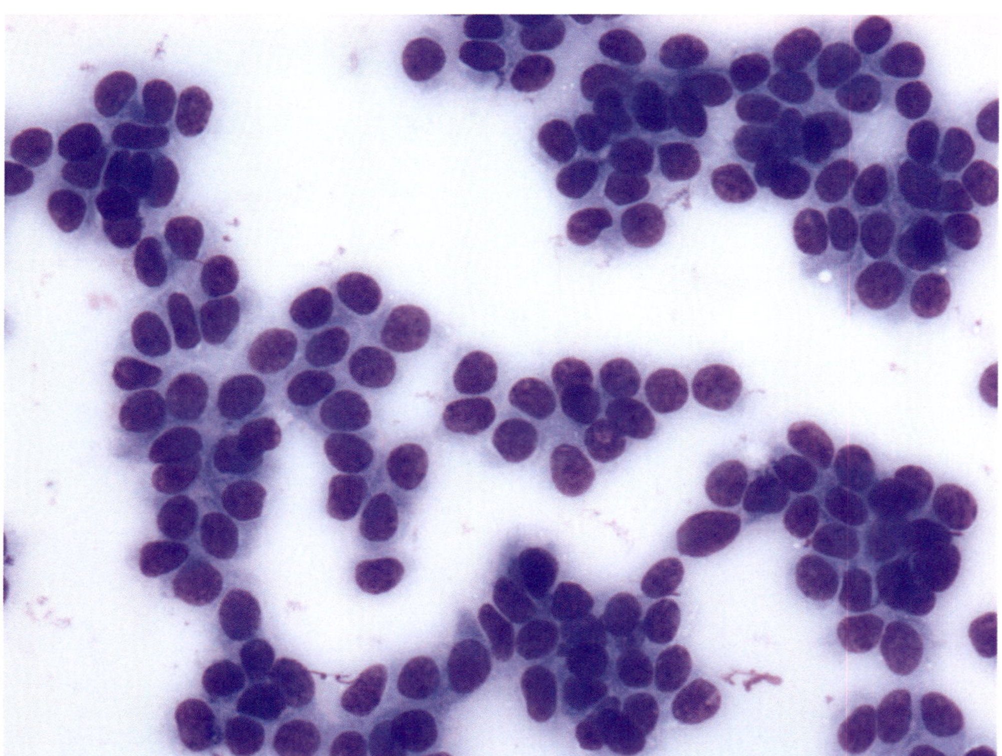

Figure 56. Basal cell tumour. Variations in nuclear size and shape do not imply malignancy.

## CRITERIA SPECIFIC TO CERTAIN EPITHELIAL TUMOURS

### CANINE MAMMARY TUMOURS

The usefulness of cytology in the diagnosis of canine mammary tumours (CMTs) is controversial. The great heterogeneity of CMTs (highly variable cell morphology in different parts of the lesion) can give rise to false negatives or, in the case of highly proliferative benign lesions, false positives. The ranges of sensitivity and specificity for differentiation of benign from malignant tumours are very broad (21–65 % and 56–94 %, respectively, depending on the study consulted). However, applying a strict cytological criterion proposed by Simon et al.,[12] these percentages increase to 88 % and 96 %, and tumour types are classified as follows:

- Adenoma: if the epithelial cells and cell groups are monomorphic and <5 % of cells fulfil more than three nuclear criteria of malignancy.
- Carcinoma: if the majority of epithelial cells and cell groups are markedly pleomorphic and >20 % of the cells fulfil more than three nuclear criteria of malignancy (Fig. 57).
- Adenoma with small number of atypical cells: if the cells and cell groups are compatible with adenoma, but 6–20 % of the cells fulfil more than three nuclear criteria of malignancy.

According to these authors, the evaluation must be carried out in at least four preparations, ideally by two independent cytologists. In this author's opinion, cytology should not be used to make decisions about the management of mammary tumours unless the proposed criteria are strictly applied.

There is no doubt as to the usefulness of cytology for differentiating between CMTs and other dermal or subcutaneous lesions located in mammary regions (lipomas, mast cell tumours) and for evaluating possible metastasis (Fig. 58).

### BASAL CELL TUMOURS

Tumours diagnosed cytologically as basal cell tumours include several histological types: follicular tumours (trichoblastoma, pilomatricoma), basal cell epithelioma, and sebaceous epithelioma, among others. In dogs, most of these tumours are benign. Therefore, differentiation prior to histological diagnosis is not strictly necessary, as a common diagnosis of tumour of basal origin can be established. In cats, pigmented basal cells, which should not be confused with melanocytes, are commonly observed (Fig. 59).

### HEPATOCELLULAR CARCINOMAS

Hepatocellular tumours are difficult to diagnose by cytology. Normal hepatocytes can be binucleated (and increase in number in hyperplasia/degeneration processes) and have a very prominent nucleolus. Therefore, a tumour cannot be considered a neoplasm based solely on these criteria. To ensure diagnostic accuracy, other nuclear atypia and/or mitoses must be clearly evident (Figs. 20 and 60–62).

Well-differentiated carcinomas are practically indistinguishable from hyperplasia. Two specific characteristics support a diagnosis of carcinoma:[7] the presence of capillaries traversing groups of hepatocytes, and naked nuclei surrounding groups of apparently normal hepatocytes (Fig. 63).

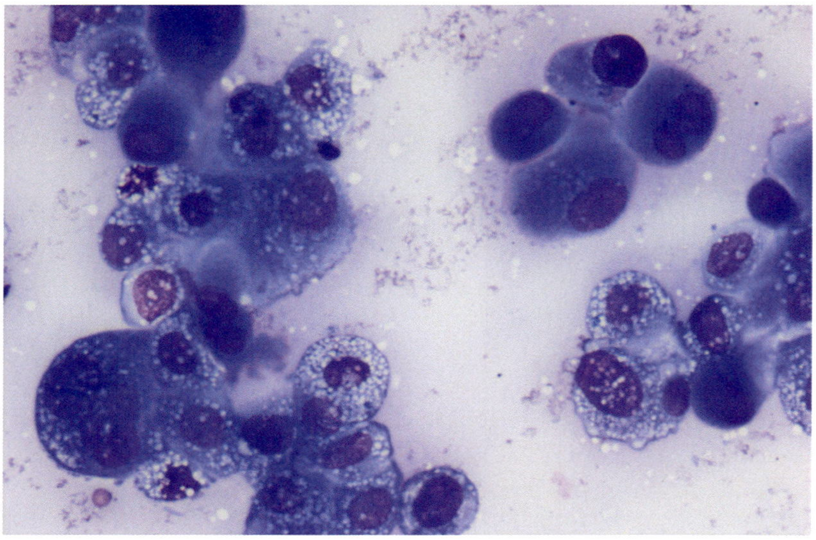

Figure 57. Canine mammary carcinoma, in which highly vacuolated cells with a low degree of atypia and cells that clearly fulfil malignancy criteria are observed.

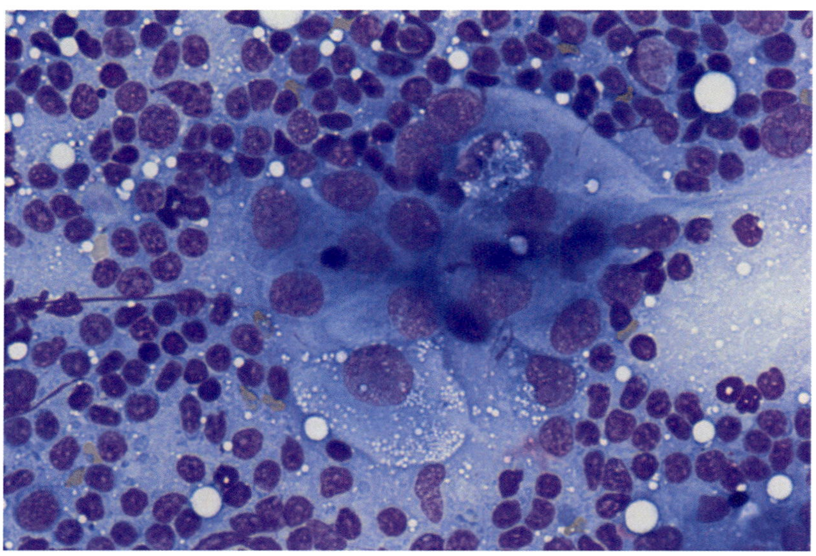

Figure 58. Lymph node metastasis of a canine mammary carcinoma.

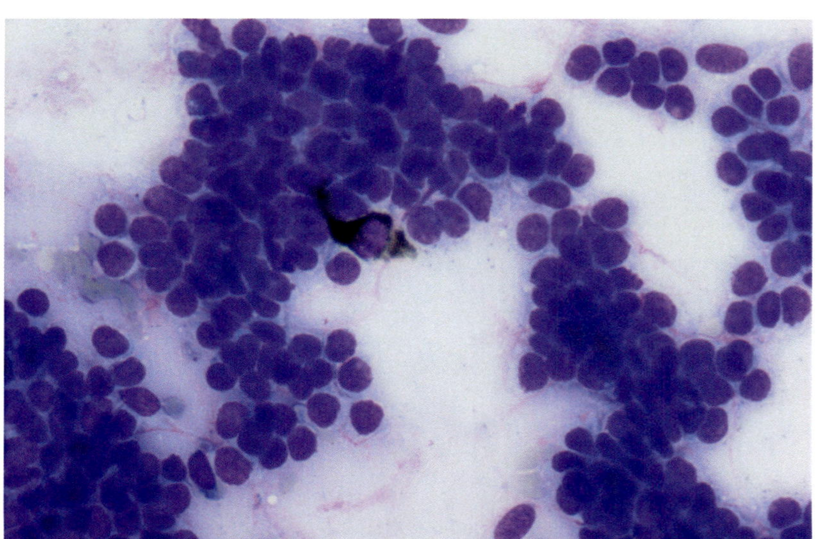

Figure 59. Feline basal cell tumour. Despite the presence of a pigmented cell this tumour should not be mistaken for a melanoma.

Figures 60–62. Poorly differentiated hepatocellular carcinomas. Nuclear atypia and mitoses (arrow) are clearly evident.

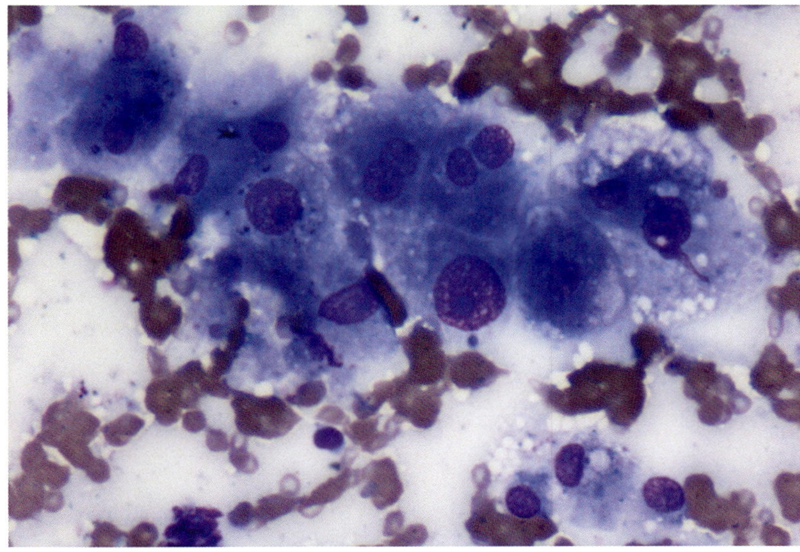

Figure 60.

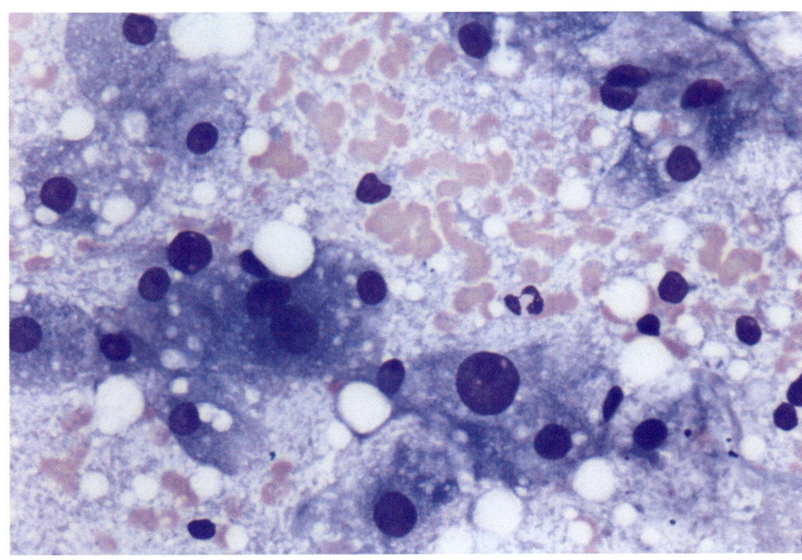

Figure 61.

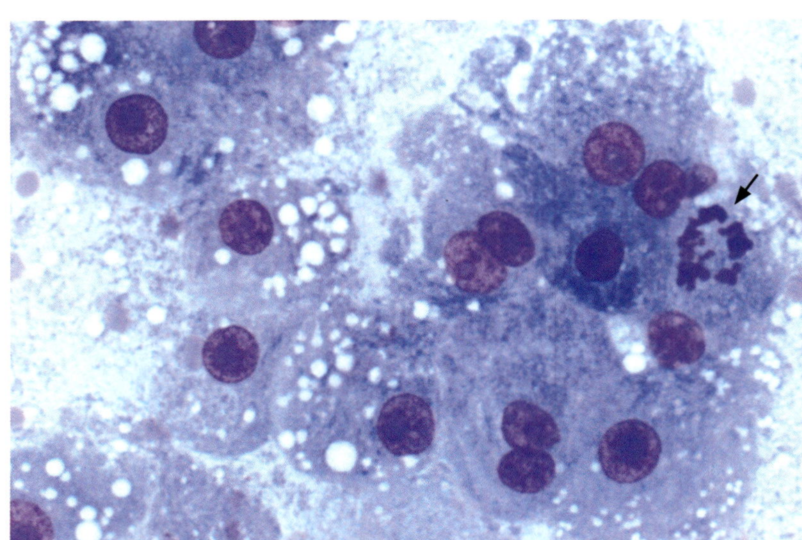

Figure 62.

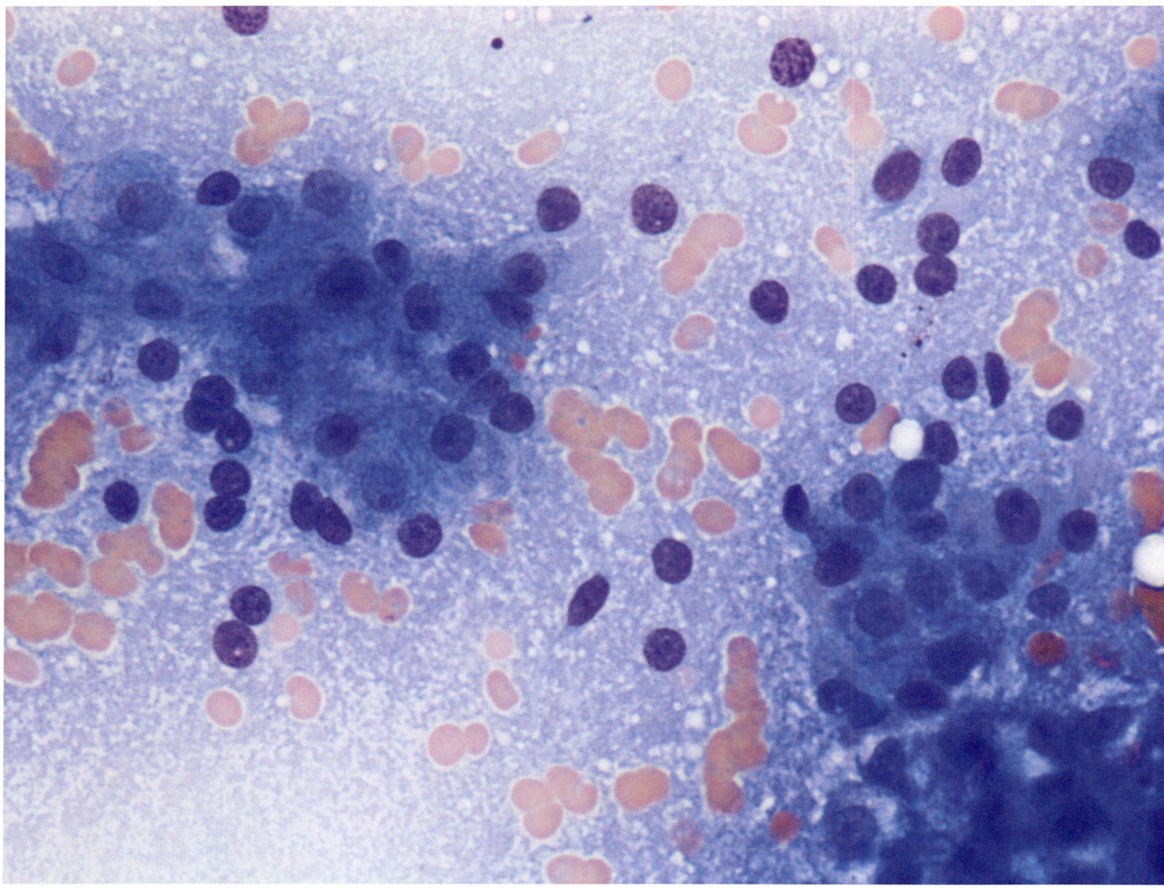

Figure 63. Well differentiated hepatocellular carcinoma. Naked nuclei are located around groups of hepatocytes without significant atypia.

## DIFFERENTIATION BETWEEN REACTIVE MESOTHELIUM, MESOTHELIOMA, AND CARCINOMATOSIS

Tumour diagnosis based on the analysis of effusion fluids is very complex; often, it is impossible to determine whether the cells are reactive mesothelial, neoplastic mesothelial, or carcinoma cells.

The intense activation of mesothelial cells is evidenced by the presence of cellular and nuclear atypia that can be attributed to neoplastic changes (Fig. 64). However, mesothelial cells are very similar to epithelial cells, and therefore the cytological picture of mesothelioma closely resembles that of carcinomatosis. Mesothelioma should be suspected if most cells exhibit very marked nuclear atypia in the absence of inflammation (Fig. 65). Conversely, carcinomatosis should be the primary differential diagnosis if groups of atypical cells are observed together with "normal" mesothelial cells (Fig. 66).

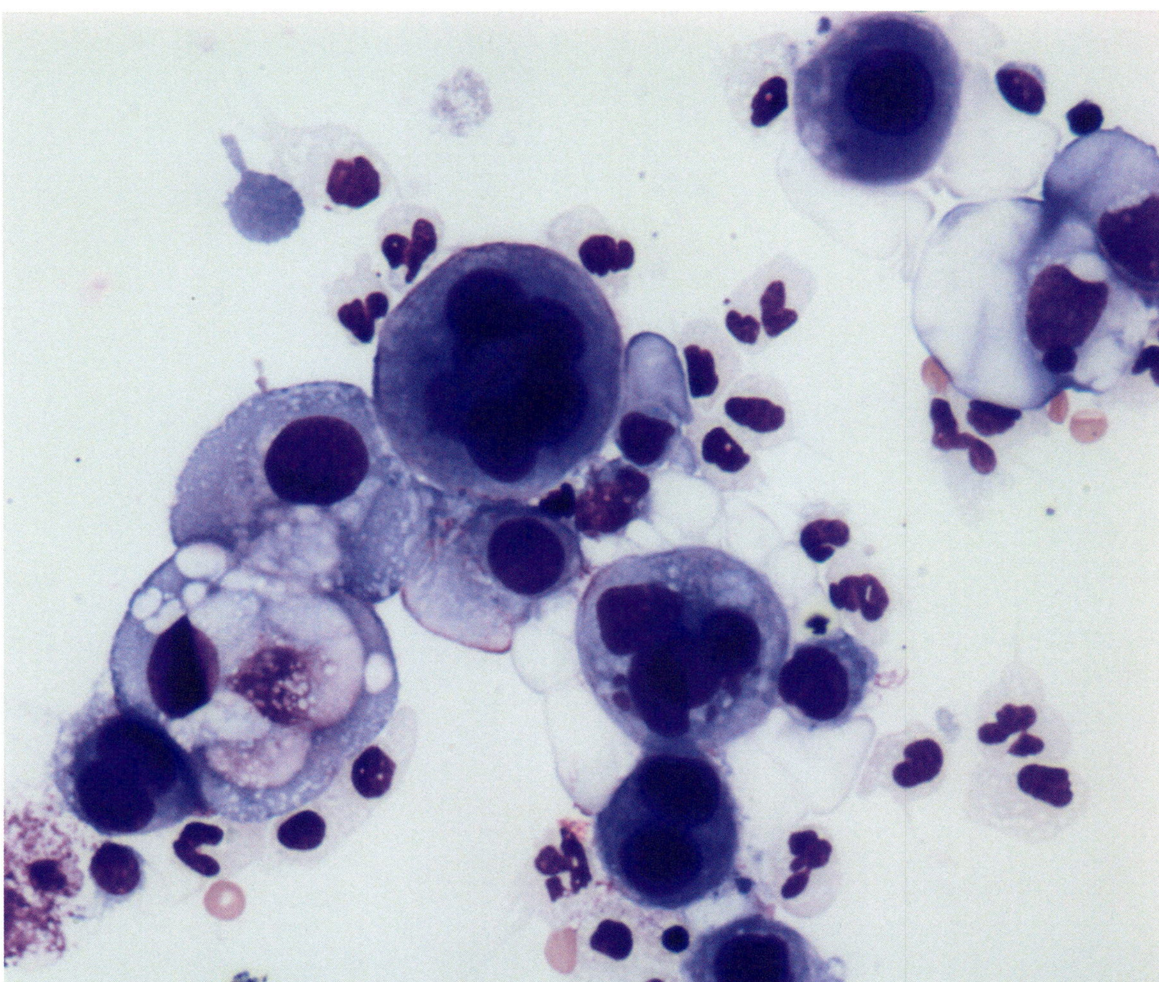

Figure 64. Intensely activated mesothelial cells (ascitic effusion). Despite the obvious atypia, this tumour did not correspond to mesothelioma.

Figures 65 and 66. Pericardial (65) and pleural (66) effusion cytology samples corresponding to mesothelioma and carcinomatosis (arrow indicates malignant group of epithelial cells), respectively.

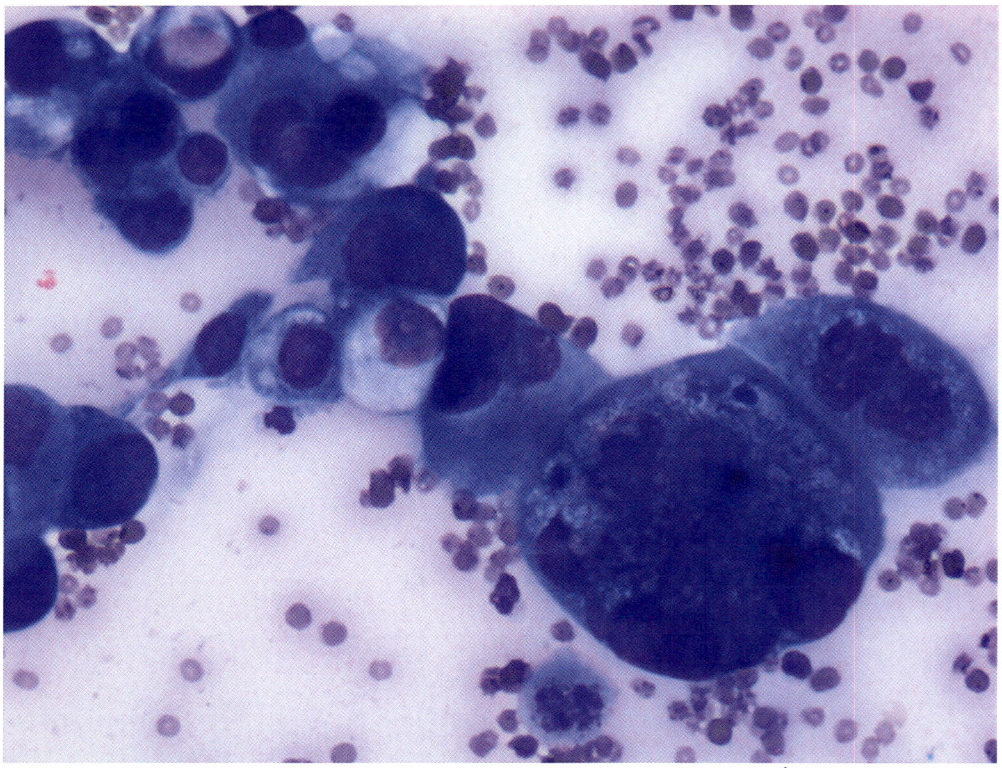

Figure 65.

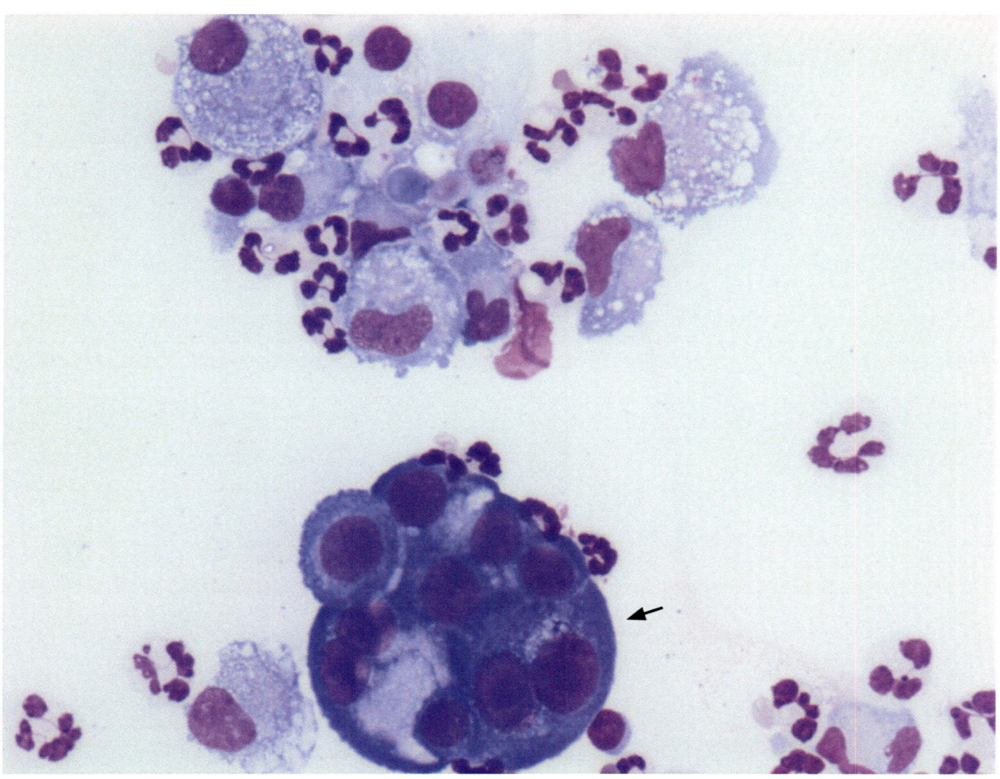

Figure 66.

# 08

# Cytology of melanoma

# Cytology of melanoma

Melanoma is an important tumour type, particularly in canine clinical practice. It is a very heterogeneous type of tumour, with variable biological behaviour. Many malignant melanomas have a high metastatic capacity and, therefore, a very poor prognosis.

Cytology is widely used for the initial evaluation of patients with suspected melanoma. While melanotic melanomas are easily recognizable, the cytological diagnosis of amelanotic tumours is one of the main challenges faced by cytologists.

## CYTOLOGICAL EVALUATION OF MELANOTIC MELANOMA

In melanotic tumours, the presence of melanin in the cytoplasm is a crucial diagnostic key.

Melanocytes (melanin-producing cells) cannot be classified as from any specific cell lineage, since their morphology can resemble epithelial cells (forming groups), mesenchymal cells (oval or spindle-shaped), or round cells. In normal conditions melanocytes are small cells (15–20 µm) with a round/oval nucleus (which can be central or eccentric), and moderate to abundant cytoplasm with moderate basophilia. The main characteristic of melanocytes is the presence of black or blackish-green pigment in the form of fine, punctate granules dispersed throughout the cytoplasm, sometimes in large amounts that mask the nucleus. Occasionally, independent granules may not be visible, but the cytoplasm may have a diffuse greyish-black hue (Figs. 1 and 2).

It is necessary to differentiate melanocytes from other cells that also contain granules or pigment.

Melanophages are the cells that are most difficult to distinguish from melanocytes. Melanophages are macrophages that phagocytose the melanin released in the dermis (pigmentary incontinence) and transport it to the drainage lymph nodes for elimination. They are observed in normal conditions in lymph nodes and skin and are associated with inflammatory processes and tumours. They are large, round, macrophagic cells. Their melanin pigment, unlike that of melanocytes, is usually distributed within the cell as intensely coloured coarse granules of varying sizes. It can be so abundant as to obscure the macrophage vacuoles (Figs. 3 and 4).

In macrophages containing haemosiderin (a product of haemoglobin degradation after erythrophagocytosis), the pigment is more brown or bluish than black (Fig. 5).

The basal cells of cats can contain melanin granules, and are thus sometimes mistaken for melanocytes.

Some thyroid tumours contain epithelial cells in which blackish thyroxin granules can be observed. In these cases, confusion can be avoided by considering the location of the lesion and the predominant cell type (neuroendocrine) (Fig. 6).

Cytology of benign melanoma typically reveals a low level of cellularity. Notable features include abundant extracellular melanin, which can form accumulations. Instead of intact cells, these samples typically contain melanin and scattered nuclei, which in most cases are masked by the abundant pigment and cannot be evaluated (Fig. 7). If the nuclei are visible, they do not exhibit marked atypia (Fig. 8).

Cytological samples of malignant melanomas generally reveal a high degree of cellularity. Typically, 2 or even 3 distinct morphologies are observed in the same preparation, resulting in a classification of "mixed cellular origin". This feature should be distinguished from cellular pleomorphism as a cytological criterion of malignancy. In pleomorphic tumours, variations in shape and/or size are observed within cells of the same lineage, while in mixed tumours cells of distinct lineages can be clearly identified. Therefore, in most melanomas the presence of cells of distinct lineages cannot be considered cytological evidence of malignancy.

Highly pigmented cells can coexist with others containing little or no pigment (highly, moderately, or poorly melanotic melanomas). Cells commonly exhibit signs of malignancy, including anisokaryosis, nuclear pleomorphism, and the presence of large and atypical nucleoli (a highly characteristic finding). While melanophages may be numerous, their presence is not diagnostic (Figs. 9–11).

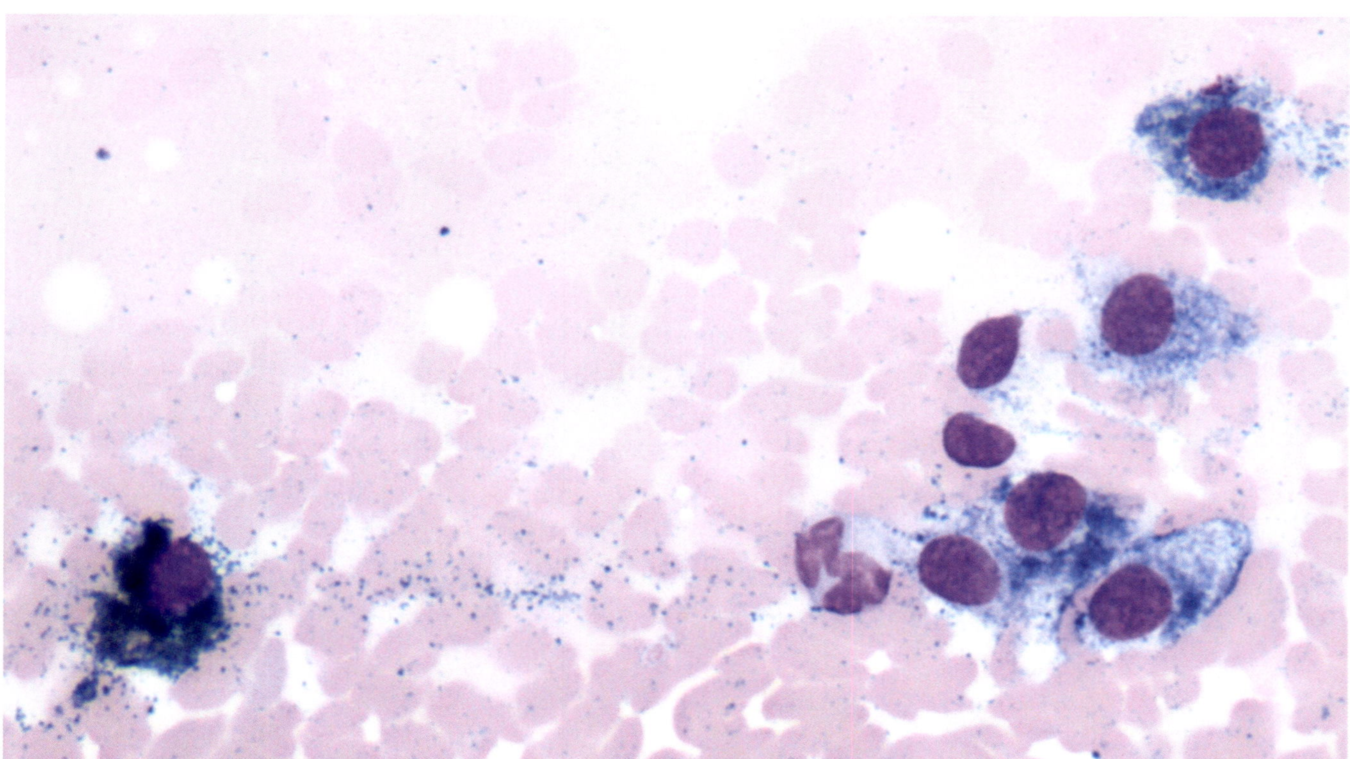

Figure 1. Melanocytes exhibiting mesenchymal morphology and containing abundant melanin, both in granules and distributed more diffusely in the cytoplasm.

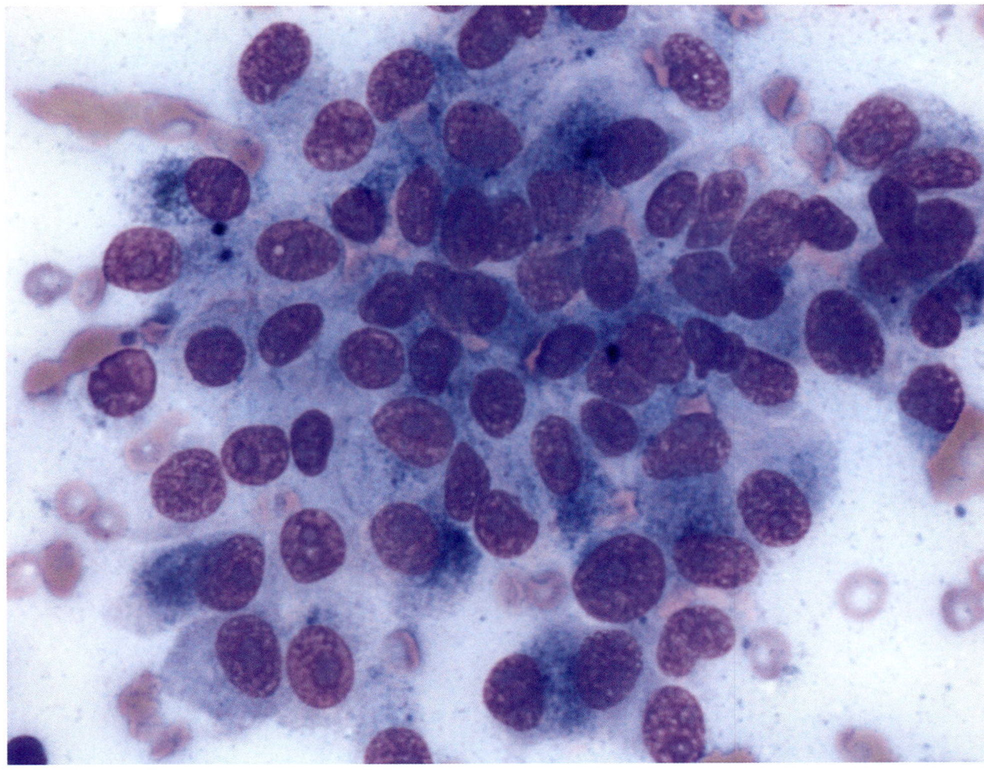

Figure 2. Melanocytes in a group. The melanin confers a diffuse hue to the cytoplasm.

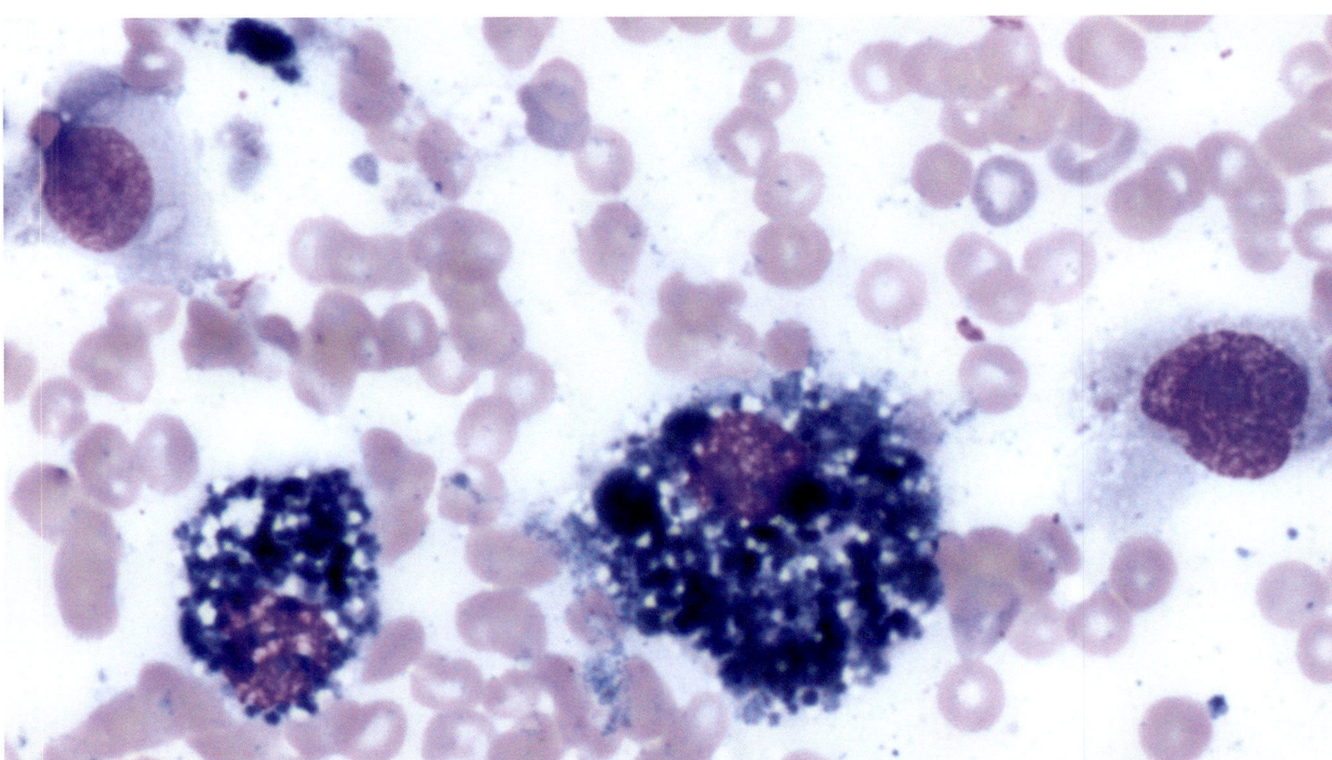

Figure 3. Two melanophages and two tissue cells are visible (amelanotic melanocytes, although in this single image it is impossible to classify them as such).

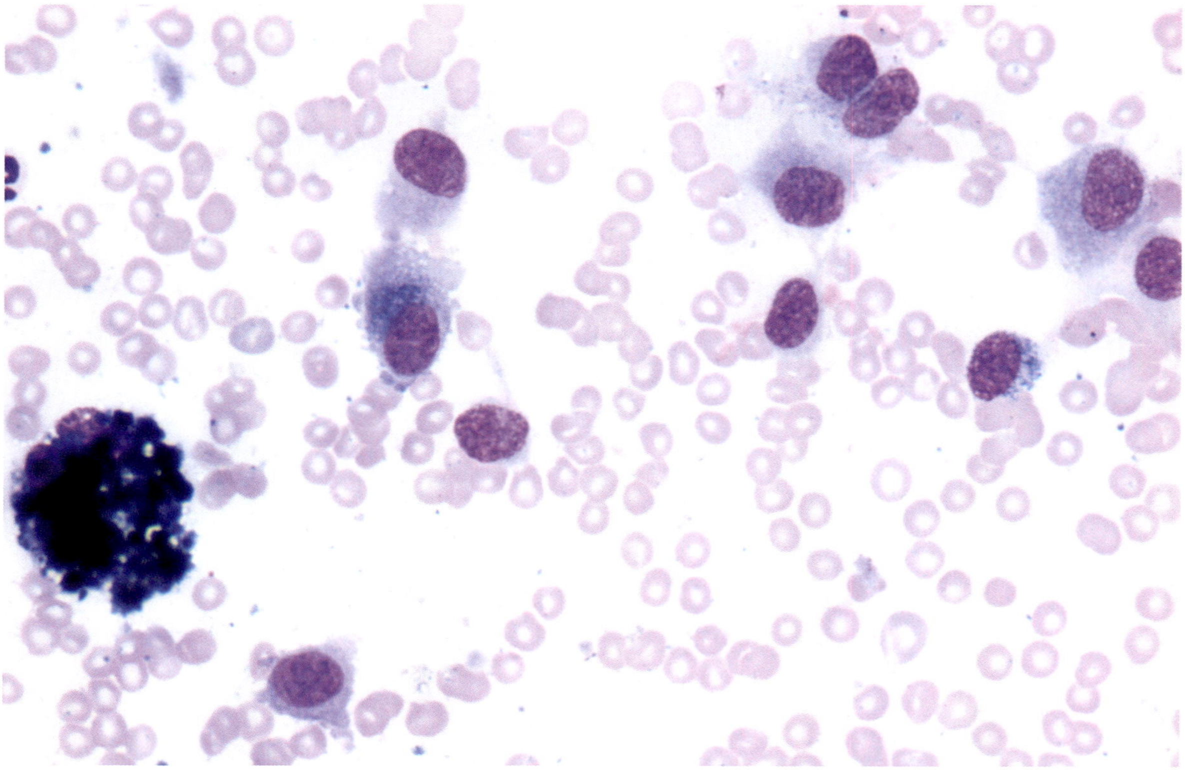

Figure 4. Several melanocytes are evident, most of which are amelanotic and some of which contain little pigment, as well as a melanophage, which is easily identifiable by its shape and the distribution of pigment in the cytoplasm.

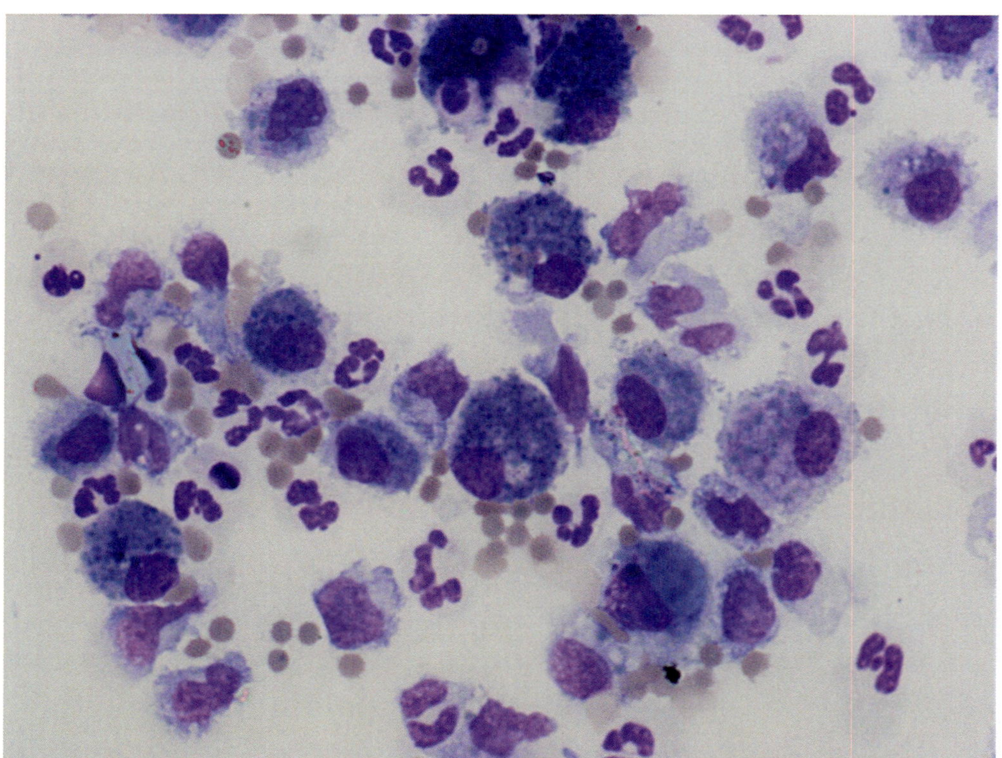

Figure 5. Note the numerous haemosiderin-containing macrophages, which should not be confused with melanocytes or melanophages (abdominal fluid cytology).

Figure 6. Group of thyroid cells containing thyroxine granules. These cells can be mistaken for melanocytes.

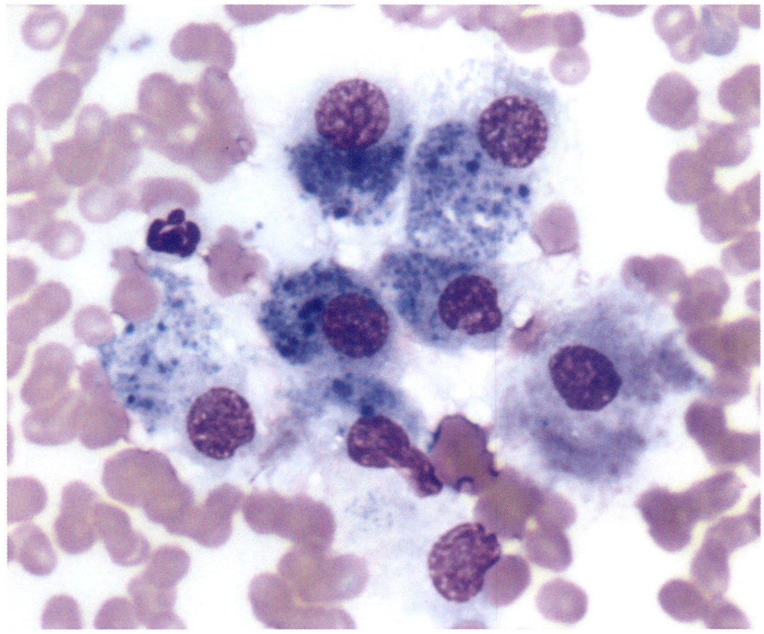

Figures 7 and 8. Melanocytomas. Samples with abundant extracellular pigment and scattered cells containing large amounts of melanin. The nuclei do not exhibit atypia.

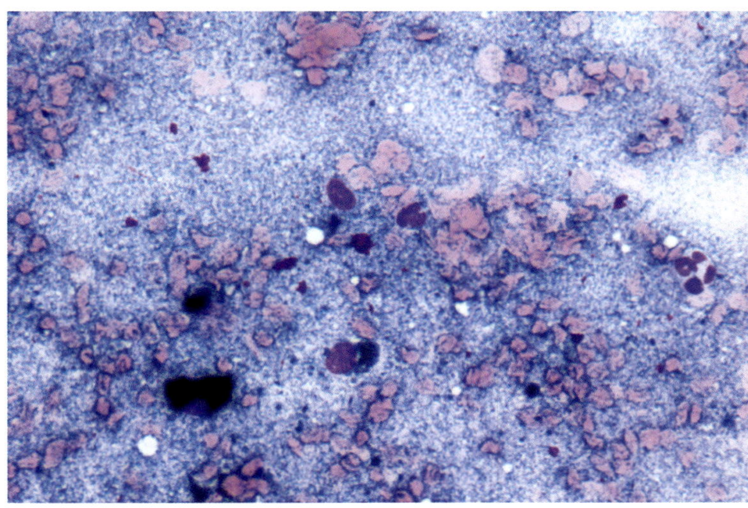

Figure 7.

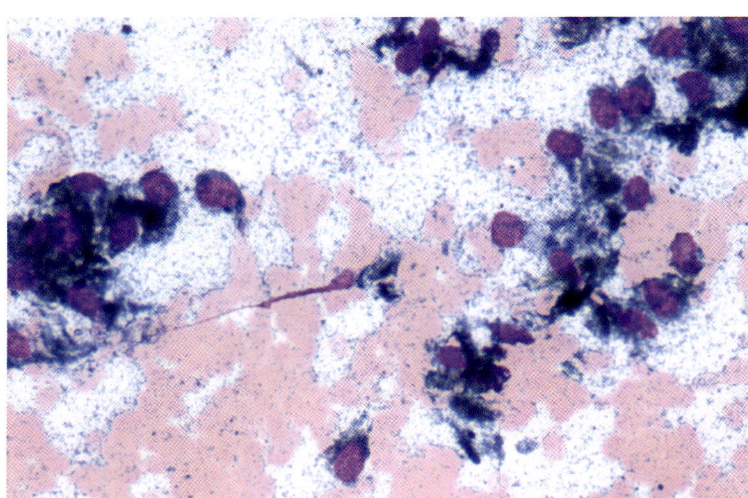

Figure 8.

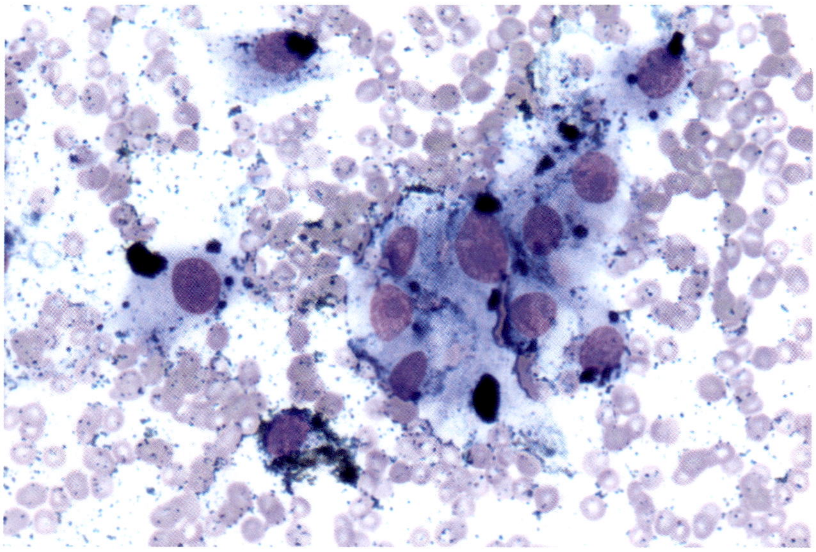

Figure 9. Very melanotic malignant melanoma. Abundant extracellular pigment, mesenchymal melanocytes, and a group of epithelial cells. The nuclei exhibit marked atypia (anisokaryosis and macronucleoli).

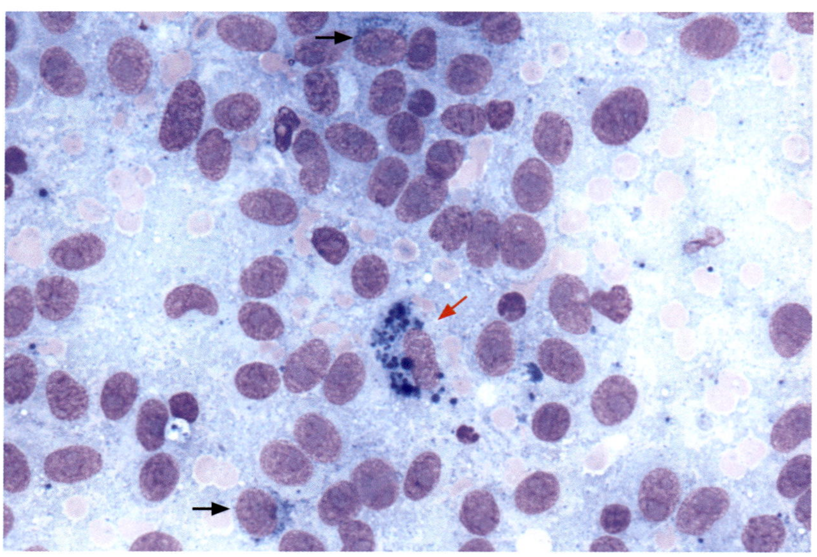

Figures 10 and 11. Poorly melanotic malignant melanomas. Few melanocytes contain melanin (black arrow). Signs of malignancy are evident. Melanophages are present (red arrow).

Figure 10.

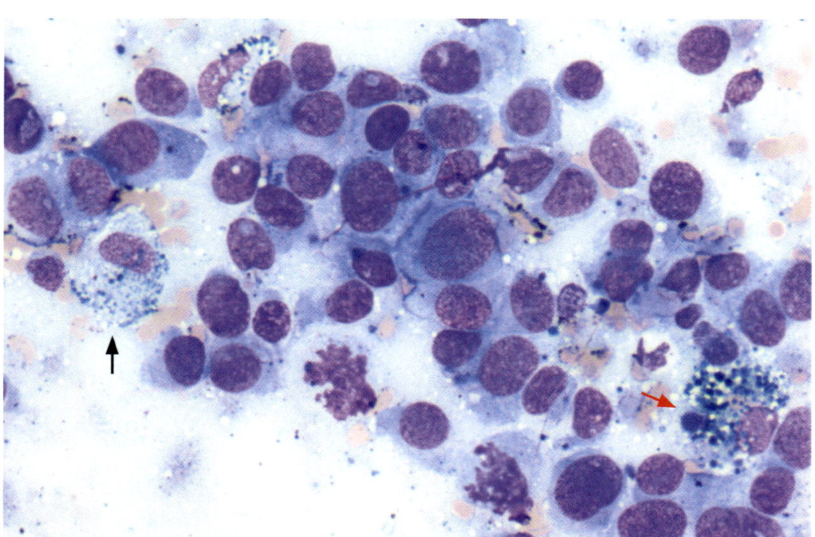

Figure 11.

# CYTOLOGICAL EVALUATION OF AMELANOTIC MELANOMA

The cytological diagnosis of amelanotic melanoma is complex. The absence of melanin prevents determination of cell origin and the fact that round, epithelial, or mesenchymal cells can be exfoliated complicates the evaluation. Therefore, the sensitivity and specificity of cytology for the diagnosis of amelanotic melanoma should be considered moderate (66.7 % and 85.7 %, respectively).[9]

If the cell population is predominantly of one particular lineage, a diagnosis of a round cell tumour (Fig. 12), such as a high-grade sarcoma (Fig. 13) or undifferentiated carcinoma (Fig. 14), is most likely.

The presence of melanophages can aid diagnosis, but is not considered definitively diagnostic.

The presence of a mixed population, in which two or all three cell lineages are evident, is the main criterion for selecting amelanotic melanoma as the first differential diagnosis (Figs. 15 and 16).

Cytological evidence of malignancy is typically very evident, and therefore it is not usually difficult to identify high-grade malignant tumours, although the cell origin may be indeterminate or ambiguous. As in malignant melanotic melanoma, atypical mitoses are common, but cytology does not allow determination of the mitotic index; histopathological evaluation is necessary to define this important prognostic variable.

Figures 12–14. Samples for which cytological diagnoses of round cell tumour (probably a histiocytic sarcoma), high-grade sarcoma, and carcinoma were established, respectively. Histology and immunohistochemistry confirmed a diagnosis of amelanotic melanoma in all three cases. The presence of some fusiform cells (lower part of Fig. 14) could have helped orient the cytological diagnosis in this case.

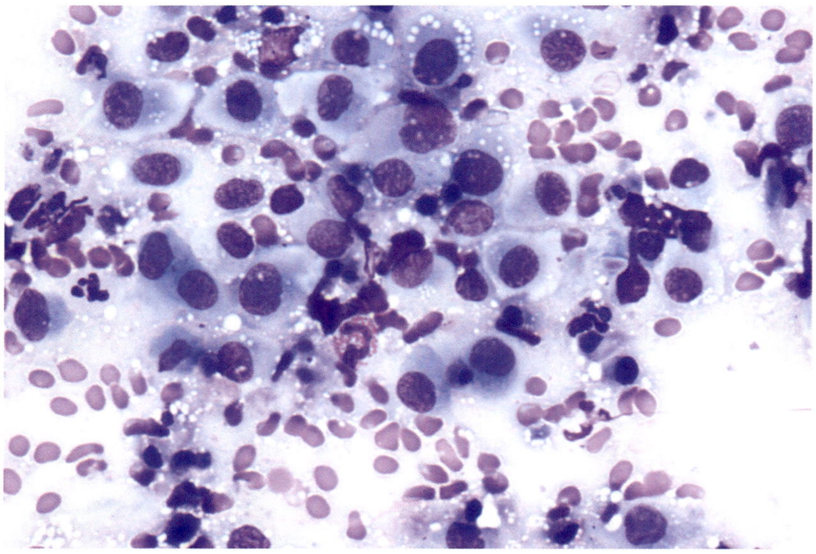

Figure 12.

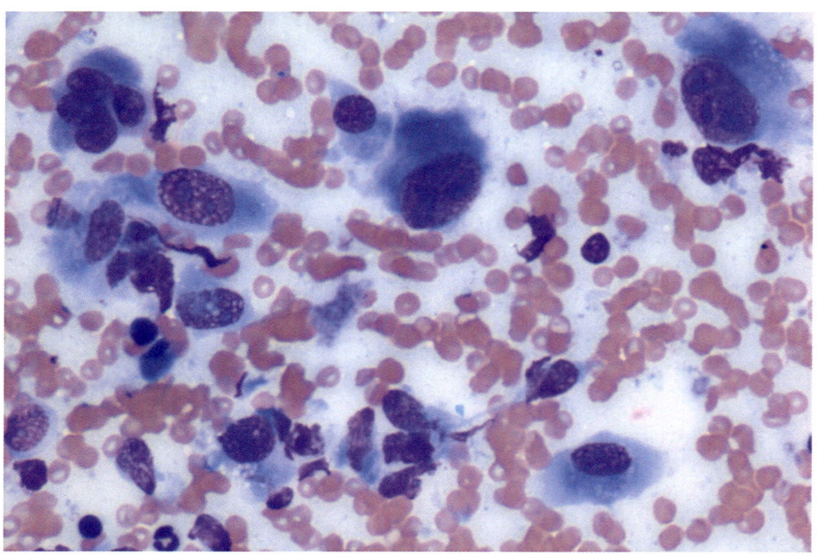

Figure 13.

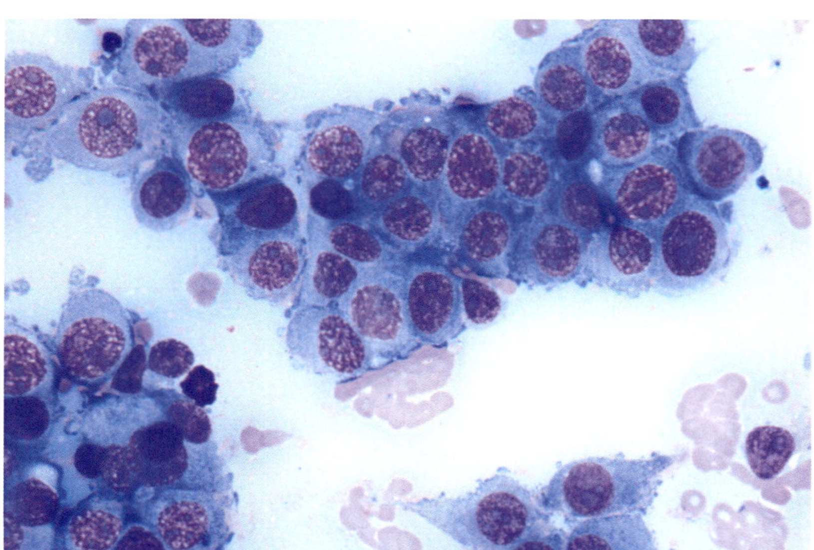

Figure 14.

Figure 15. Different fields of the same tumour sample. Based on the simultaneous presence of epithelial, round, and mesenchymal cells, melanoma is selected as the first differential diagnosis.

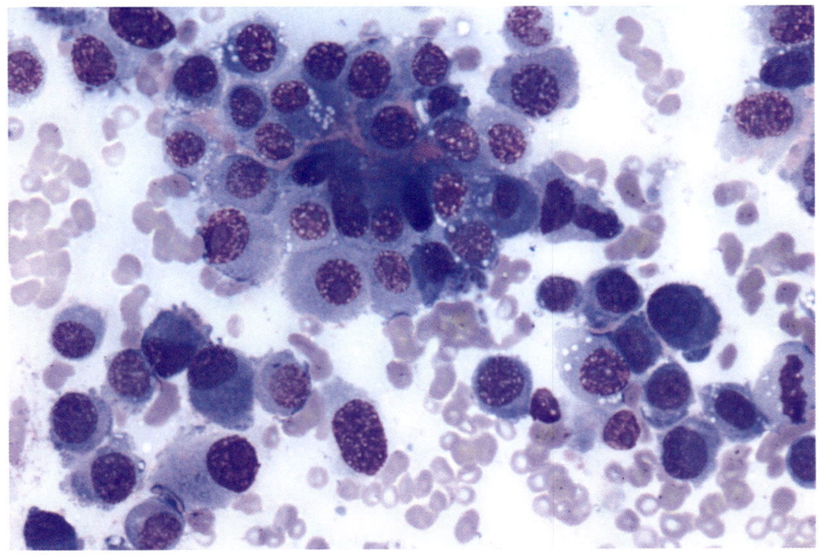

Figure 15A.

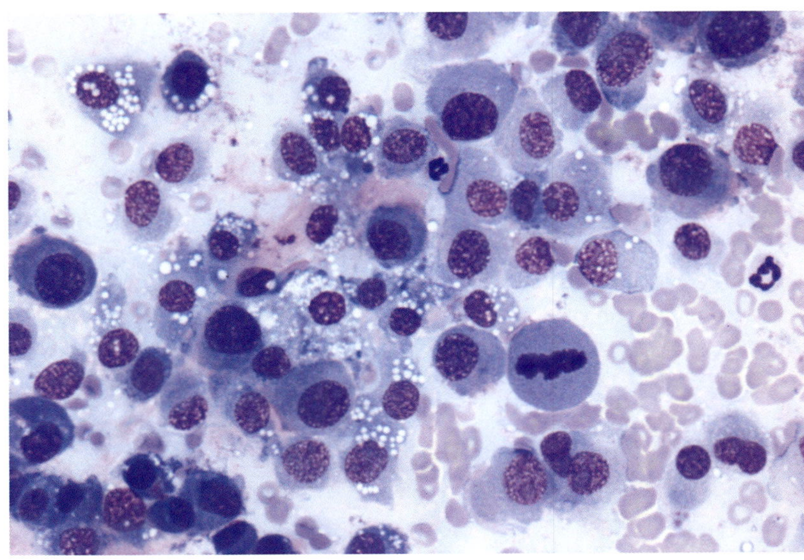

Figure 15B.

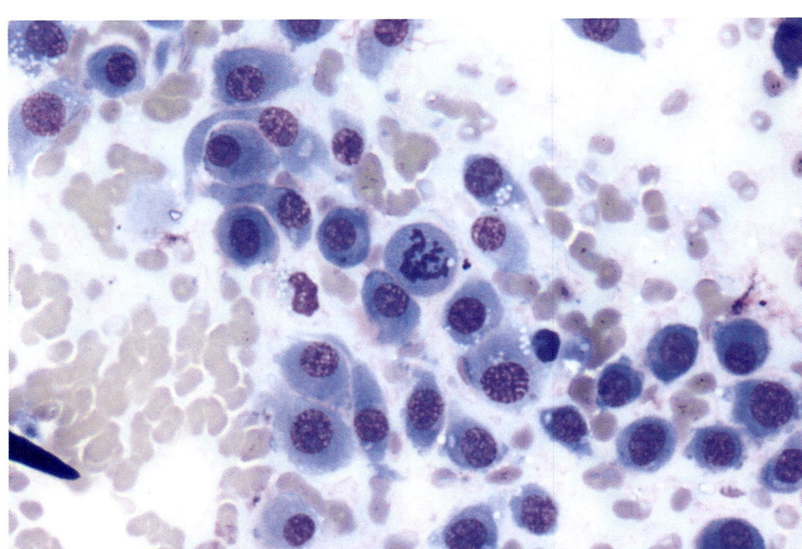

Figure 15C.

Figure 16. Different fields of the same tumour in which cells of distinct lineages are observed. The presence of two melanophages (B) cannot be considered sufficient to reach a diagnosis of melanoma, but can be considered evidence of a mixed tumour.

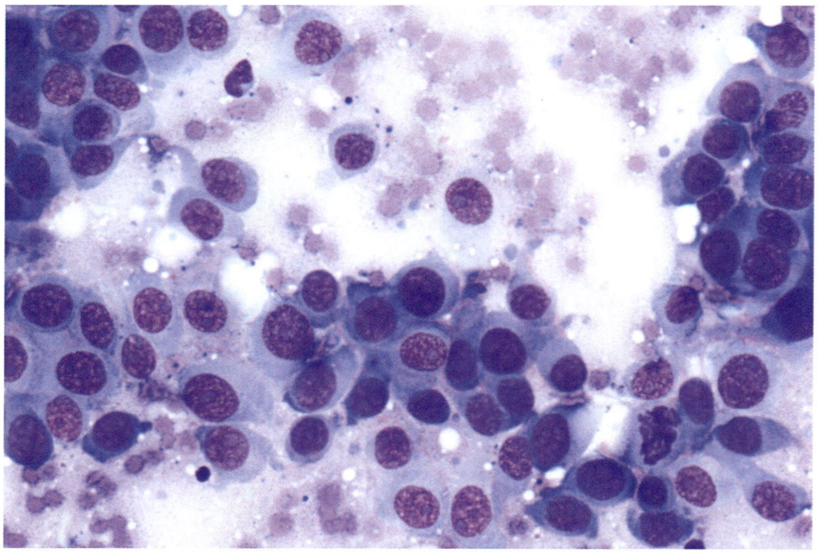

Figure 16A.

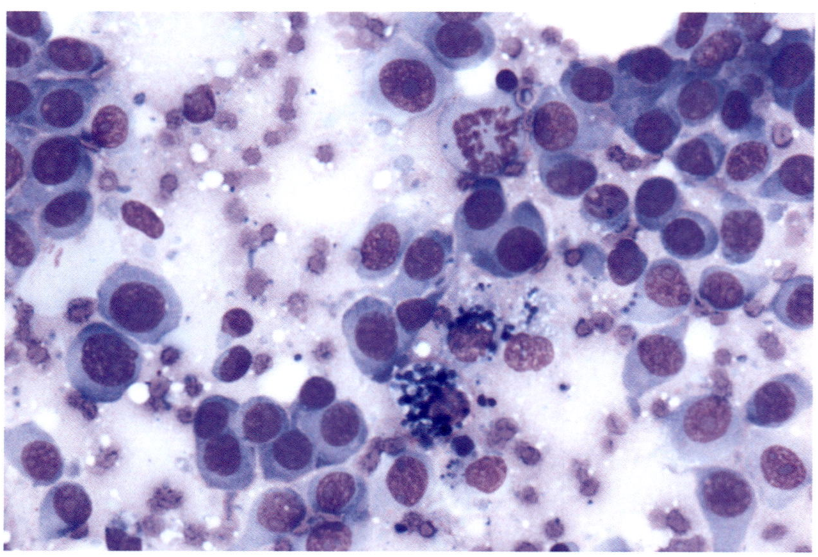

Figure 16B.

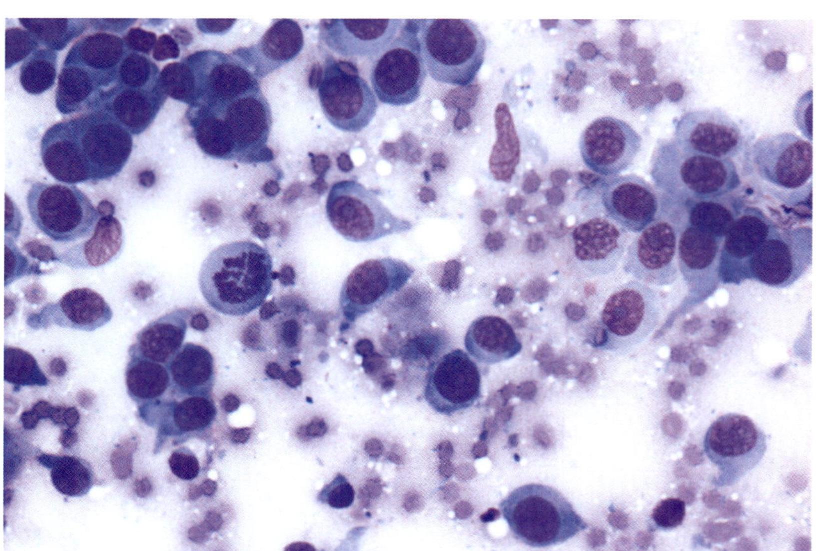

Figure 16C.

# METASTATIC MELANOMA: CYTOLOGICAL CONSIDERATIONS

Upon diagnosis of a malignant melanoma, evaluation of the regional lymph node is required, and cytology is the most commonly used diagnostic tool. However, the results are not very conclusive when compared with histopathological data, and are of little use in estimating survival. If metastatic cells are scarce it can be difficult to demonstrate the presence of neoplastic melanocytes (especially given their very heterogeneous appearance), and if the melanocytes are pigmented it can be difficult to distinguish them from melanophages, which are very common in both normal and reactive lymph nodes (Fig. 17).

The following criteria have been proposed to define lymph node metastasis of melanoma:[4]

- Nonmetastatic lymph node: few or absent melanin-containing cells (0–5 per preparation), absence of cohesive nonpigmented cells, mesenchymal morphology, and/or signs of malignancy.
- Metastatic lymph node: increase in the number of melanin-containing cells (>5 per preparation, although this threshold is usually exceeded) or the presence of fusiform cells showing signs of cohesion and/or with evident nuclear atypia (Figs. 18 and 19).
- Suspect lymph node: presence in each preparation of >5 melanin-containing cells that exfoliate individually, with rounded morphology and/or without evident nuclear signs of malignancy.

Metastasis can only be verified if the neoplastic population is very abundant and displaces, or even replaces, the normal lymphoid tissue (Fig. 20). However, it should be noted that if the neoplastic population exhibits a rounded morphology, differentiation from lymphoma or metastasis of other round cell tumours can be difficult (Fig. 21).

Tumour cells can be identified in other organs (Fig. 22). If tracheal wash is used as a diagnostic tool in cases of suspected pulmonary metastasis, macrophages containing anthracotic pigment should not be confused with melanocytic cells (Fig. 23).

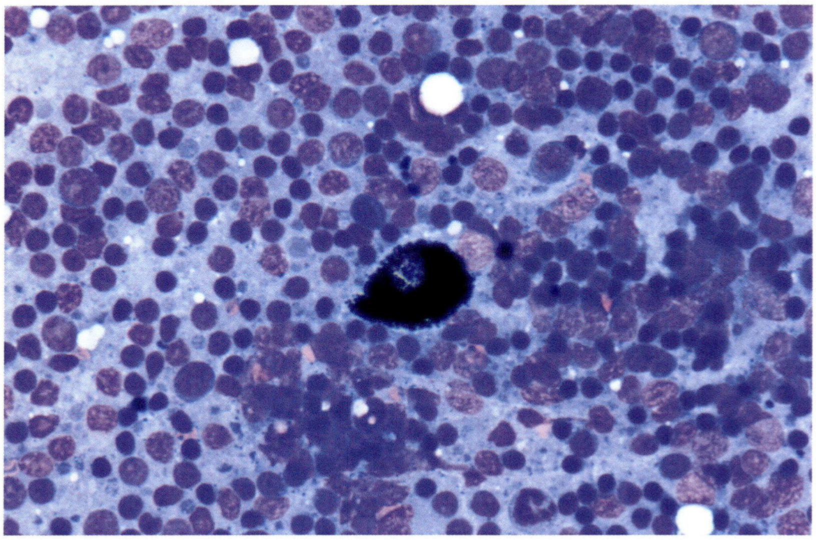

Figure 17. Reactive lymph node in which a melanophage is evident. This cell type is found in lymph node tissue in normal conditions, and does not indicate metastasis.

Figures 18 and 19. Lymph node cytology samples that meet the criteria for melanoma metastasis. Black arrows indicate melanocytes (pigmented or nonpigmented); red arrows indicate melanophages.

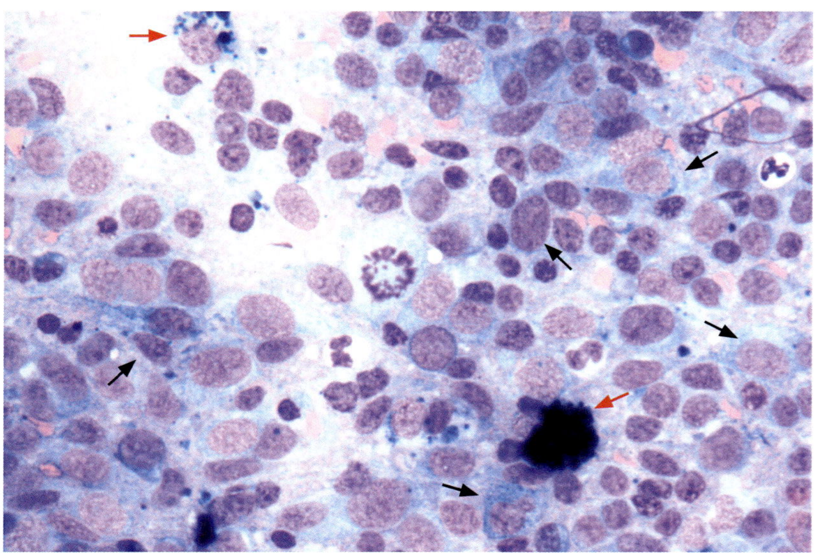

Figure 18.

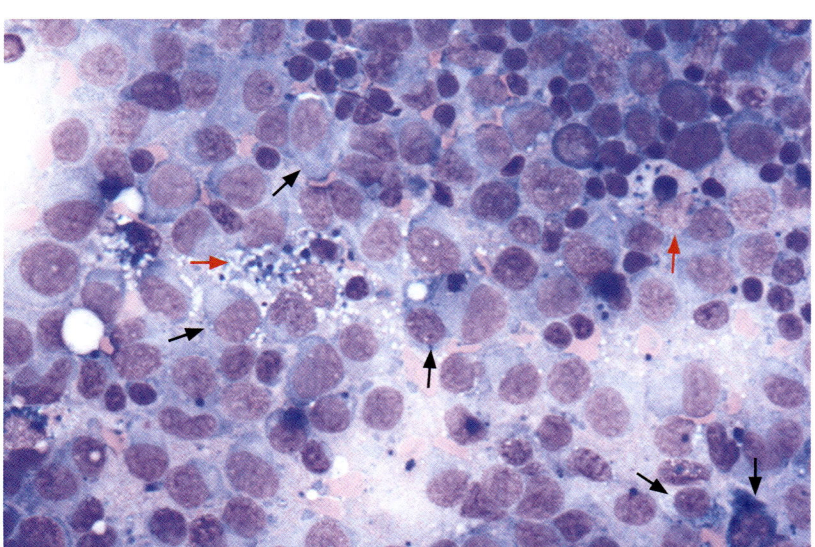

Figure 19.

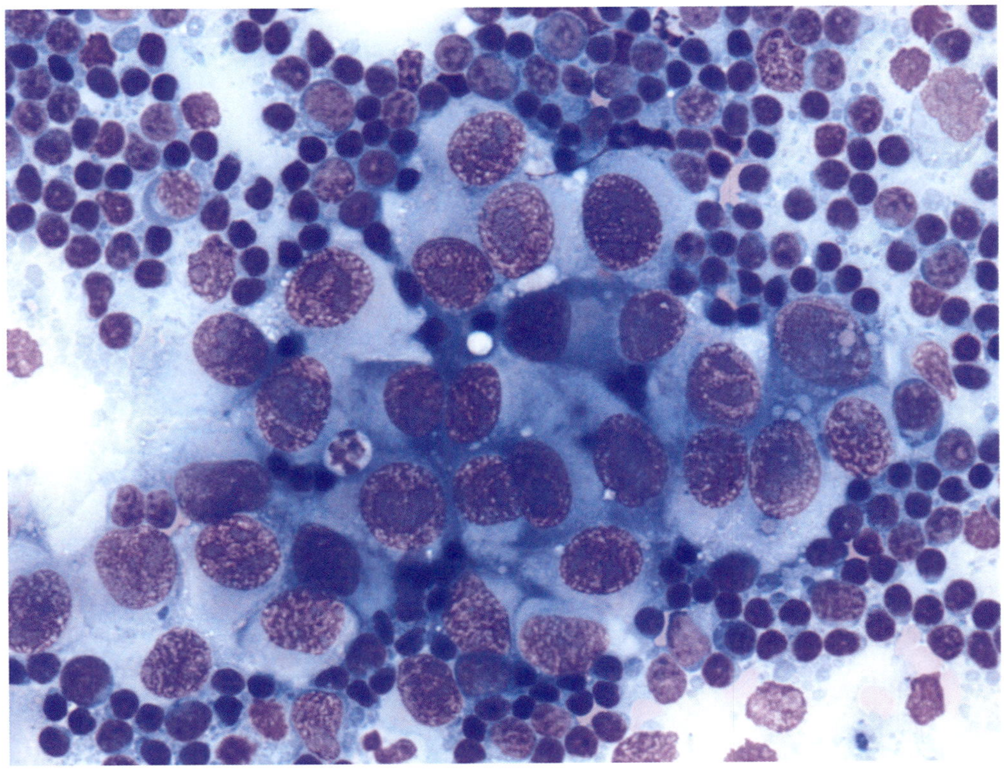

Figure 20. Lymph node metastasis of an amelanotic melanoma. Metastatic cells are distinguished from lymphoid cells based on their size, morphology, and atypia.

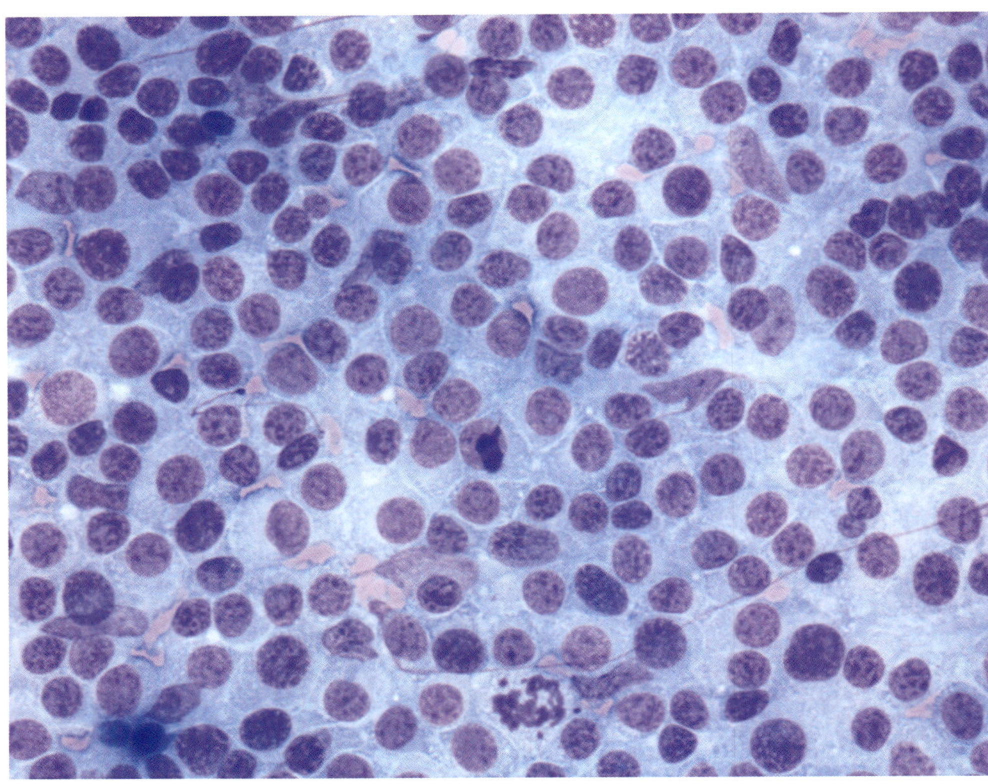

Figure 21. Lymph node metastasis of amelanotic melanoma. Cytology reveals few mature lymphocytes and a predominance of round cells, which should not be confused with lymphoblasts. In this case, the main differential diagnoses is metastasis of other round cell tumours.

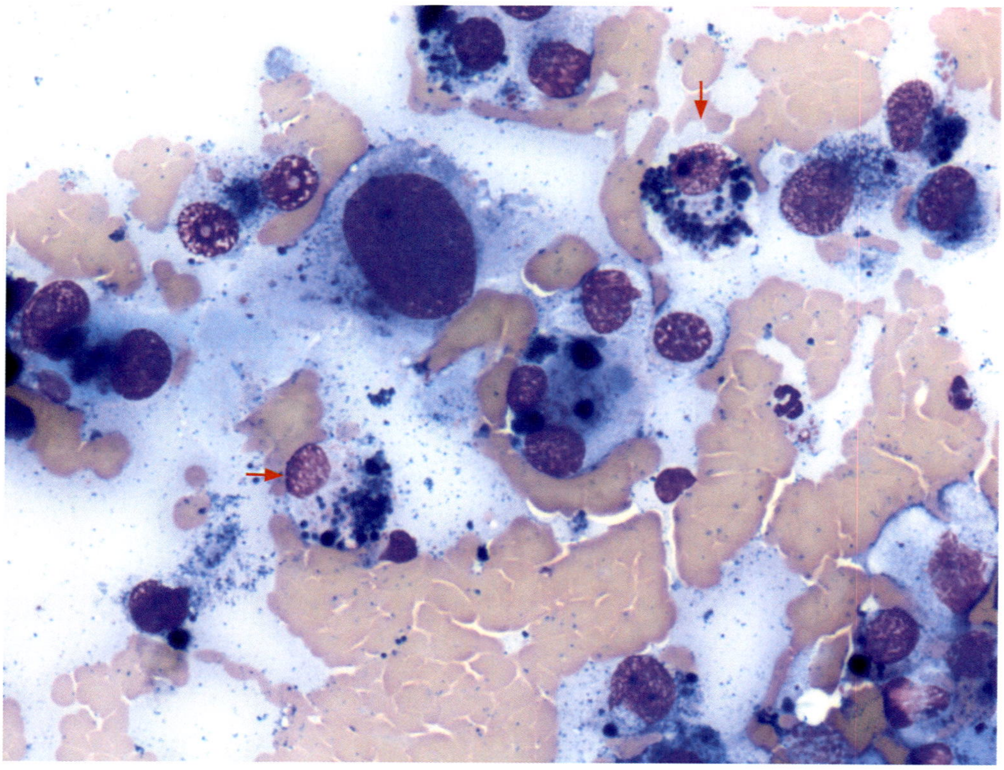

Figure 22. Splenic metastasis of an iris melanoma in a cat. Melanocytes and melanophages (red arrows) are evident. Note the giant cell with a giant nucleus.

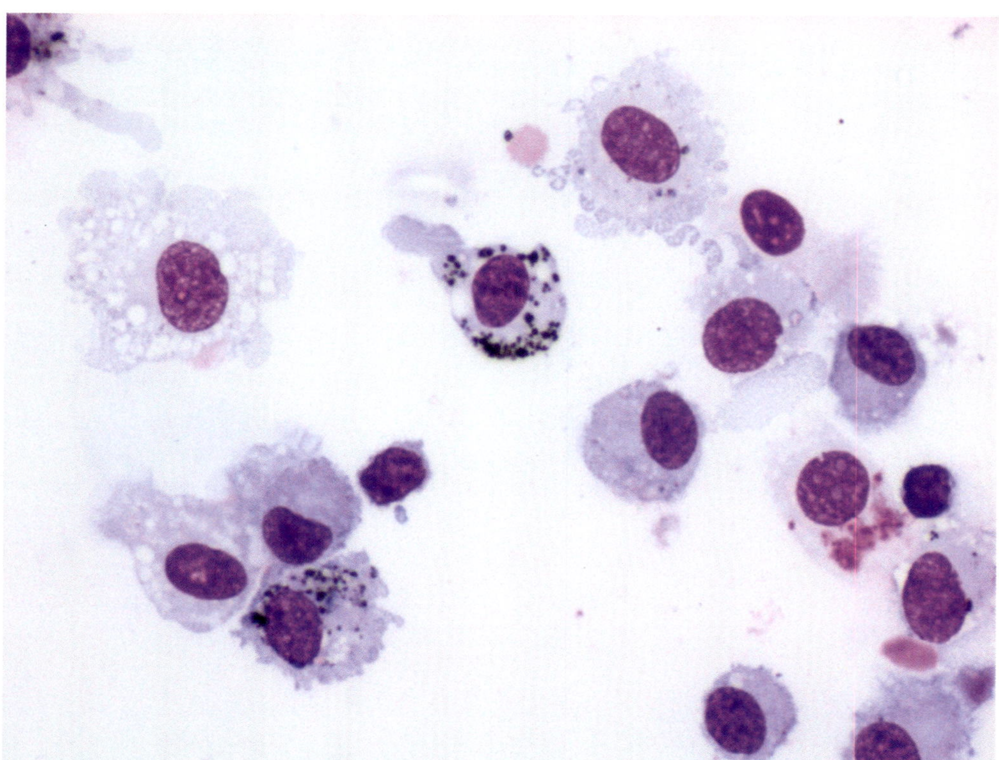

Figure 23. Tracheal wash sample. The macrophages containing anthracotic pigment should not be mistaken for melanocytes or melanophages.

# References


1. Camus, M.S. et al. Cytologic criteria for mast cell tumor grading in dogs with evaluation of clinical outcome. *Vet Pathol*, 2016 Nov; 53(6):1117–1123.
2. Caniatti, M. et al. Cytological features of canine haemangiopericytoma in FNA biopsy. *Vet Rec*, 2001; 149:242–244.
3. Ghisleni, G. et al. Correlation between FNA citology and histopathology in the evaluation of cutaneous and subcutaneous masses from dogs and cats. *Vet Clin Pathol*, 2006; 35:24–30.
4. Grimes, J.A., Matz, B.M., Christopherson, P.W. et al. Agreement between cytology and histopathology for regional lymph node metastasis in dogs with melanocytic neoplasms. *Vet Pathol*, 2017; 54:579–587.
5. Hergt, F. et al. Use of a 2-tier histologic grading system for canine cutaneous mast cell tumors on cytology specimens. *Vet Clin Pathol*, 2016 Sept; 45(3):477–483.
6. Krick, E.L. et al. Cytological lymph node evaluation in dogs with mast cell tumours: association with grade and survival. *Vet Comp Oncol*, 2009 Jun; 7:130–131.
7. Masserdotti, C. et al. Retrospective study of cytologic features of well-differentiated hepatocellular carcinoma in dogs. *Vet Clin Pathol*, 2012; 41:382–390.
8. Mutz, M.L. et al. Cytologic comparison of the percentage of mast cells in lymph node aspirate samples from clinically normal dogs versus dogs with allergic dermatologic disease and dogs with cutaneous mast cell tumors. *J Am Vet Med Assoc*, 2017 Aug; 251:421–428.
9. Przedziecki, R., Czopowicz, M., Sapierzynsk, R. Accuracy of routine cytology and immunocytochemistry in preoperative diagnosis of oral amelanotic melanomas in dogs. *Vet Clin Pathol*, 2015; 44: 597–604.
10. Sabattini, S. et al. Comparative assessment of the accuracy of cytological and histologic biopsies in the diagnosis of canine bone lesions. *J Vet Intern Med*, 2017; 31:864–871.
11. Stockhaus, C. et al. The value of cytology in the diagnosis of soft tissue sarcoma in the dog and cat. *Tierarztl Prax Ausg K Kleintiere Heimtiere*, 2003; 31:148–155.
12. Simon, S. et al. Cytologic examination of fine-needle aspirates from mammary gland tumors in the dog: diagnostic accuracy with comparison to histopathology and association with postoperative outcome. *Vet Clin Pathol*, 2009; 38:521–528.
13. Valli, V.E. et al. Classification of canine malignant lymphomas according to the WHO criteria. *Vet Pathol*, 2011; 48:198–211.
14. Vernau, W. Advanced diagnostic work-up for lymphoma cases. *Proceedings International Congress Veterinary Oncology*, Verona, 2016.

Published by Servet editorial - Grupo Asís Biomedia SL